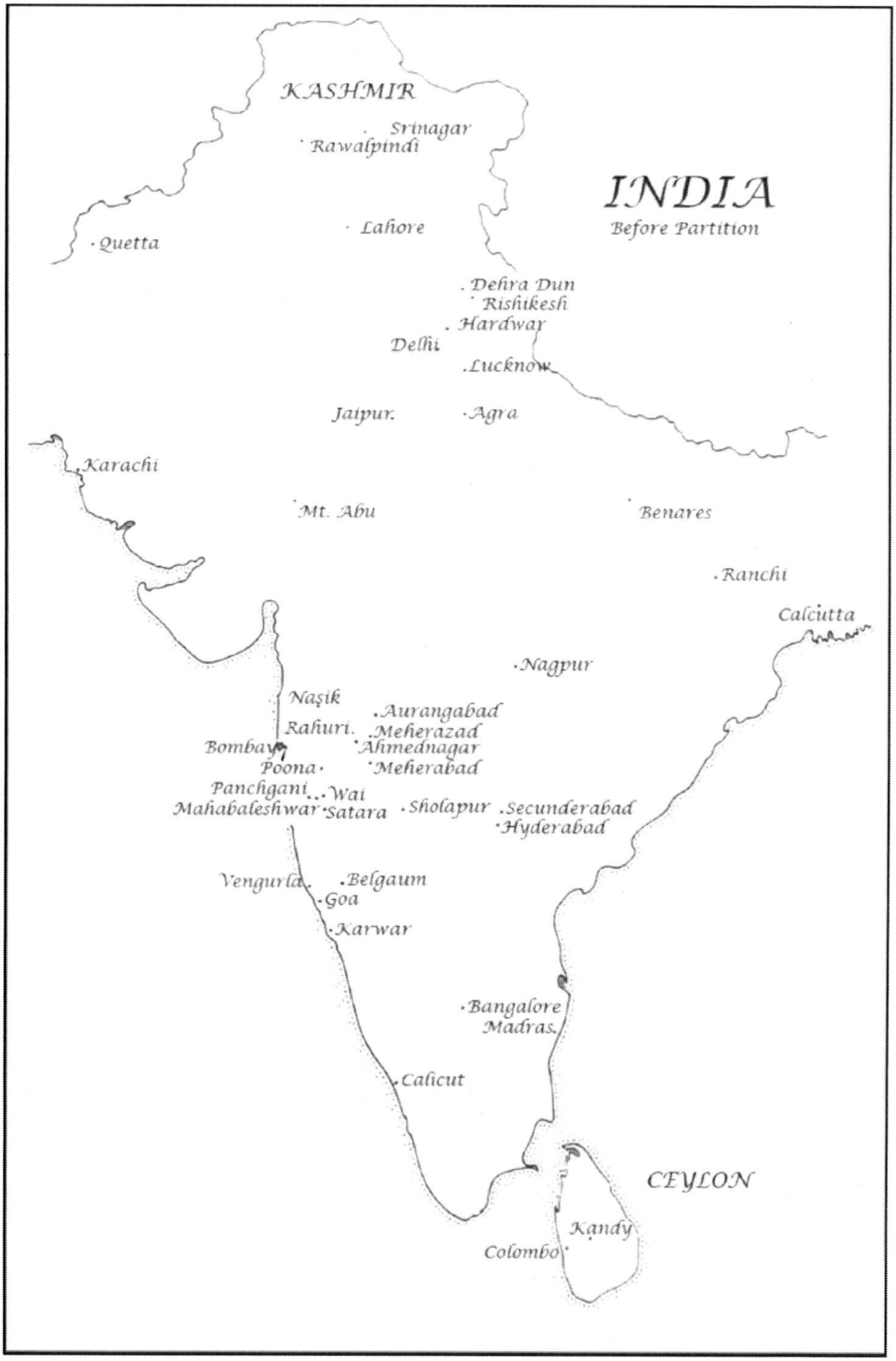
INDIA
Before Partition
KASHMIR
Srinagar
Rawalpindi
Lahore
Quetta
Dehra Dun
Rishikesh
Hardwar
Delhi
Lucknow
Jaipur
Agra
Karachi
Mt. Abu
Benares
Ranchi
Calcutta
Nagpur
Nasik
Aurangabad
Rahuri
Meherazad
Bombay
Ahmednagar
Poona
Meherabad
Panchgani
Wai
Mahabaleshwar
Satara
Sholapur
Secunderabad
Hyderabad
Vengurla
Belgaum
Goa
Karwar
Bangalore
Madras
Calicut
CEYLON
Kandy
Colombo

Slave of Love

The Life of Dr. William Donkin with Meher Baba

Bob Mossman

OCEANIC PUBLISHING

Lunenburg Nova Scotia Canada

Publisher:
Oceanic Publishing
12 Shoreline Drive
RR 1 Lunenburg, Nova Scotia, Canada B0J 2C0

www.oceanicpublishing.com

First and second printings, 2012
Third printing, 2015

Cover Photo: Meher Nazar Publications
Back Cover Photo: Slave of Love
Book Designer: Nancy Roberts
Cover Design/Map Design: Jennie Carton
Author Photo: Jason Remai

Printed in Canada at Hignell Book Printing, Winnipeg

Library and Archives Canada Cataloguing in Publication

Mossman, Bob, 1945-
Slave of love : the life of Dr. William Donkin with Meher Baba / Bob Mossman.

Includes bibliographical references and index.
ISBN 978-0-9879381-0-7

1. Donkin, William. 2. Physicians--Great Britain--Biography. 3. Physicians--India--Biography. 4. Meher Baba, 1894-1969--Disciples--Biography. 5. Meher Baba, 1894-1969. I. Title.

R489.D65M68 2012 610.92 C2012-902195-4

For Kate –

the most loving influence in our family for 37 years.

This book would not have been possible without

your support and encouragement.

We miss you.

God is not to be learned, or discussed, or studied,

or argued about. God is to be contemplated,

felt, loved, and lived.

– Meher Baba

MEHER BABA

Meher Baba was born Merwan Sheriar Irani on February 25, 1894, in Pune, India. Merwan attended St. Vincent's High School and Deccan College.

In 1913, while still in college, he met Perfect Master Hazrat Babajan, who awakened him to his spiritual destiny. After contact and training with other Perfect Masters, his own spiritual mission began in 1921. His early disciples gave Merwan the name Meher Baba – Compassionate Father.

Baba and his disciples eventually established a centre near Ahmednagar, India, that came to be called Meherabad. Here his work embraced a free school where spiritual training was stressed, a free hospital and dispensary, and shelters for the poor. He made no distinction between those of high caste and untouchables. To his close ones at Meherabad, who were of different castes and creeds, he gave training in moral discipline, love for God, spiritual understanding, and selfless service.

Meher Baba maintained silence from 1925 until the end of his physical life on January 31, 1969. Despite his silence, he led an active life, communicating with those around him, initially by means of an alphabet board, and later through distinctive hand gestures. His many spiritual messages and discourses were published in English, and include *Discourses, God Speaks, Life At Its Best,* and *Beams on the Spiritual Panorama.*

Baba encouraged people of all faiths to follow their chosen paths. He saw Hinduism, Islam, Christianity, Buddhism, Zoroastrianism, and Jainism as different rivers leading to the same goal – Divine Love.

Meher Baba travelled extensively to the United States, the United Kingdom, continental Europe, and Australia in the 1930s and 1950s.

CONTENTS

PREFACE

Dr. William Donkin, born in 1911 to a well-to-do London family, may well remain a mystery to many after they read this book.

William, who lived a life of self-effacement in India for three decades, still prompts inquiry and speculation among those who knew him and knew about him for the last 100 years.

Today's surviving family members living in England and the United States knew him in their teen years as their "favourite uncle" who tolerated their minor delinquencies such as smoking. He even cheered such behaviour on his infrequent, short trips back to England from India.

This book would not have been attempted had William been a stuffy fellow. He had a rakish, adventurous streak, probably fuelled by the exploits of T.E. Lawrence in World War I and the Lawrence of Arabia literary wildfire that swept the world when William was still a young man.

William's behaviour mirrored Lawrence's. He and a British companion barely survived a gruelling six-month trek across the Sahara Desert by camel and horseback in 1932.

Shortly after the pair's desert exploit, which created headlines, photographs in the London Times, and even public appearances to recount their experiences, William would embark on a larger, challenging, more taxing lifelong journey.

In October 1933, he met Indian Spiritual Master Meher Baba at a Russell Road home in London's toney Kensington neighbourhood. His life changed forever.

Already enrolled in medical school, he asked Meher Baba whether pursuing a medical career would benefit Baba's work in India. He graduated six years later as an orthopaedic surgeon from London's St. Bartholomew's Hospital ("Barts") and immediately left for India in July 1939.

Doctoring was not a high priority on the agenda when he joined Meher Baba's ashram. William would drive a bus, clean out latrines, and seek out God-intoxicated souls across India – a favourite pursuit of the Spiritual Master.

In the late 1940s William assumed for a short time a new role – author – when he wrote *The Wayfarers,* a book about Baba's work with the God-intoxicated or "masts." Today an online search of Dr. William Donkin will pull up his book, a painstakingly detailed account of the God-intoxicated men and women of India. It is the only literary work of its kind and some of those close to William in India say he himself took on the qualities of a mast (pronounced "must") after completing the book and was never the same afterwards.

Slave of Love has been simmering for many years. The dust jacket on Donkin's book *The Wayfarers* said enough to tickle my interest in William:

"At the age of 20 he crossed the Sahara by camel and horseback.... As a member of Alpine Club, London, he went mountain climbing in the Alps, Norway, High Atlas, Corsica.... Qualified as a doctor from 'Barts' in 1939."

And then went to India to serve a Spiritual Master.

A brief conversation about this intriguing British chap with Meher Baba's sister Mani on a trip to India in 1995 prompted her to suggest pursuing the writing project.

A cast of many accompanies William in this book. He was unique as the only Western male to spend 30 years with Meher Baba in India. On countless occasions William would serve as a frontrunner and contact person with Baba's followers in countries of the Western world.

His life in India was no cakewalk. Baba said early that he was out to destroy egos in trying to bring his followers closer to Divine Love and God-realization. William along with everyone else would be reshaped and reinvented throughout this demanding process.

Many years later there are still gaps in William's story and at least one lingering mystery. The reader will undoubtedly ask the why of William's life with Meher Baba many times along the way. Just as Meher Baba dealt with all of his lovers as individuals, different readers will form their own conclusions.

Meher Baba, on one occasion when the intake of food was being discussed among followers, said he wanted them "as thin as air."

He believed that in the end, the individual with their selfish thoughts and desires should not exist.

The final goal. Effacement …

ACKNOWLEDGEMENTS

Mani S. Irani, Meher Baba's sister, planted the seed for *Slave of Love* in October 1995. She said simply that Dr. William Donkin's life "would be a fascinating story."

Along the way since then there have been many people who have helped bring the book to life.

My wife for 37 years, Kate, encouraged me both in the early years of research and in the later years of writing. Although not a follower of Meher Baba, she was tremendously loving and giving to her partner and our children Jessica and Jonathan. She left us much too early in July 2009.

I am indebted to friends in Nova Scotia and Myrtle Beach who eased the pain of loss and helped mend my heart in the months that followed Kate's departure. I will be forever thankful to members of the Meher Baba community in South Carolina and throughout the world who were so kind.

There are of course specifics and logistics to writing a book. Louise (Garnant) Silverman read over, edited, organized, and researched and contributed footnotes for *Slave of Love* – not once, but twice when a second revision was necessary. Louise passed away in November 2012. I miss you, dear friend.

My genuine appreciation goes out to book designer Nancy Roberts and to longtime friend Jennie Carton who designed the book cover.

There were many years of waiting before the family of William Donkin finally came into my life. But when William's niece Bridget Mathieson Barry and nephews Richard and Charles Donkin and George Mathieson did, they revived the project with their friendliness; their generous support; and the Donkin Family letters, papers, and photos pertaining to William's life that they made available.

The research never ends, and someone said early on that the longer one waits the better the book. Along the way, Richard Donkin uncovered an old 1938 home movie showing William at play as a young man with his parents, twin sister Mary, and a cousin at Winterfold, the family estate in Surrey. The link http://vimeo.com/15507901 will give readers a brief look at this spirited, fun-loving young man. William would continue to be a merry prankster throughout his life.

During the lengthy research and writing, there were folks who urged me on in the project and their words were often timely and much needed. I am indebted to Sheila Krynski at Sheriar Foundation of Myrtle Beach; the late Don Stevens of France and England, long-time disciple and author of many Baba books; and to my 1995 India roommate Philip Creager for his helpful tips and contributions along the way.

My trips to England and India in the fall of 2010 would have come up empty without still more helpful input. In London, Cassie Tarquini scanned and copied photos and documents for hours, allowing me to spend a wonderful afternoon interviewing William's nephews Richard and Charles. Thanks also to archivist Glyn Hughes at the London Alpine Club and to Katie Ormerod, deputy archivist at St. Bartholomew's Hospital (Barts). Also to Hilla Talwar, who shared her remembrances about William Donkin and her life as a child and young woman with Meher Baba. They all kept me productively busy during the week's stay in London.

In India, Janet Judson and Jessica Mednick at the Meher Baba Trust Archives had uncovered a mountain of material on William before my arrival and kept me at work most mornings at the Archives during the three-week stay in Meherabad, India, in October 2010. Added thanks to Bif Soper for generously providing the photo of Lingmala Falls in India, to Gerrie Grevatt for her photo of Kitty Davy, and to longtime Myrtle Beach photographer Jack Thompson for his beautiful photo of Elizabeth Chapin Patterson and the aerial shot of Meher Spiritual Center.

The fabric of the story would be much thinner without the input of many others. Sheela Kalchuri Fenster, who in the Introduction recalls her life as a child and young teenager with her "best friend" William. The stories and support from Bhau Kalchuri (last male mandali, who passed away in October 2013); Meherwan Jessawala (younger brother of mandali member Eruch Jessawala); and Meheru Irani (last female mandali, who passed away in April 2012). Dara (Meher Baba's nephew) and Amrit Irani's hospitality, remembrances of William, and the 2010 tour of William's residential bungalow quarters in Ahmednagar, where he spent the final months of his life.

I am indebted to Debjani Ray in India for putting me in contact with Motiram Kamble, who served William as a young man and still lives in Meherabad. The interview with Motiram and the stories of his younger years with William were priceless. I thank Jal Dastoor at the Meher Baba Trust office for turning on a dime to help make the interview happen and Shridhar Kelkar, who served as interpreter during the wonderful session with Motiram.

In addition to my gratitude to the Donkin Family members, I will be forever grateful to Pat Sumner, David Fenster, Martin and Christine Cook, Sufism Reoriented, Wendy and Buz Connor, Doug Frank, and Duncan Knowles for giving special permissions to use various photo collections and for providing such high-quality, wonderful images to work with.

A retired newspaper journalist knows very little about the book publishing business. My heartfelt thanks to Nancy Roberts, David Fenster, Sheila Krynski, and Naosherwan Anzar for their creative coaching, patience, sound advice, guidance, and friendship along the way.

Finally and foremost, I thank Meher Baba and William Donkin. They are still such an inspiring, sweet, fulfilling part of my life.

Bob Mossman
Lunenburg
Nova Scotia
Canada

How true and loyal is your best friend? Would they take the blame for something you did?

I am not sure I would, but William Donkin was just such a friend to me.

Several times, I was the cause of some conflict at Meherabad or Khushru Quarters, where we both lived. We were called to Meherazad, where Baba angrily confronted us. William inevitably accepted all the blame, as if it were his fault, and never even mentioned my name to Baba as the real culprit. I could only stand there and silently thank him from the bottom of my heart. Other times, when either Adi Sr. or my mother complained to Baba about something William did – some angry word or irritable action – most times Baba would scold William, but at the same time he would wink at him. Baba gestured very discreetly to him to ignore what he was saying, that Baba was not really serious. (Adi's head was bowed and my mother wasn't paying close attention – so they never knew.)

Eruch, on behalf of Baba, would continue to berate William in a loud voice. William would stand before Baba with a broad smile on his face. At the end, Baba gestured to William, "Happy?"

William whispered, "Yes, Baba." (He always spoke in a soft voice with Baba.)

Adi was incensed. *"Happy?!* I did not bring this man here to make him happy!" But Baba embraced and kissed William on the cheek. Baba pointed to his own heart and made the sign of perfection, indicating that William had a very good heart. So I felt that William Donkin was the greatest, truest friend in the world.

I was only five years old when I first met William. He was forty-six at the time, but I never had the feeling that he was some older "adult." I spent hours in his company, listening to him and learning from him. William would patiently explain things to me, on *my* level.

William loved animals; he was a true naturalist, always "studying," observing, drawing, and painting nature. (He was a great artist.) He tamed some wild baby foxes once, for example, and learned the names of all the local flora and fauna.

He couldn't stand noise from the servants or from the Sarosh Cinema in Ahmednagar, but the ceaseless chirping of sparrows and crows above his house at Meherabad delighted him. (And he could mimic their calls perfectly!) Most people would consider the cawing of crows an annoyance, but William once collected me from my home at 5:00 a.m. so that I could listen to them. "If you hear their voices in the morning," he told me, "it feels like they are singing for God."

He was a stickler for cleanliness. Hygiene-wise, I've never found anyone in the world as particular as he was, except perhaps for Mehera.

Most importantly, William's devotion to Baba was very, very deep. His devotion to Baba was in his actions. When Baba gave him some order, not to do something, for example – no matter how difficult it was, William obeyed 101%. He was willing to make any sacrifice for Baba.

It was an example I tried (and failed) to emulate.

At darshan times, when devotees waved sticks of incense in front of Baba, William used to watch from afar and comment to me, "It smells good, but if it goes in the lungs it is as harmful to you as smoking. Poor Baba has to suffer with breathing that smoke. He will get sick; he has allergies. But even though Baba is suffering, he doesn't complain."

I asked him, "If smoking is so bad for your health, why do you keep a cigar in your mouth all day long?"

"Did you ever see me smoke it?" he countered. "I never light it. But you're right. Even putting it in the mouth is bad, so I'm trying to stop. But it's an old habit of years."

So I felt free to question William, to argue and discuss things with him.

At the time Baba dropped his body, William was a source of great comfort. I was weeping that day, of course. William told me, "Sheela, God came on earth and gave us the chance to be with him. We are so fortunate. How many people are there in the world? Who had the chance to stay with him? We did! So don't forget this.

"Physically, we cannot see Baba, but internally, he is always with us. We have to *feel* like that. Baba has dropped his body, but it doesn't mean that he has left us. He is here. He's here. Never forget this."

William's words helped me tremendously to become inwardly strong.

Through Bob Mossman's book, I hope more of William's great strength of character and purity of heart will be revealed to those who came to Baba after he dropped his body and who never had the chance to meet William Donkin.

Sheela Kalchuri Fenster
Meherabad
India

1

New Beginnings – Meeting the God-Man

William Donkin wrote and published one book in his life, *The Wayfarers* – a book that has been overlooked by most of the world for more than 60 years.

This is not surprising. The publication was about God-intoxicated people. A strange undertaking for an upper-crust Englishman who attended prep school in Kent and later Rugby School, which was made famous in the popular 1940 movie *Tom Brown's School Days.*

Donkin went on to graduate in 1939 from London's famed medical school, St. Bartholomew's Hospital, commonly known as "Barts."

The Wayfarers was first published in 1948 – nine years after William Donkin moved permanently to India – and it is still in print today.

The God-mad or -intoxicated, known as masts (pronounced "musts"), were an unusual lot. And Meher Baba was not sold on the day's popular measure of mankind:

"It is important to remember that the average man himself has not really any balance of mind. The average man has only an appearance of balance, because he can often effect a provisional adjustment between the warring elements in his mind."[1]

The God-intoxicated men and women that Donkin met and learned about through his life with his spiritual master were, he believed, living in another zone – a cut above himself and most other ordinary beings of the world.

Ramju Abdullah, a colleague of Donkin's wrote in the forward to *The Wayfarers* in one long sentence, "The simplest way for man to get nearer to God is to get nearer to those who have already achieved the cherished proximity to Divinity … and who have established direct contact with spirituality by transcending the limited scopes of ordinary understanding, reasoning, knowledge and experience, within which man has instinctively trapped himself, and from which he finds it difficult to emerge because he always insists upon looking outside – be it for help and knowledge, or for freedom and peace."[2]

William and his twin sister Mary, born on November 14, 1911, in Wimbledon, England, were the youngest of four Donkin children. When William and Mary were 11, the family moved to a stately home and property in Surrey.

The Donkin men – William's grandfather, father, and his older brothers Bryan and John – were all in the engineering field. That sounds staid, but they were also adventurers. Most of the Donkin family were able mountaineers and members of London's Alpine Club. William and his brother John would become members in 1936, joining their father and older brother.

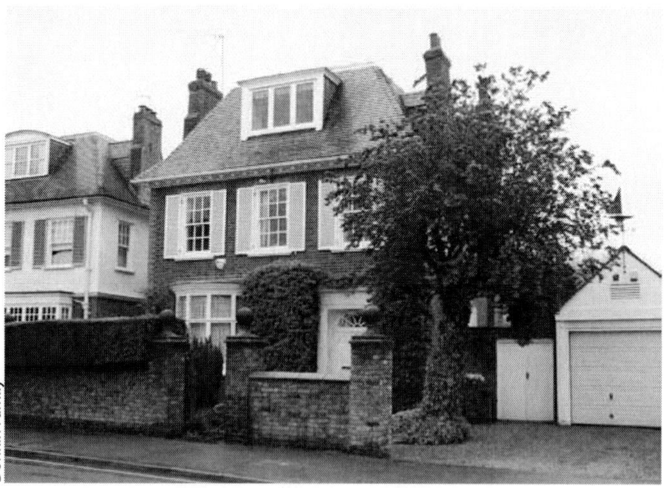
Donkin Family

A modern-day photo of the house in Wimbledon where William Donkin was born.

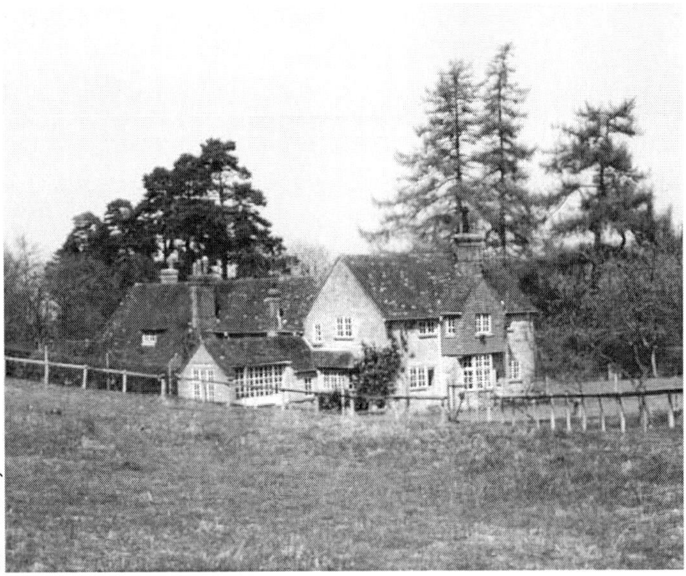

Donkin Family

Winterfold, located on a large acreage in Surrey, was purchased by William Donkin's father in 1922. A small old structure was eventually remodelled and expanded into this rambling home. William left his family life and the beautiful rural surroundings of the Donkin estate to live in India in 1939, but it was to Winterfold that he returned on his visits to England.

The club was then located at 23 Saville Road. Their mountain climbing trips to the Alps, Norway, High Atlas, and Corsica would be frequent.

One member of the family – William's father's distant cousin – had been killed in a climbing accident in the Caucasus in 1888. William Frederick had been an accomplished photographer, and his collection of striking climbing photos hung on the walls of the Alpine Club many years after his deadly fall. One photo shows a small, stone-walled bivouac shelter clinging to the side of a mountain-face. This would have been the last overnight stopover for William Frederick, a fellow British climber, and two guides, who all perished after leaving the campsite. While some of the group's belongings were discovered at the bivouac site almost a year later, their bodies were never found.

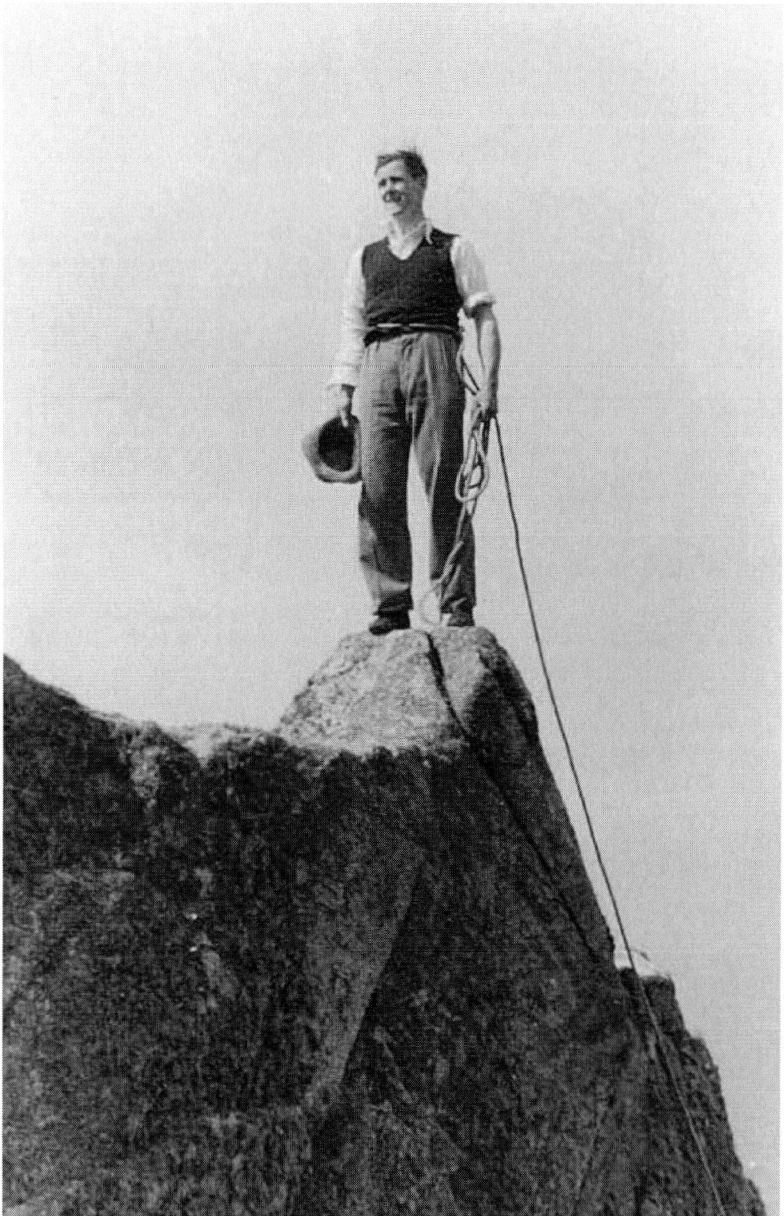

Donkin Family

A happy William stands atop a conquered mountain pinnacle. His immediate family and ancestors were all avid climbers and members of the London Alpine Club.

Our William's adventurous dreams started early and went beyond conquering cold mountain ranges of Europe. In 1932, at age 20, he and companion Norman Pearn crossed the Sahara in the hottest months – May to September – covering the first 1,400 miles by camel and the last 300 on horseback. Norman Pearn would become a well-known Middle East explorer, later writing the book *Quest for Sheba: In the Footsteps of the Arabian Queen.*

William's father, Sydney Bryan, investigated Pearn's character deeply before giving his blessings as well as financial help to the trip. He wrote letters to people who knew the Pearn family and even went as far as contacting Scotland Yard to verify that Pearn was not an unscrupulous character.

Sydney Bryan also found out all he could from his own contacts who knew Africa about the route the two young men would take. Most said the men were foolhardy to attempt the desert crossing, spelling out numerous dangers ranging from marauding bandits to dying of thirst or starvation.

William and Pearn had scouted out the territory together the year before on a shorter trip and thought they knew what they were getting into. Once on the longer journey they quickly found out the warnings were well founded. The Sahara experience was gruelling.

"As we understood that six days under such conditions of heat was the limit to which a camel could go without water, every moment was precious.... Each of these days we moved for 12 to 16 hours without halt.... Rest was mostly taken by day, although we could not extend the midday siesta very greatly, since the heat and lack of sufficient food were telling on the camels."[3]

A letter home to William's family describes the desert life:

"Wounds do not heal easily here since when I fell from my camel 4 weeks ago the slight abrasion is only just healing now.

"The other night a five-inch, blood-sucking spider gadded up me, round my neck and down my front, causing much consternation among us all.

"The Arabs catch desert rats, mice, lizards of all sorts, sand fish, etc. the throats of which they cut and we roast them

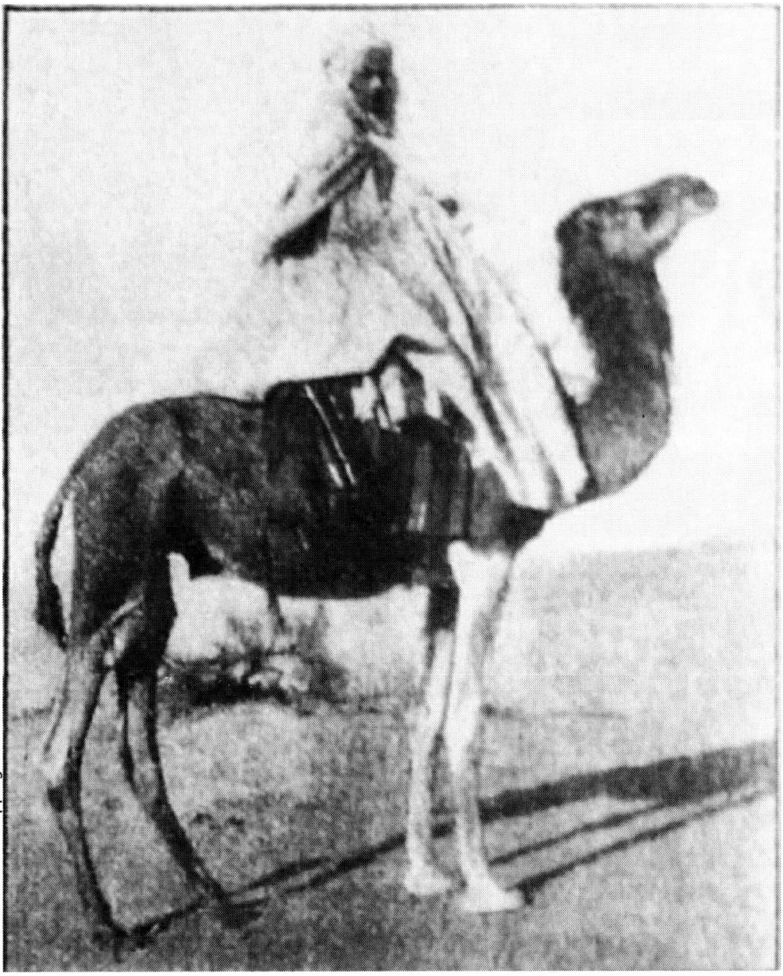

London Times newsclipping

William Donkin as a young man on his Sahara adventure.

in the fire and eat them. They are not bad, though hardly worth the killing since they are so small."[4]

William's five-page letter included several sketches he had made of the desert landscape.

Donkin and Pearn tasted fame briefly from the publicity their adventure attracted, both before their journey began and on their return to London. An article in *The London Times* announced the men's appearance at an upcoming lecture. A photo showed a nomadic William in full Arab dress on a camel.

William's Sahara trip may well have touched a chord within him that would soon set him on the major challenge of his life – living with Meher Baba in India. It would be an adventure he would never turn away from, even when severely and endlessly tested. The desert trip may have helped prepare him for the rigours of life he would face in India years later.

Like a sailor on the sea for months, whose life is filled with sunrises and sunsets, in crossing the Sahara, William witnessed vastness and beauty, along with desert journey hardships. There are even hints of a future medical career in the precise observations he made on the trek:

"We crossed the boundary between Southern Algeria and French West Africa. Visibility was good, and we had a very fine view of the plain, utterly flat and barren, the tanezruft dissolving into the calm hot sky.... Two days later we found evidence of more substantial vegetation of former times in the shape of multitudes of fossilized twigs and branches, and ... great fossilized tree trunks.... There were signs of a more recent fauna in the quantity of fragments of the shells of ostrich eggs."[5]

In the fall of 1933, with the newspaper and lecture experiences of his Sahara trip well behind him, William, about to enrol in medical school at Barts, found himself at a busy London street corner one evening. Will Backett*, a fellow Englishman who had met Meher Baba in 1931 on his first trip to London from India, describes the scene involving William at the London tube station:

"Dr. William Donkin's first contact with Baba occurred one rush hour at Liverpool Street Station, one of London's large terminus [*sic*].

"Evening papers at the bookstall were in great demand and he impulsively chose *The Occult Review***, which he had never seen before and which included Spiritual Master Meher Baba as the subject of one letter to the editor.

---

* Will Backett was an early English disciple of Meher Baba, who called Will and his wife Mary his archangels.

** *The Occult Review* was a British illustrated monthly journal published from 1905 to 1951 containing articles and correspondence by many notable occultists of the day.

"Communicating with the *Review* editor, he was given the address of an office at 50 Charing Cross, which he visited for more information on Meher Baba.

"Immediately on entering the office, one unforgettable afternoon, he said he was searching for spiritual healing, and at once was assured that he had come to the right place, as that was Baba's work."[6]

William may have been being very astute. The term "spiritual healing" was part of the written message Baba had delivered the year before on sailing into New York. "Spiritual healing is by far the greatest healing, and that is what I intend to give," Baba told newspaper reporters on May 19, 1932, while aboard *SS Bremen.*

William would have found a mimeographed booklet at the Charing Cross office titled *Shri Meher Baba, The Perfect Master – Questions and Answers.* The publication was put out by the Baba-affiliated Circle Editorial Committee in 1933. It contained a brief biographic sketch of the Indian Spiritual Master along with detailed answers from Baba on specific spiritual questions.

Shortly after, in October of that same year, William met the God-Man personally in London.

This was not Baba's first time in London. In 1931, he had made his first trip to England from India on the *Rajputana.* The ship also was carrying the famous passenger Mahatma Gandhi*, on his way to that year's Round Table Conference in London. Gandhi and Baba knew of one another. Baba recognized Gandhi as a great soul, but said he would achieve a higher degree of spirituality if he gave up politics.

William was understandably nervous in October 1933 as he climbed the front steps at 32 Russell Road, the home of Kitty Davy** in London's Kensington district. The atmosphere was charged in the home where Baba was receiving people in personal interviews.

---

* Mohandas Gandhi (1869–1948), the well-known pacifist, was the political and spiritual leader of India during the Indian independence movement.

** Kitty Davy was an early English disciple of Meher Baba. She lived with Baba in India from 1937 to 1952 and assisted in running the Meher Spiritual Center in South Carolina from 1952 until her death in 1991.

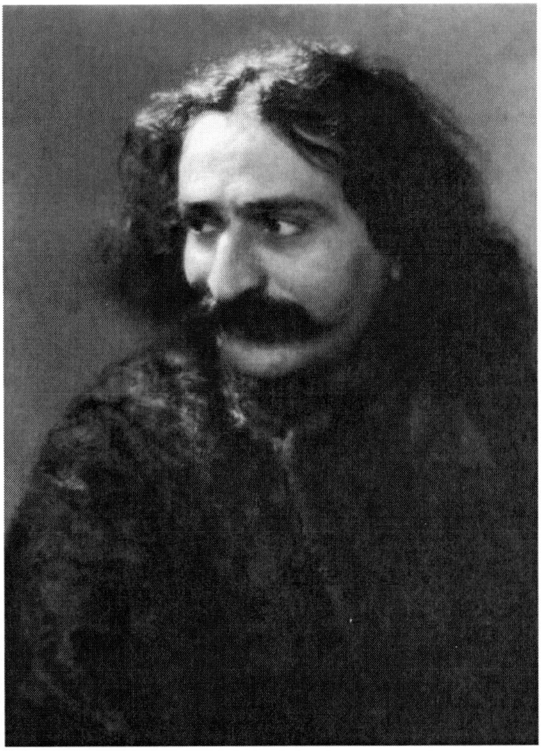

M&C Cook Collection

London portrait photographer Kinye Imai took this picture of Meher Baba on Baba's first visit to England in 1931.

Later William would briefly describe the meeting. He shook hands with Baba and was introduced. William said he was not aware of any other human figure in the room, just a feeling of being surrounded by a "great light." The encounter affected him for days. In sublime shock, the young medical student probably did not know the magnitude of what was ahead of him.

Baba would be quick to tell his followers that his charted course for them was no picnic. In *The Narrow Lane* – a small book about Baba – the inside cover page quotes Baba as saying, "The lane that leads to Me is narrow, and only men and women of great daring enter it."

Eliminating an individual's ego was the major thrust of Meher Baba's philosophy.

In Baba's work with the masts, or God-intoxicated of India, he was trying to shift these spiritually advanced wayfarers to a level where they could assist Baba and render some sort of universal help to mankind. On the other hand, with the followers who lived in the world, Baba would either lead them gently by the hand and/or brow-beat them into a higher spiritual state. To achieve this greater spiritual awareness, much had to change and be given up in the selfish, ego-centred lives of Baba's followers. William Donkin would soon learn this first hand.

When they first met in London, William asked Baba about the career path he had chosen:

"Is taking surgery a good idea?"

"Yes, you should pursue that. I will also need a surgeon in India," said Baba. Six years of medical studies is not a light undertaking for anyone.

In many letters that would follow between Baba in India and William in London, he was encouraged to continue his studies and strive for excellence. It is fair to say that William was in his "honeymoon" phase with Baba, as he was coaxed along during the medical school years.

In the first years after they met, Baba maintained constant connection to William in London through a two-way written correspondence. Meher Baba made a point of keeping in touch with those he met in the West and often did so through Westerners who had moved to India to live at his ashram.

Kitty Davy, in whose London family home Baba had met his first Western followers, was part of a group of Westerners who were called in December 1936 to live with Baba for a number of months in Nasik*, India.

---

* Nasik is on the Godavari River in a very beautiful and fertile area known as the "green belt." Nasik is considered a holy city with many forts and temples, and it is said to be where Lord Rama stayed when he was in exile. It is in the Western Ghats of Maharashtra on the edge of the Deccan Plateau. The Western Ghats is a mountain range that runs north to south along the western edge of the Deccan Plateau, separating the plateau from a narrow coastal plain along the Arabian Sea.

William and Kitty became better acquainted after October 1933. On one occasion in London before her 1936 departure to India, she invited William over to the family's Russell Road house for tea. The two also met at the Circle Editorial Committee office at Charing Cross and had lunch afterwards.

Baba demanded proper conduct from his followers. Both Kitty and William would have been aware of his rules of behaviour, although Kitty admitted in her book, *Love Alone Prevails,* that Westerners did not at first grasp how serious the rules were. The written correspondence allowed Baba's followers the opportunity to express their personal feelings, however, as well as describe the demands presented by living with Baba.

Kitty forthrightly apologized for not writing sooner in an April 15, 1937, letter to William from the Meher Retreat in Nasik:[7]

"I did not feel in the letter writing mood and I cannot write artificially to you of all people.

"Thank you so much for your many letters – the last of which is by me now.

"It has been a bed of roses for me up to now, and I have been supremely happy all the time, but alas – the thorns have begun for others as well as for myself.

"Baba forgives, but that is no compensation for the betrayal of trust and one's own weakness that one feels. It is torture and being me I cannot throw things off easily. How I wish I did not brood – but I will go on trying and repeat and repeat.

"'Think only of Baba. Be happy and don't worry.'

"So take warning – if you come out here. Remember Baba sees the future and knows full well by his orders how to avoid dangers and don't disobey. As Purdom says 'become immersed in Baba's orders.' Love is not sufficient until we are more perfect in it than we are now.

"Will – excuse my mood – but I am in the thick of it – in the attempt to throw it off, but Baba has to bring these things up out of our subconscious so that we really see ourselves as we are and don't live in a dream.

"It is essential to the elimination of the ego....

"Best wishes. Your letters make Baba so happy.

"Love, K.L.D."

William was invited to meet with Baba personally during his school years in the 1930s, when Baba travelled to Cannes on the French Riviera. In addition to bringing the Western followers who lived with him in India, Baba also invited a number of other Western devotees from abroad to join him.

While William was pleased to be a part of the group and to be able to spend time with Baba at a stately home on the Mediterranean, he quickly got a taste of Baba's often unusual requests. Baba asked William to search for "a perfect boy" in England. Before and after this, Baba sent others on the same search.

In 1924, Baba had established the Prem Ashram school in India at his Meherabad headquarters. The Prem Ashram was a free school that was open to all castes and faiths and drew students from faraway places, mainly from other parts of India and Iran.

Youngsters from all religions (including Christianity) attended the school, which became one of Baba's efforts at destroying barriers between different faiths of the world and also breaking down the caste system prevalent in India. The search for the perfect boy was one of the recurring directives Baba gave in connection to the school. He said his work with a perfect boy would help the youth of the future.

William accepted the challenge and found a youngster that he recommended to Baba, but the boy proved unsatisfactory for Baba's purposes. This strange chore was to be the first of many unusual requests and jobs William would face in his life with Meher Baba. William would find himself driving a busload of Baba's close followers across India. Then suddenly his role would change to working with Baba cleaning latrines. Between these jobs, Baba would assign him only a smattering of medical duties.

2

Early Life and India at Last

It is uncertain just how William's early childhood in England prepared him for the seesaw life with Meher Baba. The gruelling desert adventure at age 20 would certainly have made him adaptable to change.

As a youngster growing up in London, the background of his parents might hint that their children could readily accept an unorthodox lifestyle.

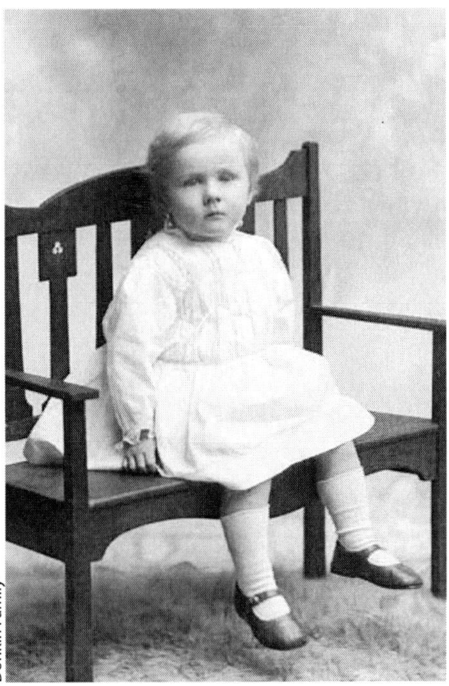
Donkin Family

A childhood photo of William Donkin

William's father, Sydney Bryan Donkin, was an accomplished, successful, inventive engineer and businessman. While he seemed conservative to an outsider, those close to him saw him as kind, not stern.

Sydney Bryan loved climbing mountains perhaps even more than his engineering pursuits, and he passed this passion on to his three sons.

William's mother – Phoebe Smiles Donkin – had a liberal background. She graduated

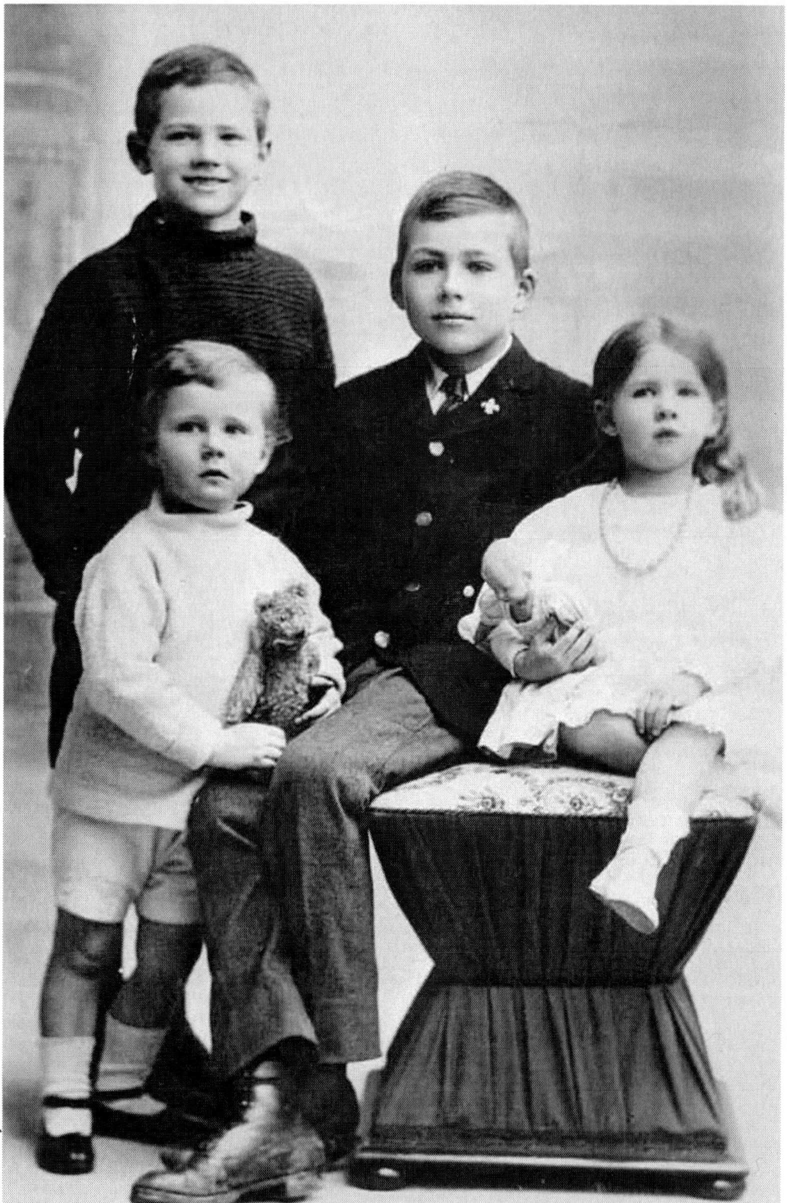

Donkin Family

A 1915 photo of William and his twin sister Mary with older brothers Bryan, seated, and John.

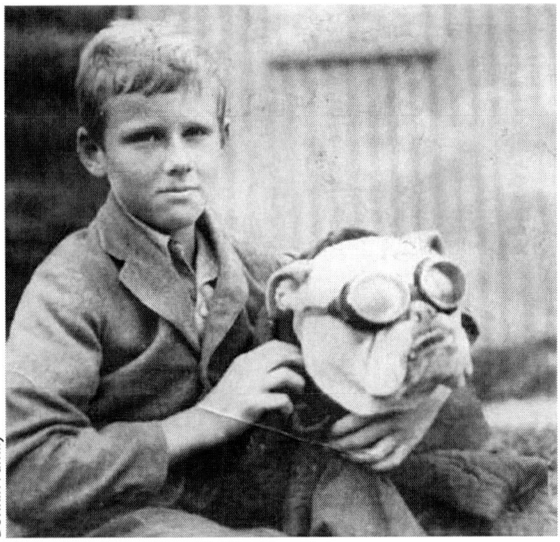

Donkin Family

William as a young boy exhibits a sense of humour with the family dog. Humour would be a part of his character throughout his life.

from the Slade School of Art and was a dedicated advocate of the philosophical teachings of Jean Rousseau. She was the grandniece of the well-known Scottish author and reformer Samuel Smiles*.

William's mother penned observations of William as a toddler and youngster. When William was a little over a year old, her comments, found in the Donkin family papers, included, "William Donkin born November 14 at about 12:30 p.m. one of twins with sister Mary). Weighed about 7 pounds, was a fair baby. Very energetic and lively. Later on he seemed less strong and now over a year later is less able to stand than his sister. But seems more wide awake intellectually. He is less shy than she is."

Another entry when William was 10:

"William became delicate in 1914 and had a succession of operations for glands.... He draws very well and took the prize for drawing last term. He has a fondness for little literary facts and should be able to write. He might make a good architect. He sings well. He is small for his age and pale and rather thin,

* Samuel Smiles was an author and reformer whose most famous work, *Self Help,* was based on a speech he gave for the Mutual Improvement Society, published as *The Education of the Working Classes.*

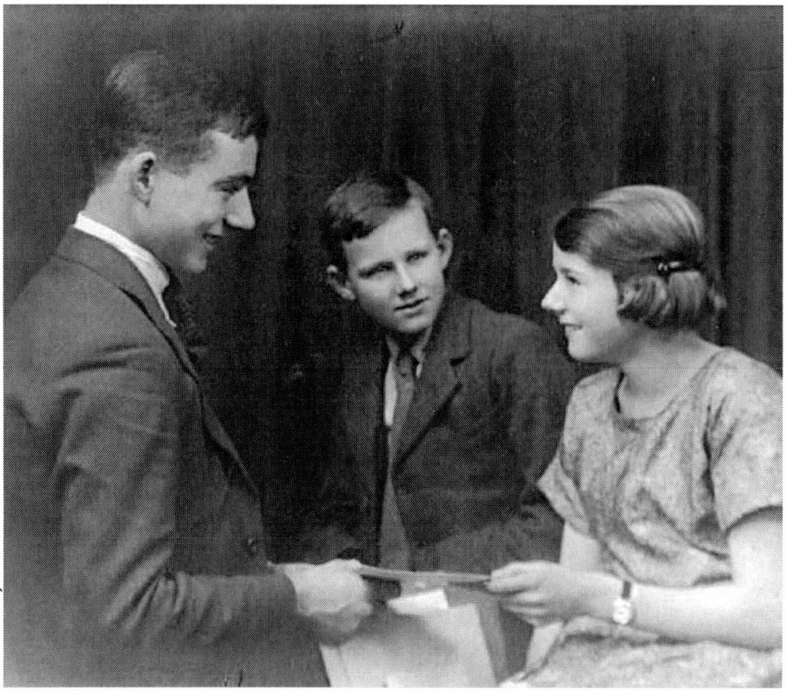
Donkin Family

William and his twin sister Mary are shown in discussion with their oldest brother Bryan in 1921. The family would have been living at the Winterfold estate in Surrey, England, when the photo was taken.

but he always keeps well. He is very fond of flowers and showed his love for them long before he could speak. If one gave him a flower in his pram his whole face lit up and he loved listening to the school children singing long before he could speak. He is very interested in French and does well at it."

The four Donkin children enjoyed a lively and interesting upbringing in the large family house and estate in Surrey called Winterfold, which their father purchased in 1922. The property was ample in acreage, had an outdoor tennis court, and the house included a darkroom where the children would develop their own photographs. There were early indications that William harboured inclinations beyond photography, however.

One of his unique pastimes as a youngster was extracting roadkill from country roads, which he would take home and dissect. While this may have been done with a peculiar sense of fun by the youngster, it also is an early indicator of his interest in anatomy and medicine.

An account of William's years as a student at Rugby School also reflects that mischief was very much on his mind and a part of his makeup – a trait he would foster and enjoy his entire life. He reportedly got suspended from school because he stole another student's trousers. In a further prank, William returned to Rugby School in disguise several days later and treated his classmates to a dinner out to get back into everyone's good graces.

William's decision to respond wholeheartedly to Meher Baba's call was conveyed to his parents shortly after he met Baba in 1933. While the artistic, free-spirited mother may have accepted her son's leanings, his father soon indicated hopes that his son would get over the attraction to the "God-Man."

Baba had told followers who came from the West to Nasik in India in December 1936 that their stay there would be a honeymoon with him. He had made the retreat as comfortable as possible according to Western standards. Baba also warned them that their lives would be much tougher when they moved from Nasik to another location in India.

Baba decided to extend the honeymoon phase for the Westerners in Nasik with a trip to France later in 1937. Kitty Davy was also part of the Nasik group that travelled to Cannes with Meher Baba for a four-month stay midway through the year.

She wrote to William from Cannes, "What are you thinking about it all? Are not Baba's ways strange? I have never felt him work so intensely as he is doing now. Sometimes I wonder if I can stand it; but of course one can, as Baba never gives you more than you can stand.

"Love, Kitty"[8]

Kitty added the following footnote to her letter: "Do send me your address ... I feel so lost without it."[9]

William lived at a number of different addresses in London while attending medical school, including the flat his father maintained there for his own work days in the city.

While William was reluctant to put his feelings about Meher Baba into words to other followers, Kitty would have seen his letters, as Baba asked her to answer the letters from the British followers on his behalf.

William was invited to stay with Baba in Cannes in late September. His visit would be short because of his medical studies, and his time there was also interrupted with other Baba-related travels.

His excitement at being invited to visit Baba in Cannes is reflected in this letter:

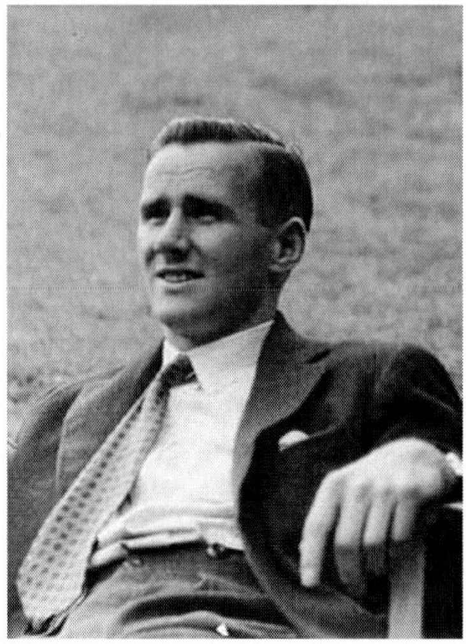

Donkin Family

William strikes a casual pose during his 1933–39 medical school years in London.

"Dearest Baba:

"1,000 thanks – you're a peach, to say the least of it. How I am longing to see your ... beautiful smile again.

"If you the man are so marvellous, how much more unbelievable must the Infinite you be....

"Love to you dear One, now and ever.

"Yours Will. Donkin"[11]

On William's arrival in Cannes, he and Kitty both became involved in the hectic search of trying to find a perfect boy, after William's selection of a boy in England was rejected. The new search involved William and Kitty making separate trips to Paris to find boys through the Spanish Refugee Association. Neither of the boys selected met Baba's approval, and William had to make sure the two boys were returned to Paris. William also was asked to return a maid to England that Kitty had brought with her; the maid did not meet Baba's approval.

The larger group left Cannes in November. During her return to India, Kitty again wrote to William from aboard the ship *Circassia,* and again on December 8, 1937, after some of the Western group took up residence with Baba in Meherabad:

"Not only does Baba interest himself in the smallest details of our own life – its health, food and general activities – but also the whole of the management ... is also in Baba's hands. Every detail on the domestic side he plans and arranges."[12]

Another of Kitty's letters to William on January, 18, 1938, echoes her struggle to come to terms with Meher Baba's orders:

"Talking of inhibitions always makes me think of Margaret [Craske]*. She always said Baba's work was to break down. That he was like a mouse – nibbling away all the time.

"Baba in a lecture on love said 'Love gives and never asks.' So why want to be loved at all? It is that thought that is uppermost in my mind at the moment. Don't want love or the experience of love and then you can't mind if it is withheld, but the difficulty is when you can't express it spontaneously or not finding yourself loving less.

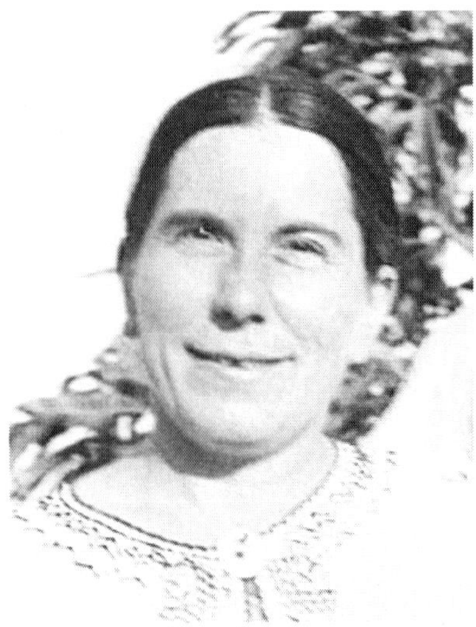

Kitty Davy

"But my answer to this is that love is and cannot be just feelings ... feelings come and go ... grow hot and cold. So there must be a stage beyond, and the transition period is not too pleasant. This is private. It's just what seems to be happening at the moment. I try hard to think of Shakespeare's words: 'To thy own self be true.'"

The personal contact with his new Spiritual Master that Cannes afforded certainly helped further cement William's

* Margaret Craske was a British dancer (dancing briefly with the Diaghilev Ballet) who was a well-respected dance teacher and one of the 20th century's leading authorities on the Cecchetti method. She met Baba in 1931 and dedicated the rest of her life to him.

loyalty to Baba. While there was a lapse in his attendance at medical school between 1937 and 1938 and some indication that he considered dropping out, Baba emphasized to William the importance of completing his studies. He would be sustained by letters to and from Baba in India for another sixteen months before completing his six years at Bart's.

Upon graduating from medical school, William's diary entry on his departure from London for India in July 1939 reflects his enthusiasm:

"I left London on July 7 or 8; I forget the exact date now.... There was quite a party at Victoria [Station] to see me off and to send their wishes to Baba."

Not content to ride the train to catch the boat to India in Marseilles, William decided to ride a bicycle part of the way.

"I arrived at Clermont-Ferrand* [by train] on Sunday afternoon, and it was not until the following afternoon ... I managed to buy a second-hand bike. Rather short in saddle, but OK. Paid 200 francs for it with new front tyre and pump. Cycled from there to Marseilles – about 200 miles or so – beautiful hills....

"The boat trip from Marseilles to Bombay [Mumbai] was uneventful. Pleasant, but a bit boring."

On arriving in Bombay, William's reticent character was evident. This trait of avoiding the limelight in public situations with Baba would continue and it is rare to find him in photographs and films of gatherings.

"At Bombay [Baba followers] met me on board, and covered me with flowers round the neck and with bouquets to carry. It made me feel perhaps a little self-conscious, but it was nevertheless a very pleasing way of welcoming me to India; the jasmine has a wonderful scent."

William kept a personal, detailed diary starting with his departure from London in July 1939 until after the war in 1945. It includes his early life with Baba, work with the God-intoxicated masts, interaction with Baba's Eastern and Western followers and his wartime years in the Indian Medical Service (IMS).

---

* Clermont-Ferrand is a city in the Auvergne region of France.

William faced a mishmash of characters on landing in India in 1939. Baba did not shy away from turmoil in personal relations and often used the interplay between personalities of followers to wear down and destroy personal egos.

There were usually a number of fellow Western followers living in India. Their tenures with Meher Baba could be weeks, months, or years. Sometimes they would arrive in India expecting to stay months – even years – then suddenly be sent back home after a few weeks. No Western male follower stayed continuously in India as long as William Donkin.

While his skills as a physician were sometimes drawn upon in response to medical needs of Baba's Western and Eastern disciples and followers, William was also expected to respond immediately and without argument to many other non-medical job requests and whims of his Master. For years, Baba had encouraged William's regime of intense medical training in London, and on William's arrival in India, Baba often just as insistently expected him to ignore the medical talents he had brought with him.

William was bright enough to understand that Baba was employing tactics to destroy his ego; but like many other Baba followers in India and elsewhere in the world, he would have pondered the natural question, "Why? What's the point?"

Elimination of the personal, selfish ego of his followers was a relentless part of Baba's work. To achieve God-realization or Divine Love – he insisted – the individual ego must go.

Baba was a strong proponent of evolution. But while other advocates of this origin of the species trace man from earlier primates, Baba's explanation plunges much deeper into nature's realm.

Man (through the evolution of the soul's consciousness through various forms), he insists, evolved originally from stone. This most limited life form progressed onward through "kingdoms" of seven stages: stone or metal, vegetable, worm, fish, bird, animal, and eventually human.

Once the soul evolved fully to humankind (full consciousness), the next process, says Baba, is reincarnation and "involution." The soul then goes through thousands of incarnations to eventually pass through the seven stages or planes of involution before achieving God-realization and Divine Love.

Many of the masts Baba contacted and William Donkin wrote about in *The Wayfarers* were on these higher planes of the path. They were in total communion with God.

By the time William met Baba in 1933, the Spiritual Master had already attracted a small worldwide following of people living outside of India who were drawn to him and his messages. Oddly enough, he had achieved this by not saying a word. In 1925, six years before his first trip to the West, Baba had begun to observe silence, and he continued this practice for 44 years.

The reasons he gave for starting and maintaining silence were straightforward:

"You have asked for and been given enough words – it is now time to live them."

This statement refers to the past human manifestations of God, including Buddha, Jesus, and Mohammed. He said these God-realized beings had spoken the truth, and in the modern age few people were listening to the messages of Divine Love and brotherhood these God-men had given during their tenures on Earth.

Baba insisted he would teach nothing new. His role, he said, was simply to awaken mankind to age-old truths.

Baba's followers, from all walks of life, came to him with plenty of egotistical baggage – both personal and professional. Baba himself said his Western followers in particular were "hard nuts to crack" and that Eastern followers were more inclined to the spiritual life and obedience.

Adaptability had to be a quick study for the Westerners. The trained physician Dr. William Donkin would soon learn to drive a bus full of followers and look after domestic pets in the ashram; London music teacher Kitty Davy would slave in the ashram kitchen; successful American businesswoman Elizabeth Patterson* would chauffeur Meher Baba; and talented British

* Elizabeth Chapin Patterson was one of Baba's early western mandali and founded the Meher Spiritual Center with Norina Matchabelli at Baba's direction. She was one of the first women insurance brokers and was an ambulance driver for the Red Cross in World War I. She was the driver in Meher Baba's 1952 car accident in Oklahoma.

ballerina and ballet instructor, Margaret Craske, would dance only for Baba at his beck and call.

The followers who stayed with Baba and were dedicated enough to be called mandali (disciples) took all of Baba's orders on the chin and cheek, and were expected to turn the other cheek and to do so cheerfully.

William stayed in India permanently and became one of the mandali. Kitty Davy remained a faithful mandali, and on Baba's orders, would move to the United States to help Elizabeth Patterson run the secluded 500-acre Meher Spiritual Center on the coast of South Carolina. Margaret Craske remained a steadfast mandali, and after World War II went back to her career as a ballet instructor, moving to New York City to teach. A number of Margaret's students would become Baba followers and a few even met Meher Baba in the 1950s.

Early on, Baba said the male mandali would run things in the East and the women would be in charge in the Western world. He would not let men dominate women any more than he tolerated mistreatment of Untouchables by Brahmins in India.

On William's arrival in India in September 1939, he was still very much in the honeymoon phase. After his tour of Bombay*, William travelled eastward to Poona**, the city where Meher Baba was born. From there William went on to Ahmednagar***, a city of 250,000. The Meherabad ashram is about nine kilometres from "Nagar."

Shortly after arriving there, William's diary relates his reunion with Baba:

---

* Bombay (now Mumbai) is a collection of seven islands located approximately at the centre of the west coast of India and is home of a structure known as the Gateway to India. Bombay is one of the most populous cities in the world and is the commercial capital of India, although in 1939 it was struggling with economic depression as was the rest of the world.

** Poona (Pune) is one of the largest cities in India, located on the western edge of the Deccan Plateau. It is considered the cultural capital of the state of Maharashtra and is home to many colleges and universities.

*** Ahmednagar, a city in Maharashtra state, is on the Sina River about 75 miles northeast of Poona. The largest district in Maharashtra, Ahmednagar is known for sugar, milk, and bank co-operatives. Due to scarce rainfall, Ahmednagar often suffers from drought.

"It was good to see him again after so long. He certainly looks better than he did in Cannes when I saw him last. Baba ordered me to take care of my health and incur no hardships, physical or mental, not to worry and to tell him of anything which is on my mind or worrying me.

"Secondly, I am not to worry about thoughts, good or bad, but I am not to 'put the bad ones in action.'"

For the most part Baba's women and men followers lived a completely separate existence in the ashram. He did not allow the men and women to have much contact or get to know one another. William's first few days in India were spent playing games that included a Chinese card game and Ping-Pong – a favourite game of Baba's that he played with Eastern and Western male followers. Baba would humorously dictate the game rules to his advantage. Marbles was another favourite, and at one point William was made "secretary of marbles" in Meherabad.

Baba had a habit of making up comical nicknames for male followers such as Lamppost, Popeye, and Barsoap. William longed for a nickname, and Baba would, on occasion, call him "Peachy," because of Baba's order for him to eat three peaches a day. William's most popular nickname became "Don" during his time in India, although he would over the years be given other nicknames that included "Donkey" and "son of an ostrich."

This light-hearted side of ashram life was often darkened with talk of war. Speculation was voiced about when England and the United States would declare war on Germany to check its aggressive stomp through Europe. In August 1939, William wrote, "Baba is quite enigmatic over the political situation. On Friday on reading the paper regarding Poland and Germany, I said it looked as if another crisis and perhaps war was on the way. He gave me a quick wink, which I think meant – no war yet."[13] In less than a month Germany would invade Poland, and on September 3, 1939, Britain's Neville Chamberlain declared war on Germany.

Ashram activities continued despite the world upheaval. Although Meherabad was considered home base at this time, Baba was often on the move. William soon became part of the nomadic journeys.

Hunting masts, driving a bus packed with devotees, dealing with mechanical breakdowns, getting stuck in the mud, packing and unpacking a mountain of luggage on the bus roof, and getting constant new directives from their Spiritual Master became daily challenges for William and others. After leaving Meherabad, the bus caravan first stopped off at Nasik, where Baba had changed the original ashram for Westerners into a mast retreat. After a short stay there, the group moved to Bombay and later to Bangalore in the south where a more permanent colony was planned.

Of his initiation for the trip William wrote, "Today, I have been practising driving the Chevrolet bus, which if the present arrangement stands, I am to drive ... starting on August 9, with a full complement of ladies. It will be an interesting drive – even if tiring."

William's diary description of the bus trip to Bangalore reflected continuous misfortunes:

"Burst one tyre on the way. I was very tired and after tea and bread and butter, the first meal since 8 a.m. that morning ... [we] set off in the bus to the station – 12 miles off. Filthy bad road, and me very tired already. We got back at midnight, slept fitfully on the stone floor 'till 5 a.m. Then off at 6:30 again.

"There is no doubt that Baba likes to make one exasperated and tired in order to work on one. At home he says I eat when I like and things are easy, but when tired, it is not easy to control emotions and he will make me, he says, mentally and spiritually strong."

William's bus-driving duty was complicated by Baba's order that Mehera* was not to see any men, including any of the male mandali. Kitty Davy recalls the awkward arrangement in the "Blue Bus," as the vehicle was affectionately called:[14]

"Later when Donkin joined them ... and helped Elizabeth with the driving of the Blue Bus, Baba sat in front with them, and a curtain was hung so that if Baba wanted to communicate with Mehera, he would draw the curtain aside so that Don [Baba's nickname for William] or whoever was there couldn't see

* Mehera was Baba's most beloved female disciple. She joined him in 1924. Baba said she was the purest soul and that she loved him as he should be loved.

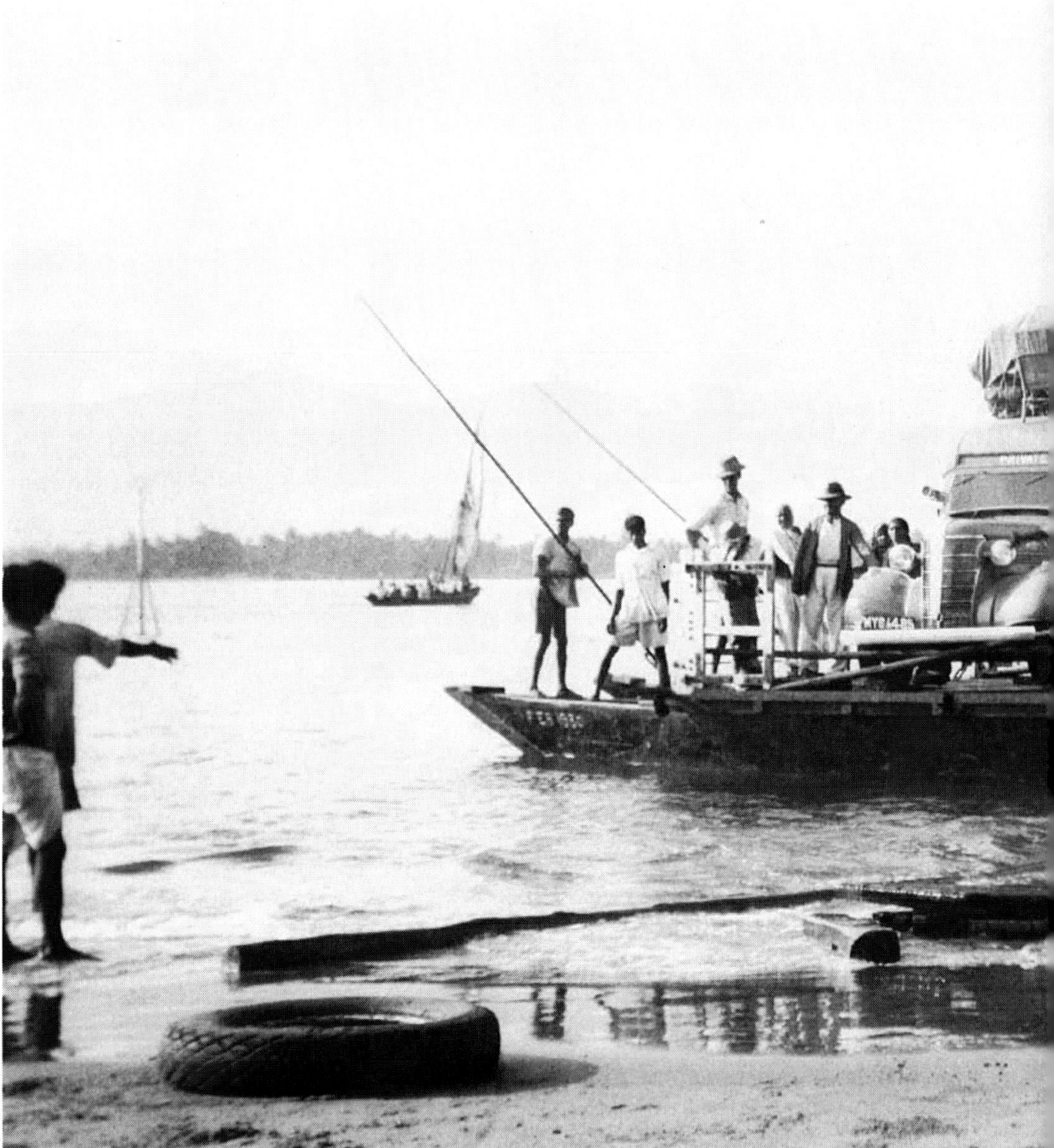

Elizabeth Chapin Patterson Photo Archives

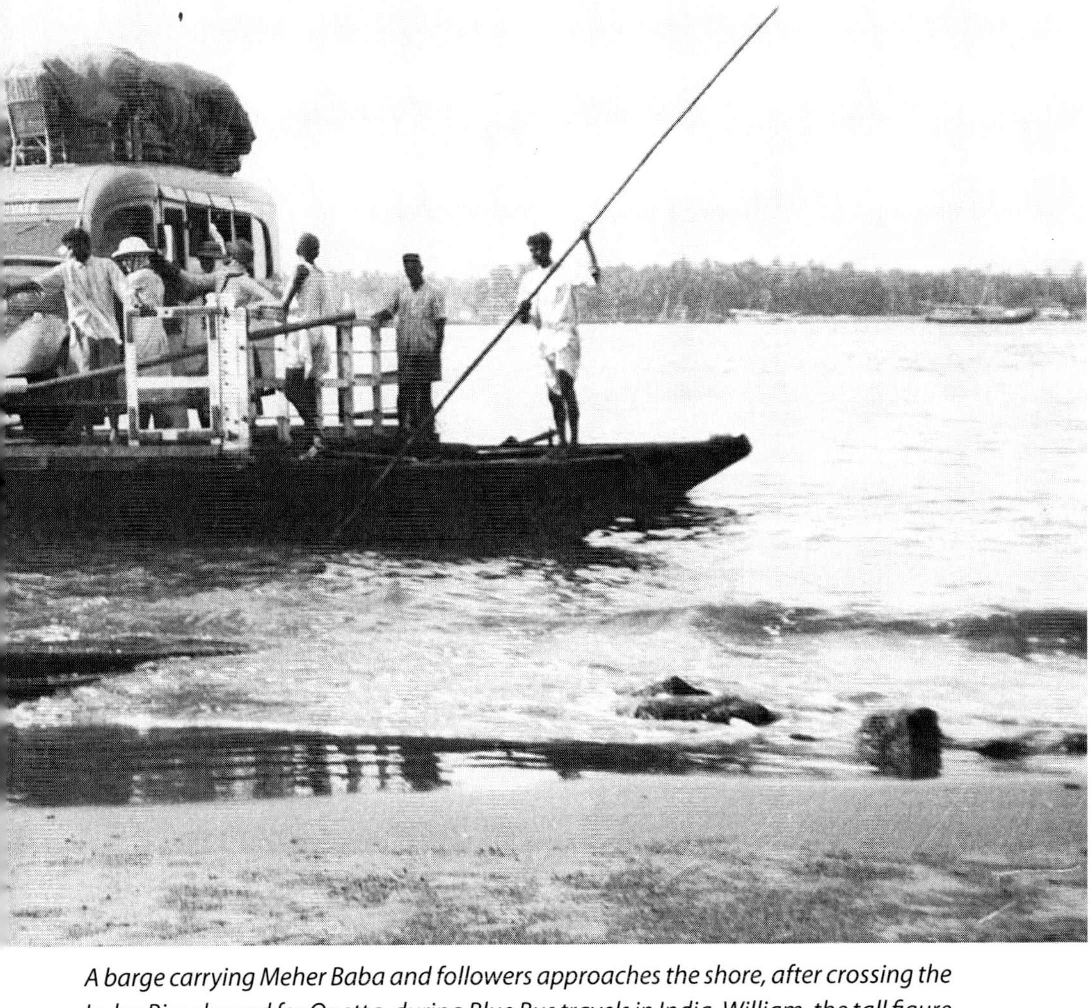

A barge carrying Meher Baba and followers approaches the shore, after crossing the Indus River bound for Quetta, during Blue Bus travels in India. William, the tall figure wearing the hat on the left of the photo, referred often to breakdowns and other calamities involving the Blue Bus in the personal diary he kept from 1939 to 1945.

Mehera. Baba made sure all the men were out of the way whenever Mehera entered the bus.... No chance ever for Mehera to see the [male] mandali face-to-face."

This procedure with Mehera was not a passing whim of Baba's. Keeping her from seeing men and keeping men from getting glimpses of her would be a continuous practice for almost 30 years.

William and others, whatever their thoughts and inclinations, would soon discover the essence of what Baba had once told them:

"Give up yourself; serve others, not yourself; and above all love Baba."

A tough order.

But William was already aware of and had heard about Meher Baba's service to others – especially the poor and weak. On many occasions Baba would bathe groups of lepers and the poor for hours, giving them fabric for making clothes and a small amount of money or grain.

The mandali had to give and give and then give more of themselves. And never expect to be given anything in return. "Except my love," Baba constantly reminded them.

William had felt enough of a surge of Baba's love when he met Baba at Kitty Davy's parents' home in October 1933 to pursue the medical education that he thought would help him be of service to Baba. At one point during his studies, he dropped out of medical school, but later went back and stayed the course when Baba urged him to complete the degree to qualify as a doctor.

The early 1930s were trying times for many in the world. The heartbreak and terrible aftermath of the World War I lingered and the stock market crash of 1929 and great Depression that lasted through the 1930s prompted many people to look inward for healing in response to the chaos.

As William joined Baba in 1939, the world was again on the brink of another global war. A number of people, including William, were willing to respond to Baba's call.

On many occasions, particularly the evenings, followers would gather and listen to spiritual discourses from Baba.

Maintaining his 14-year silence, Baba would relay his thoughts using an alphabet board.*

Bhau Kalchuri, a long-time mandali member who passed away in October 2013, wrote in Volume 7 of *Lord Meher,*** about one of the discourse sessions:

"Baba asked the mandali, 'Where is God? – Where is God?'

"Donkin replied 'In Baba – Baba is God.'

"For a moment all were taken aback. Donkin's answer was so simple, so natural.

"Baba then spelled out, 'If you take me as your master and believe me perfect and one with the Infinite, if you believe this in all faith, then Don's [William's] is the only correct and logical answer.'"

William may have walked away from this session feeling lofty and wise, but if Baba got wind of superior feelings – inflated egos among his followers – he would be quick to inflict a lesson to humble the person.

William related a follow-up query to the "Where is God" question that Baba asked at the same discourse session:

"Then he [Baba] asked where was God not to be found. We all said nowhere, or words to that effect, and then Baba said God was not to be found in the ego.... He said, God was everywhere and therefore the ego had no existence but was illusion."[15]

During the group's stay at Bangalore William was sent to the local hospital to gain experience working as a doctor in India:

"I have today been to the hospital. I am to work in an honorary capacity to get experience. I start work tomorrow."

Shortly after their arrival in Bangalore a Western follower, Nonny Gayley, fell ill. Nonny, the widow of a US attorney, and her daughter Rano, an artist, were both living in the ashram. They had met Baba at the home of Kitty Davy's parents the same week as William in October 1933.

Nonny died of heart failure on October 13, 1939. This was the first time that Baba had been present at the death of

---

* Shortly after beginning silence, Meher Baba began communicating through words formed by pointing to a wooden board with letters painted on it. One of his mandali would read the board out loud.

** *Lord Meher* is Bhau Kalchuri's multi-volume biography of Meher Baba.

one of his followers. His response to Nonny's passing struck William deeply:

"We went quickly to [Nonny's] bedside with Baba. She had stopped breathing. Baba pressed the eyelids to close them with his own fingers.

"Baba said she had come to Him; and that it was the first time He had been present at the death of a disciple. Even when His father Sheriar died Baba was away in Europe.

"Baba wanted Nonny to be cremated, and he said she would be buried on the hill at Meherabad, near Baba's tomb* with the words 'Nonny, Baba's Lover' engraved on a monument, where her ashes were laid. He said of Nonny that she was one of his greatest lovers.

"Somehow death when Baba is around doesn't seem to matter. She had a very easy death and life just seemed to creep out of her body, ever so gently, no doubt Baba's work."[16]

William, who was attending the 64-year-old American when she died, recalled that her last words were, "What beauty, what beauty!"

Rano Gayley recalls her relationship with her mother:

"Nonny wanted to be pals with me, but also wanted me to respect her. She was the antithesis of me – feminine and delicate. Her relationship with Baba was always separate from the rest of ours. Baba never tested or teased her, perhaps because of her past births, or her short connection with Baba in this life. Baba always handled her as something fragile that might break – but Baba's wish was her pleasure."[17]

In addition to hunting for masts while in Bangalore, Meher Baba was also trying to purchase a 500-acre tract of land outside the city where he hoped to establish a centre (university) for spirituality. William was one of the followers involved in meetings with the Mysore State prime minister in an effort to obtain the property.

Plans were also in motion to bring the masts housed at Meherabad to Bangalore. At the same time followers were

---

* Baba's tomb (or Samadhi) had been built at Meherabad in the 1930s at Baba's direction. Meher Baba was interred there after he dropped his body January 31, 1969.

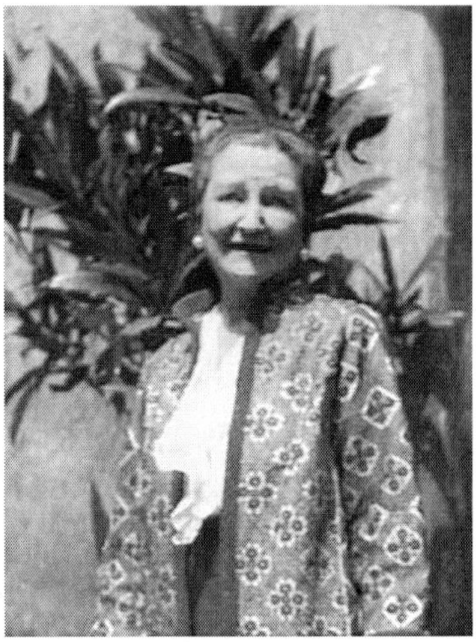

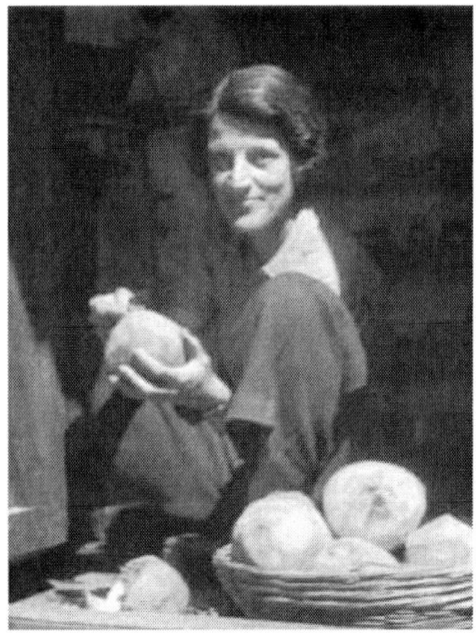

Western women Nonny Gayley, left, and her daughter Rano met Meher Baba in October 1933 in London at the same time as William Donkin. Nonny would spend the last six years of her life in India and Rano spent more than 50 years at the ashram.

looking for more masts in the Bangalore area and as far away as Bombay.

Baba said he was most happy when working with the masts, although much of this work remains a mystery to this day. One favourite mast, Mohammed, who first met Baba in Rahuri in 1936, was brought to Bangalore from Meherabad. The mast (who called Baba "Dada") would be part of the Baba community for almost seven decades.

William had been paired with Dr. Nilu* through correspondence even before his arrival at Meherabad. The personal and working relationship between the two men would create many opportunities for Baba to whittle down the egos of both physicians. On one occasion, a follower suffered a terrible toothache, and Baba sent both William and Dr. Nilu to the patient. The outcome of the doctors' visit is described in *Lord Meher*:

* Dr. Nilu met Baba in 1925, joining him after finishing his medical studies. He died from injuries in Meher Baba's 1956 car accident in Satara, India.

"Donkin with much difficulty extracted two teeth.... Later in the day after seeing [the patient's] condition, Baba became furious and scolded Donkin and Nilu.

"'Who told you to pull out his teeth; are you doctors or barbers,' said Baba.

"To describe a doctor as a barber in India is the same as calling him a butcher. Baba later explained to the two physicians, who felt terrible, that he had been working on another level when he scolded them."

This would not be the last dressing-down of the two men. In the future Baba would often refer to them as a "pair of barbers" when they were not behaving according to his wishes.

All of Baba's followers faced his rebukes on occasion – some more than others. Newer followers, such as William, who had been with Baba for only a few months at the time of the tooth-pulling, felt the bite of Baba's criticisms more than the Easterners who had been with him from the outset in 1922.

3

Meher Baba and Living in Bangalore

Meher Baba's road to God-realization is a detailed story in itself. The short version of it is that 19-year-old Merwan Sheriar Irani, a seemingly regular college-enrolled teenager, was awakened to his spiritual status by the female Perfect Master Babajan in Poona in January 1914.

Following this, Merwan spent a total of seven years in contact with Babajan and four other Perfect Masters.* He stayed the longest with Upasni Maharaj, until starting his own following and ashram (with Maharaj's blessing) as Meher Baba.

Each of the Perfect Masters had worked on Merwan, "bringing him down" from the ecstatic state he had slipped into after Babajan kissed him on the forehead. Merwan's experience with these Perfect Masters is comparable to the experience of the masts that he later contacted.

After his experience with Babajan, Merwan had changed so radically that his parents were unable to understand him and barely coped with him living under the same roof. He did not return to school and after a while tried a few occupations. When these did not work, he ran his father's toddy shop. Finally he gave this up and drifted off to be dealt with by the other Perfect Masters.

* Baba said there are always five Perfect Masters in the spiritual hierarchy, and when the Avatar comes they help him realize his status. In Baba's time, they were Babajan, Upasni Maharaj, Sai Baba (of Shirdi), Narayan Maharaj, and Tajuddin Baba.

All of these Perfect Masters later relayed to their own followers that their spiritual knowledge and prowess had been passed onto Merwan, who would soon be known as Meher Baba or Compassionate Father.

By the time William met his Master in the fall of 1933, Baba was on his third trip to England and had visited the United States in 1931 and 1932. On his trip to California in 1932, movie stars Mary Pickford and Douglas Fairbanks had entertained him at their Pickfair estate. While in Hollywood, Baba met Gary Cooper, Tallulah Bankhead, and other stars. He also made several side trips to countries in Europe during these tours, usually staying with Western followers or in nearby hotels.

Baba's return to India in the late 1930s indicated that the whirlwind world tour phase would give way to a more stationary period in India – at least temporarily. The Bangalore colony was part of this new phase. When not mast-hunting or working in the hospital in the city, William was involved with others in planning the new spiritual centre a short distance from Bangalore.

Baba experienced opposition from a group of protesters at this time, but still had the Mysore prime minister's support for the establishment of the new centre. Just four months after his arrival in India, William's increase in duties created more opportunities for criticism from Baba. Oddly enough, he welcomed the stormy sessions:

"Baba ticks me off quite a bit now, which I am glad about. I feel I like to be treated like the other boys and have the corners rubbed off; besides it makes me love Baba much more," wrote William in a November 8, 1939, diary entry.

Another entry indicates William was a quick study in Baba's desire to destroy personal egos. He seemed determined to roll with the jabs and learn from the brow-beating:

"Baba is looking very handsome these days with shining face and eyes. He was very pleased when I did my first appendix a few days ago, and said He was proud of me.... Baba sometimes praises me in front of the others and blames me in front of them, I think the latter is the better compliment from Him."

Without experiencing Baba's love, it is tough to fathom what William was getting from Baba to sustain him. Baba's relationships with his disciples and followers were very much on an individual basis. He did not employ a cookie-cutter approach in his spiritual mission. He insisted that this had to be the case because each follower's existence was tied to their own past incarnations. The sanskaras (impressions) they had picked up through different lifetimes influenced the relationship they had with Baba – each on a unique individual basis.

Baba insisted on complete honesty from his followers. When he asked British disciple Kitty Davy what she wanted from her relationship with him, Kitty replied, "I would like to increase my capacity to love." Kitty, who spent 16 years living with Meher Baba in India before coming to the United States to help run Meher Center, would be a close mandali for nearly 70 years.

While the reticent William Donkin never openly publicized what he wanted from life with Baba, it is certain he and Baba discussed their relationship often. William may have quickly become like Baba's Eastern mandali, who were content simply to love and serve their Spiritual Master. Baba wrote several books in the forties and fifties including *God Speaks,** which he said on one occasion was written for intellectuals. Most of the close mandali admitted they had never read the books and felt no need to do so as long as they were living with Baba.

William was quickly learning about the many quirks of living in the ashram, particularly the strict rules of conduct that existed between followers of different sexes.

The male and female members of the ashram were segregated. For William and Dr. Nilu, treating female patients was a complicated, second-hand, proxy experience:

"Doctors Donkin and Nilu could not directly treat the women staying in the ashram in Bangalore, since all the men were forbidden from seeing the Eastern women. Rano [Gayley] would report the health [situations] and the doctors had to prescribe medicine without seeing the patients."[18]

---

* *God Speaks*, published in 1955, was the only book dictated by Baba on the alphabet board. It presents Baba's description of creation, the soul's journey, and what Baba calls "The Divine Theme."

William was also observing mast activity at the time at the Bangalore ashram. He describes one mast who was found in the forest outside Belgaum* as having "a filthy turban, and very bright eyes indeed. He looks about 40 years old. He loves flowers, tobacco, and tea." Many masts were chain smokers and were often plucked from squalid surroundings to meet with Baba.

William continues his description of this particular mast and Baba's relationship with him:

"Every day Baba covers him with flowers and feeds him. Baba says he is very advanced, between the fifth and sixth plane.... He likes Baba to sit near him, and is much quieter than when he first came."[19]

William, who often dried the masts after Baba bathed them, explained that masts found it painful coming to Baba:

"He is like fire to them and burns them by His very high spiritual state."

William was learning procedures at the local hospital, administering to medical needs of ashramites, observing mast activity, and driving the Blue Bus, but there was still time for fun. On one occasion Baba asked his followers to fill in forms stating their work and amusements. He asked for suggestions for ashram recreational activities. William describes the outcome:

"I suggested a game such as badminton, cricket and as a joke marbles in the compound. Of course Baba voted for marbles, and I have now been made secretary of the marble club, with a budget of 10 rupees per month. Baba is [club] president."

Donkin's twenty-eighth birthday on November 14, 1939, was another light-hearted occasion. But the games and laughter were often peppered with war talk and war-related work.

"Baba says the war will go on for another year at least.... We in the house are to make 4,000 bandages; the other house to make 1,000. As today is my birthday and yesterday Chanji's [a follower, who was Baba's first secretary], the mandali were allowed 10 Rs. of sweets."[20]

---

* Belgaum, in Karnataka state, borders on Maharashtra and Goa. It is in the foothills of the Western Ghats and has a cool climate with numerous rivers, hills and dense evergreen forests. It was the site of a major British military installation.

The war was certainly on William's mind. His article "Order out of Chaos" in the December 1939 issue of the *Meher Baba Journal** reflects his attitude:

"Happiness cannot be achieved by economics. Civilization means something more than complex material life, good education, good health, and good food.

"Man must be free and in the West as it is today he is not free, but is pursued by his insatiable appetites and crushed by the weight of his inventions.

"Even war offers some hope of breaking the cords that bind him. But in the present war, whether one or the other party wins with flying colours, or whether at the end of a protracted and devastating struggle, delegates from all nations put their very heads together to elaborate another Versailles, a lasting peace can never be achieved without the guidance of one who, through his spiritual state, can impart genuine wisdom to the outline of a new world order."

The establishment of the new spiritual centre on the outskirts of Bangalore was not going smoothly. Vegetation had not been cleared from the site, and the prime minister was being asked to intervene to coax the work along.

William continued to take emotional upheavals from Baba in stride:

"It is really a privilege to be ticked off by Baba. I have such a deep feeling of satisfaction and love from Him, when He does it; even though specifically it is no joke."

In addition to the mast Mohammed, a second favourite mast, Chatti Baba, was initially brought to Bangalore. Getting him there was not an easy venture.

Baba was becoming quite well known in India as a Spiritual Master. To avoid attention in his travels Baba often insisted that followers not divulge his identity. He said to simply refer to him as an uncle or elder brother.

William says that at one point while escorting Chatti Baba to Bangalore, the group stayed in a hotel. Baba fed and bathed the

---

* The *Meher Baba Journal*, a monthly magazine, was published from 1938 to 1942 by some of Meher Baba's mandali who formed the Meher Editorial Committee.

mast. William related the unfolding predicament with Chatti Baba and the difficulty the Baba group encountered in keeping a low profile:

"He ran out of the hotel. With great difficulty they got him back and he began throwing earth over himself in the hotel compound. Then Baba started throwing buckets full of water over him, clothes and all, and that calmed him down a bit.

"He would not often look at Baba, and would always stand up when Baba was there.... Baba says he is on the sixth plane.... He has very clear eyes."[21]

Most of the excursions away from the Bangalore colony involved mast-hunting in the surrounding countryside. At one point there were at least six masts staying at the ashram compound which was called The Links.

As December 1939 progressed the new spiritual centre was finally shaping up for an official opening – the laying of a foundation stone, since there were no buildings yet. The centre site occasionally brought forth some startling discoveries:

"This evening Padri* brought back a nine-foot python from the Byramangala** site. They say there are lots of them there. The other day he brought back a huge black scorpion from the site too – some place!"[22]

Part of the original construction included a large, grey polished granite foundation seat with the words engraved and painted in gold:

Foundation Seat of the
Meher Baba Universal Spiritual Centre.

William drove the bus to and from the centre site on opening day. He made five trips (a total of 250 miles) carrying mandali men and women.

---

* Padri (Faredoon N. Driver) was Mehera's cousin and one of Baba's earliest mandali (joining in 1922). He became a homeopath and Baba called him one of the pillars of Meherabad. Baba gave him the nickname Padri because of his lanky, priest-like stature.

** Byramangala is a scenic village with a panoramic landscape and lush greenery that is 24 miles from the city of Bangalore.

While there was a great deal of pomp involved in christening the new centre, activity at the site would for various reasons remain dormant for decades.

A group opposed to Baba conducted a protest during the opening of the new centre. Baba welcomed opposition to his work, and it came from various factions of the population as a regular occurrence. In addition to the protest group at the centre opening, there was a man called Colonel Irani, who was Mehera's maternal uncle and a continuous critic of Meher Baba. He had given two anti-Baba lectures in Madras.

William's diary mentions that Baba continued to encourage emotional turmoil within his group of followers:

"There's no doubt, Baba can be very irritating at times; pretending not to hear what one says, or teasing one about nothing rather unjustly.... All of it because He wants to try to upset us, for His own reasons of course. These little games of moods, which He plays with us, are really very funny, when done to someone else."

William's insight into Baba's way of working was being fine-tuned. He recognized that being made to look the fool, however painful, certainly ground down the ego. It of course helped that all were in the same boat and the same tactic was employed on all of the mandali.

"But it makes Baba all the more loveable. His moods change so fast from one individual to another, and from one instant to another, and as time goes on one gets a solid feeling of His greatness in all things, which grows on one day-by-day and binds one faster to him."

Baba was relentless in his attempts to destroy the small selves in all his followers. His methods were at times tactless, but he warned his followers early in their relationship that life with him was no cakewalk.

His habit of demanding complete honesty from his followers and asking them at inopportune times in front of others, "What are you thinking?" brought discomfort over and over to many close to him.

Adi K. Irani, Baba's long-time secretary (after Chanji), relayed one incident when a woman follower brought her daughter to Baba for his darshan (audience). Adi relays Baba's quick question to him when the daughter bowed down:

"Adi, what are you thinking?"

He responded that it was so nice to see Baba's followers bowing down to him. On another similar occasion involving the same young girl, Baba again asked Adi, "What are you thinking?"

Adi replied as before, but later admitted privately to Baba that he had been having thoughts of other than sisterly love toward the young woman.

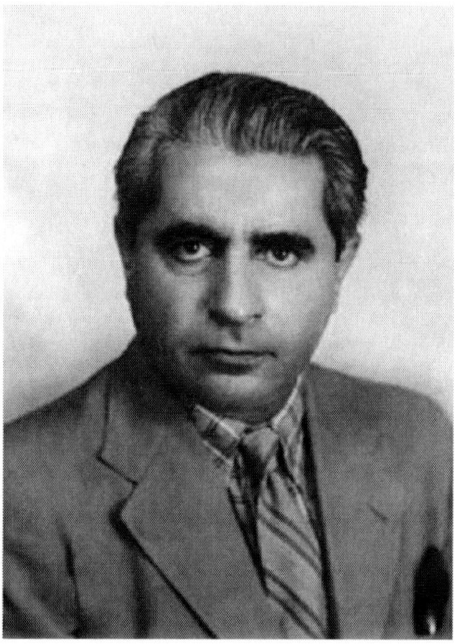

MN Publications

Adi K. Irani (Adi Sr.)

Adi says it was very difficult being put on the spot in front of others with "What are you thinking?" but the courage to give the honest answer brought great approval from Baba.

It was in Bangalore that the women mandali first heard the Cole Porter song, "Begin the Beguine," which would later become very important in Baba's work. Margaret Craske had brought the record with her when she came to India from England.

"For some days, it was played like other records," Mehera remembered.

"Then all of a sudden, Baba liked it so much and had it played every day. In fact, he said: 'Play this record every day at such and such a time, when I come to be with you!'

"One day he said, 'Now every one of you must learn this song.'"[23]

Even after the official opening, construction problems at the new spiritual centre continued throughout the group's stay in Bangalore. This situation came to a head in mid-February 1940, when Baba broke off his relationship with the contractors. The mandali decided to try to carry on the building work themselves.

At this point Baba split up the group, disrupting any individual comfort zones that may have formed. Some remained at Bangalore, others went to nearby Byramangala to work on the centre, and a few returned to Baba's headquarters in Meherabad.

"Most of us think this is a sign that Baba will leave for Meherabad with all of us in June, or before, and this is his way of starting the move," said William at the time.

Meher Baba's birthday was celebrated February 18 that year* and William's diary description of his Spiritual Master written the next day reflects his mood about life with Baba, seven months after his arrival in India.

"He was looking radiantly noble with hair let down for once, and really glistening. He was a fine sight to look at. His phenomenal strength of character and his sort of mysterious spiritual beauty and radiance, very much visible as he sat on His couch.

"Baba's face in repose is such a fusion of spiritual bliss and serenity and a sort of dragging sadness, which gives such dignity and grandeur to the face that really surpasses the scenery of nature, both in its amazing hold on the onlooker, and its rapid changes."

William and Dr. Nilu were, like Adi Sr., not immune from Baba's jabs concerning their feelings about the women visiting the ashram. William conveys an incident in his February 27, 1940 diary entry:

"Yesterday morning Nilu and I had a bit of a crisis with Baba. He had been 'poking' us over Nargis (Dadachanji), so we had some straight talk back. A straight talk with Baba is very refreshing; he never evades anything, and never harbours bitterness."

During this period Baba was fasting for periods of time on different combinations of milk, honey water, and lemon juice. He continued his work with the masts, "pandering to their slightest whims," according to William.

---

* Baba's birthday (February 25) would be celebrated according to the Parsi calendar, which meant it would fall on different dates each year in our standard (i.e., Gregorian) calendar.

The description of what became known as "the mast hotel" given in William's book *The Wayfarers* shows the eccentric detail that went into catering to the masts:

"Baba was constantly attentive to their wishes, and did all he could to keep them amused. A tea shop was designed and executed with elaborate carelessness, to conform to the preferences of masts for derelict houses of refreshment.

"Tea, paan*, cigarettes, and beedies [Indian cigarettes] were at all times available, free on demand to any of the masts.... The atmosphere was genuinely suggestive of the meaner sort of restaurant to be found by the score in the poorer parts of the teeming cities of India."

William says that Chatti Baba was the dominant figure in the mast hotel and also a favourite of Baba's. This mast lived a regular life before becoming God-intoxicated. He had worked as a station master, which was reflected in his ashram behaviour. He would tap out Morse code messages with the hook that held his window open, and at irregular hours of the night or day he would shout orders in English or Tamil to imaginary railway subordinates.

Baba said little about his work with the masts, but he was careful on the mast-hunting excursions to be sure the mandali knew the difference between God-intoxicated individuals and the simply insane. The mandali were usually told to be on the lookout for a person who neglected his/her own welfare and attracted a following of devotees in their particular areas.

Finding such individuals was, in the beginning of mast-hunting work, very much a trial-and-error game; the first mast community Baba had set up a few years earlier in Rahuri in 1936 had become known as "the mad ashram."

"The Rahuri Ashram was principally for mad people, ordinary insane men from the towns and villages of the surrounding country," William would later write in *The Wayfarers*. "There were a few genuine masts and a few God-mad, but the greater number were mere psychotics of one kind or another, with nothing spiritual about them."

---

* Paan is a spiced chewing mixture wrapped in betel leaves.

Rahuri was strategically located about 30 miles north of Ahmednagar, just a short distance from Meher Baba's headquarters at Meherabad. The town was also situated on the road to Nasik, where the following year Baba would establish the early retreat for the group of Westerners invited to India.

Baba may well have opened the doors at Rahuri to both the simply mad and the God-intoxicated/mad in order to have inmates available who would reflect the difference between mad and mast. This helped the mandali improve their mast-hunting abilities, and even the insane who were brought to the ashram were not given short shrift. Everyone was treated equally.

"Baba's work – his visible and external work – was to shave, bathe, clothe, and feed each inmate as soon as he arrived and each day to scour the ashram latrine, and to bathe and sit in seclusion with a certain number of the old inmates. In this way he would throw every ounce of energy into doing every sort of menial task, and was, in very fact, Master of all, and servant of all."[24]

William was still struggling at medical school in London when the Rahuri Ashram opened. To write his book on the masts he used recollections from the other mandali who were there from the ashram's beginning. He did, however, experience the final year of the ashram. It was moved to Meherabad in 1937 and kept open until 1940.

The number of inmates at Rahuri had dropped from 40 to 20 before the move to Meherabad. William's gleaned description of the group's train trip to Ahmednagar, gives one a glimpse into occasional outlandish travels with Baba. "The mandali, 20-odd mad men, five or six masts, a gazelle, a peacock, a sheep, a white rabbit, some geese, five dogs, three monkeys, and two pet birds were all crammed in one compartment, and sat cheek-by-jowl with tin trucks, packing cases, tables, chairs, and the inevitable medley of domestic and culinary equipment."[25]

Baba's attention to the inmates of the mad ashram began to dwindle with the group's move to Meherabad, when his concentration shifted toward finding more genuine masts. But before the mad ashram closed and the inmates were returned to their home villages, Baba did spend a few brief weeks with them.

William responds to a natural question in the closing chapter on the mad ashram in *The Wayfarers*:

"The question is, of course, did these mad folk improve at all, and become more normal, as a result of their contact with Baba, and if they did not; what then was the use of the ashram?

"I think the question is a fair one, and the answer is, perhaps, not entirely satisfactory."

William did not think Baba's main purpose was to improve or heal the mental infirmities of these inmates. He attributes an improvement to the natural way the ashram operated:

"Their improvement might, of course, be put down to the strongly integrating force of Baba's individual love for them. Love does work miracles, and Baba did give them more selfless love than any ordinary mortal could have given them."

Even before the mad ashram closed, other small satellite genuine mast ashrams were being established in Ajmer and Jubbulpore*. This simultaneous activity started before William's arrival in India and his stay at the Bangalore ashram.

In finally meeting Chatti Baba at Bangalore in 1940 and interacting with him, William was able to assess what Baba said and apply it to his own experiences with the advanced mast:

"Baba has said clearly that in his contacts with genuine masts, they help him and he helps them. They love him and he loves them. And he agrees that the speculations of his disciples about the significance of his work are correct to a certain point; but beyond that he does not extend his explanation."[26]

Baba told the mandali that what each mast did for him was a private matter between him and the mast. He said his mast work was similar to the operation of the Meherabad School in the mid-twenties, but because of the advanced states of the masts, they usually know what they are doing for him, and therefore provide greater help to him.

---

* Jubbulpore (sometimes spelled Jabalpur) in Central India is known for the Marble Rocks – a gorge on the Narmada River – and the Dhuandhar waterfalls.

4

Back to Meherabad – the Long Way

After eight months in Bangalore, the group finally packed up to leave for Meherabad on April 1. At the first overnight stopover, both William and Kitty were reminded of the importance of following Baba's orders. Kitty quickly made sandwiches for everyone.

"The male mandali were not allowed to mix with the women, but Kitty noticed Don [William] standing outside by the bus and thought he must be hungry. She quickly made him a sandwich and went to give it to him. Don was grateful for the kindness, but just then Baba came and told Kitty, 'Make Don a sandwich too.'

"'But I have already,' Kitty beamed – proud of having anticipated Baba's wish.

"'Who told you to give Don anything?' Baba asked. 'Only I give things to people. Who do you think you are? Do you feel sorry for Don?'"

Kitty never did it again, and whenever she saw William, she looked away.[27]

The Blue Bus journey overland from Bangalore to Meherabad was strange and meandering rather than direct. The bus, built to accommodate 17 people, carried 36 people in total, and the 20 men riding in the front of the bus were ordered not to look at the 16 women in the back of the bus.

Arnavaz Dadachanji,* a close woman mandali member, recalls an incident involving William on the journey. Baba had just cut up a watermelon and given those on the trip small pieces to relieve their thirst.

"Although he was usually quite dignified, Dr. Donkin was finding the India summer excruciatingly hot, and in an attempt to lower his body temperature, he placed the empty watermelon rind on his head like a hat! This sort of silliness eased the difficulties of travelling in hot, cramped quarters for long periods."[28]

Baba travelled separately in Elizabeth Patterson's car. In addition to the overcrowded bus, there were five cars making the trip. The stops along the way included Jog Falls, which has a drop of 950 feet. The group finally reached Karwar, a seaside town on the Kali River, on the evening of April 4. William relates the stopover experience:

"All the women went to the 'Grand Hotel' with Baba – not so grand, old and dirty – and we men in the rest house alongside. This Karwar is a divine place. Jungle-covered hills falling into the sea, sandy bays and rocks, headlands and trees over the beach, island out to sea."

William went for a swim the next morning in the river above Jog Falls. Baba quoted Persian poetry to the group in the morning, during which William admitted he was only half awake. The gist of the translation is, "It takes time for the runner to gain speed; it takes time for the sleeper to awake; and it takes ages for one who has been spiritually asleep to be spiritually awakened."

Baba was very taken with the Karwar area and the coastline area to the point that he took the entire group to the island of Anjadiv** a mile or two off the coast.

"[This is] where Vasco da Gama first landed in India; a very tropical island about a mile long, half a mile broad with two springs of water."

---

* Arnavaz Dadachanji was the niece of Baba's first secretary Chanji. At Baba's order, she married Nariman Dadachanji (her cousin) and lived with him in Bombay until his death, after which she lived with the women mandali in Meherazad. She wrote the book *Gift of God.*

** Anjadiv Island is the largest of a chain of islands off the town of Karwar in Goa. It is a home to the Indian Navy and has remains of the Portuguese occupation from the fifteenth century to 1961.

Later the same day Baba said he wanted to buy the island (from the Portuguese) if possible. William, Norina Matchabelli*, and Elizabeth were dispatched to visit the Governor of Goa to explore this possibility.

William's diary mention of "having to buy a suit," reflects the formality of the planned visit to the governor.

It would be almost a week before the audience with the Goa governor could take place. In the meantime, the group visited Old Goa, the Church of St. Francis Xavier, and the tomb of that saint.

During the tour, they met a Catholic man who was writing a book about the place.

"He spoke good English and talked to us, but kept glancing quickly at Baba," writes William. "Afterwards Baba told us we were all blind, and we didn't see at the time that he was Baba's agent – a very advanced conscious agent."

Baba told the group that the Catholic man would leave the next day. Elizabeth ran into him then and he told her he was leaving at once and had an urge to go to a cold country, because he felt on fire.

Mast-hunting continued in the Goa area in early April.

Although Baba said he loved the area and its spiritual atmosphere, the bid to acquire Anjadiv Island proved unsuccessful.

"Yesterday Norina, Elizabeth, and I went to see the governor, on Baba's order about the island off Karwar.... He said no renting or concessions could be given to anyone – it was law. A shrewd old boy, I thought, but polite, kind and decent," said William in his April 13, 1940, diary entry.

Baba continued his quest for "a perfect boy" on many of his travels, and Goa was no exception. A 15-year-old orphan was found who spoke Portuguese and some English. The boy was working as the servant of a local priest.

"We had some trouble getting him, having to argue with the priest, sisters, and brothers ... but he came with us the next

* Norina Matchabelli was co-founder of a perfume company with her husband Prince Matchabelli. Before joining Baba as a devoted mandali, she was a stage and screen actress, mime, mystic, and publisher.

morning. Nearly all the village was there to see him off, as he was the most popular boy of the village – bright and intelligent. Much sisterly weeping when he left."

The group departed from Goa on April 15 taking the boy with them. William said everyone was happy to be on their way.

"We were glad to leave – too sticky and smelly. The hotel smelt of fish, wine, and Phenyl disinfectant."

The next stop was Khanapur, where Baba took the men to bathe in the river.

"I had a good swim, Baba watching us, and the Goa boy had a swim too. Swims OK. He's a bright lad."

Although the caravan was constantly moving, Baba did on occasion take time for a spiritual discourse.

One of the questions posed was "What is spirituality?" Baba gave a detailed answer using his alphabet board, and William transcribed it into his diary:

"It is the undoing of what you have been doing since ages. You always thought of selfish motives of eating, preserving your life, and attending to every need with zeal.

"All these lives you have made a habit of looking to yourself. If the slightest thing goes against your habit you are upset."

Baba said it was necessary to go against one's acquired nature to undo these habits and one had to focus on others rather than oneself.

"This is called Love. But it needs character, poise, perseverance.

"Poise. What is poise? That state of mind where nothing excites you, nothing upsets you. Then only can you help others. Then only can you make others happy.

"That means Love.

"Thinking not of yourself, but of others."

Masts often attached themselves to the group along the way. If they proved suitable they were included for a while. After leaving the Goa area the group went on to Belgaum and then Amboli, a British hill station in the Western Ghats near Goa offering a view of the coast.

"Baba used to sit on the bungalow veranda at Amboli to dictate his letters and other work there. The night before we left, Jampa, the Belgaum mast, was very noisy and restless and at 2:00 in the morning he broke the window and pulled away part of the frame."

Because his disruptive behaviour made him too difficult to look after, the mast was left behind in Belgaum. A diary entry at the time shows Baba was also wrestling with problems among his followers.

"Baba lectured all the ladies this morning about controlling emotions. He wants us to get angry, but to control it – to hate but to transfer the hate to love; to maintain poise always, that is spirituality. The women, He says, make such a fuss over small things. They have no courage to control their moods."

The party then moved onto Panchgani*, arriving there the afternoon of April 28. Baba then ordered Norina and Elizabeth to go back to Belgaum by car to see a site that was being offered by a school principal, who was devoted to Baba, as a possible centre for Baba's work.

"We did the 110 miles in three hours. Rotten road to it, but lovely place, with a stream running through the land ... very good water and plenty of trees ... about 36 acres in all.

"Returning that day, we set out the following one for Mahabaleshwar**, some 30 miles over the foothills of the Ghats – a twisty but beautiful route."

William sympathized in human terms with the pressure on the main vehicle in the party:

"The bus got very tired and almost petered out on the way up to Mahabaleshwar – 4,400 feet above sea [level]. After all it's carrying 28 people now, and full of luggage inside and out, and is only designed for 17. So it certainly deserves God-realization."

Panchgani and Mahabaleshwar were to play a major part in the life of Meher Baba. He and his followers on future visits

---

* Panchgani is a scenic hill station that was used by the British as a summer resort. It is known as "Mecca of Maharashtra." Baba and his companions went there many times over the years. Baba had a cave dug there in which he and various mandali would at times stay in seclusion.

** Mahabaleshwar is a hill station on a vast plateau surrounded by valleys on all sides, with many spectacular vistas, located about 125 km from Poona in Maharashtra State. It is a popular holiday and honeymoon spot and an important place of pilgrimage for Hindus.

would stay at Florence Hall, a part of the estate there belonging to the Aga Khan.*

Hotel Grenoble was chosen to house the women mandali and Baba.

"The next day Baba took the ladies out for a longish walk, and in the evening I went for a walk along the edge of the ghat. I was picked up on the way and taken to 'Arthur's Seat' some eight miles off, from whence there is a first-class view of the ghat cliffs and a 4,000-foot drop – very fine indeed."

After only two days in Panchgani, Baba and company then left for Ahmednagar – the city closest to his Meherabad ashram.

On the way, there was a brief stopover in Poona, Baba's birthplace. Here everyone went to Bund Gardens to see the tree under which the Perfect Master Hazrat Babajan would sit looking out over the river.

William describes another set-to he had with Baba during the journey that reflected the importance Baba placed on responding to orders even earlier than asked:

"Baba buttered me up in front of the others in Ahmednagar.... Two days before, however, He began poking me saying, why wasn't I ready to start – when it wasn't yet 6 a.m., at which time I had been ordered to be ready.

"I got a bit peeved with Baba, and later He 'ticked me off' for having gotten ratty. Baba always tries to upset one in one's worst moments, which with me – later with Elizabeth – is in the early morning."

Throughout Baba's lifetime he was strict about time, and many followers learned quickly to report a half hour earlier than when they were asked. Baba also demanded an instant response when he called someone, to the point that if a man had been shaving when Baba called, the disciple was to come to Baba even with his face still lathered. Several mandali members changed from wearing drawstring pants to elasticized

---

* Aga Khan III – Sultan Mahommed Shah (1877–1957) – was the forty-eighth Imam (priest) of the Shia Ismaili Muslims. He was one of the founders and first president of the All-India Muslim League, and was President of the League of Nations (1937–38).

waistbands so there would be no delay if they happened to be on the toilet when Baba called.

These demands were again designed to whittle down one's ego and sense of decorum. It would seem appropriate to clean the shaving soap off of one's face before coming before Baba, but often if one did, Baba would ask, "What took you so long?" He would not accept any explanation for the delay if it involved a personal decision which took extra time or precedence over an immediate response to his order.

The tough routine discouraged some followers enough that they did not stay with Meher Baba. His attitude was that this was part of the Spiritual Master/disciple relationship. On many occasions he would say to the follower, "If you cannot live here according to my wishes and orders it is better that you pack your things and get out!"

Often, however, even on these ego-breaking occasions, Baba would send another follower to fetch the departed one back to the fold. When this happened Baba would ask the follower for his/her forgiveness, embrace them, and urge them to stay.

Forgiveness was a mainstay of ashram life, and Baba at times placed himself in situations where he appeared to be the follower rather than the Master to teach others forgiveness.

The mast Chatti Baba was not always a willing participant in sharing Baba's work, and on more than one occasion this mast complained directly to the mandali that he was not up to the task. Shortly after the entire group moved back to Meherabad from Bangalore, France fell to Germany. Baba said Chatti Baba had a spiritual connection to France, and its collapse had caused the mast to be "overwrought with despair."

Baba on one occasion told the mandali that there was no equal to Chatti Baba in the entire world, and that he was "a very high mast of the sixth plane" and inestimable for the help he gave in Baba's work. While the descriptions of the mast may be long-winded and taxing, the fact that he was a favourite among the hundreds of masts that Baba contacted over the years supports deeper exploration.

Whenever Chatti Baba had to move from one place to another in India, the mandali were constantly nervous. The mast was usually transported on a train rather than in the bus/auto caravans that the other followers took. Chatti Baba often repeated his wish to return home, and on many occasions would refuse to return to the train on stopovers while travelling through India and Ceylon (Sri Lanka).

"The moods of this great man were extraordinary, and would fluctuate from a sunny expansiveness, to a truculent attitude without apparently much provocation," William would later write in *The Wayfarers.* "He was like a child, quick to change for a very little thing, but he had a bewitching enchantment about him that made him loved by all. The other important masts have all had their charm and some sort of disposition that made them attractive, but there has been no one who has so unanimously commanded the affection of others."

When the group finally staggered into Meherabad, Chatti Baba renewed his habit of pouring earth over his head. This was followed by a bath when "about 200 buckets of water were poured over his head." At this time he also developed an insatiable appetite and repeatedly complained about not getting enough to eat.

As Baba was always willing to please the masts, at one point Chatti Baba was even allowed to bathe Baba with 10 or 12 buckets of water. He always referred to Baba as his big brother, and on one occasion said, "My big brother still has a bit of work to do in the world, but I haven't the strength to do such work myself."

On bitter cold January nights, the mast would remain outside stripped to the waist when the mandali were sleeping inside under three or four blankets.

While Chatti Baba longed to return home to Negapatam*, to the point of being constantly miserable, he did advise a follower to stick with Baba when the follower was thinking of leaving the ashram life.

"You want to leave, don't you, but what's the good of it? All the world is in Baba's power, so where will you go. Serve him now; he is the Ocean."

---

* Negapatam (now Nagapattinam) is a city in Tamil Nadu on the east coast of India, overlooking the Bay of Bengal. It was the main seaport under the British, with fishing being a major industry.

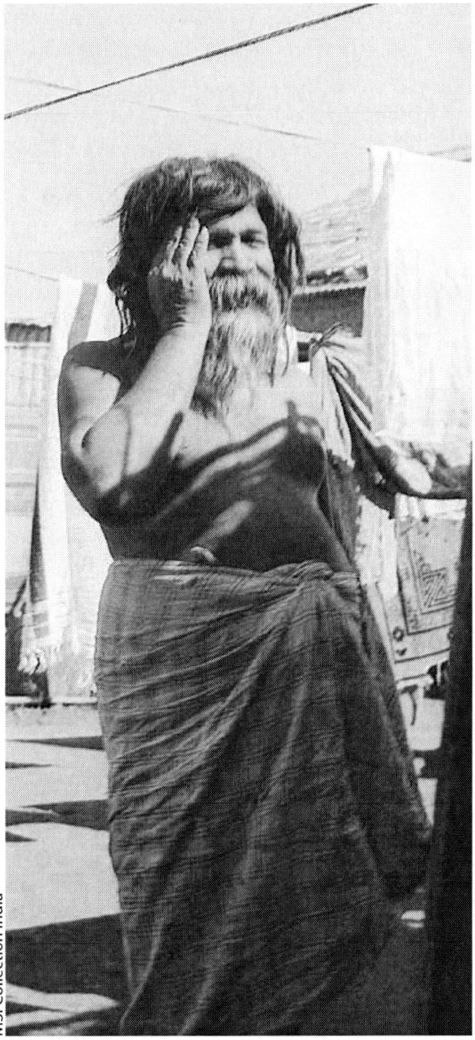

MSI Collection India

Chatti Baba was one of Meher Baba's five favourite masts. William and other disciples faced many challenges dealing with these God-intoxicated individuals. They cared little about their living conditions and material needs. The masts were often held in high esteem and revered by the people in the communities where they resided.

But finally in 1941, when the group was again off on tour in Panchgani, "Some inner crisis brought about a break in the intimate contact between Baba and Chatti Baba." One day he simply walked away from the compound, telling those who pursued him that he "must now go away." He agreed to stay another week, but again on the eighth day walked away from the compound.

"Some of the mandali followed him in a taxi and decoyed him into it by promising to take him at once to Negapatam. They drove back to Panchgani.

"Baba, who was then in seclusion, came out to see him, but Chatti Baba refused to get out of the car, wept aloud, and told Baba he was very, very tired, and that it was time for him to go."

Baba fed Chatti Baba by hand in the car, and shortly after two mandali packed their bedding rolls to accompany him back to Negapatam.

"A grey veil of melancholy closed about the hearts of those watching Chatti Baba's departure, for this old man whom all had come to love so deeply, had left them. They felt, as Baba must have felt infinitely more deeply than they, that someone irreplaceable had gone out of their lives."

William said that Chatti Baba was unique. Years after he had been separated from Baba, the mandali and even Baba himself often recalled "with delight his little ways, and especially the lightness and captivating spell of his laugh."

Meher Baba travelled to Negapatam on three occasions – once in 1941 and twice in 1942 – to contact Chatti Baba. Details of these meetings remain a mystery, although the last meeting in 1942 was reportedly ominous.

In true nomadic fashion, there was another quick turnaround at Ahmednagar and Meherabad, and within days William found himself back in Bangalore briefly. Then he returned to Meherabad and again was dispatched back to Bangalore. All of this took place in a four-day period.

Before William returned to residential life at Meherabad, he stopped briefly in Ahmednagar, where Baba and he were told of the accidental death of Buasaheb* in Poona.

"On being told this, Baba showed no emotion. Buasaheb was Baba's first disciple."

William was told to convey the news of Buasaheb's death to followers in Bangalore. He travelled first to Poona by car with a few other disciples and then onward by train to Bangalore.

---

* Buasaheb (which means barrister) was Baba's nickname for his first disciple, Behramji F. Irani. In 1914, Baba taught the illiterate young man to read and write Persian. Later Baba made Buasaheb the superintendent of the Meher Ashram.

The war was advancing dramatically at this time and Baba was monitoring the global conflict and offering his own unfolding predictions – including, surprisingly, his own death.

"Apparently a week before May 27 Baba gave out to everyone that on May 27 He would die. On that day He was, of course OK and he explained on that day Leopold of Belgium had surrendered.... This was what Baba had meant by his death.[29]

On June 11, 1940, Italy declared war on Britain and France. Although William had been going regularly to Browning Hospital in Bangalore and performing operations there, the mast compound at The Links was being shut down and a number of disciples were sent to Meherabad and elsewhere in India.

"I have had a little note from Baba saying that I shall stay here with the mandali in Bangalore until July end. Now ... it seems the masts are being disbanded – so that phase of Baba's work is over," William wrote in his diary.

5

Mast-hunting, Intense Training

During the period of upheaval in Europe, Meher Baba gave indications that he would break his 15-year silence in August 1941. He also outlined a plan to go with a small group of followers to set up a compound somewhere on the Russian border.

William's entry in his diary indicates that the mandali were learning to take a few of Baba's statements with a grain of salt:

"We all felt this message of Baba's to be rather too vague and we don't believe the date he gives at all – so we'll see."

On June 20, while still in Bangalore, William learned that Baba and a small contingent of his followers left Meherabad for Calcutta to hunt masts.

"I have been ordered by Baba to come back with Padri to Meherabad when Byramangala [spiritual centre] work is finished." Strangely, the new spiritual centre would not be fully utilized for over 50 years.

Baba's June Calcutta trip brought another favourite mast into his fold and under his influence. Karim Baba, whom mandali members called "the tiger man," received the nickname because his presence provoked in one "a mood of admiration mixed with fear." True to form, like many other masts, Karim Baba was clad in the filthiest of clothes, always chain smoking, and adorned with pieces of chain here and there on his body.

"Despite these strange and sordid accessories and the filth of his body, his superb face, and his eyes that shone like burnished swords made one forget everything else."[30]

Another mast ashram was immediately set up at Ranchi, which is 200 miles northwest of Calcutta. Baba referred to

Karim as the spiritual chargeman of Calcutta, and two of Baba's mandali – expert mast handlers – were sent to retrieve him. To their surprise, Karim Baba co-operated, agreed to go to Ranchi, and even accepted a change of clothes.

The Wayfarers description continues:

"Now Karim was a renowned figure in Calcutta and though he was perhaps not known to the small coterie of rich, whose horizon is by their office, club and house, he was greatly esteemed by the poor and middle-class masses of Calcutta."

The disciples were understandably nervous about the mood of the crowd that had gathered as Karim Baba was being clothed:

"Such masts are held in very great respect and are believed to hold the material and spiritual welfare of a place in their grasp, and the inhabitants are inclined to view their removal as a threat to the prosperity of their home town."[31]

Fortunately the crowd of about 100 remained in "a mood of inquisitiveness and astonishment only, for they could hardly believe their eyes that Karim Baba, who had sat on that one stretch of pavement for six years, was now being taken away by complete strangers."

Karim Baba's behaviour on the train trip from Calcutta to Ranchi, related in *The Wayfarers,* shows this mast to be the most bizarre that William wrote about. Karim, when using the toilet in the train, removed two or three coins from his stool, washed them thoroughly under the tap and tossed them in his mouth and swallowed them. "It was found later that Karim Baba would scrutinize his stool each day, and that on intervals of three or four days he would pass a few coins in this way, and would repeat this extraordinary manoeuvre of washing and swallowing them."

William tried to offer insight:

"One who finds such behaviour incompatible with his ideas of how a spiritually advanced man ought to behave should read Baba's explanation in Chapter One [*of The Wayfarers*] of the indifference of these God-intoxicated souls to dirt, and to the things of the world in general."

William's writing of *The Wayfarers* took place between 1946 and 1949, a number of years after he first came into contact with Baba's five favourite masts. Referring to Freud and other "depth psychologists," he offered his own interpretations of normal/versus abnormal in comparing ordinary men to the masts:

"Although [a normal man] may present a prim façade to the world, and even to his own conscious mind, he is, whether he likes it or not, impelled eventually by shameful primitive urges.

"The average man tries to veil his basic impulses from his conscious mind and from the world; but a mast, the wellsprings of whose being are intoxicated by Divine Love, who cares for no one and nothing, and who knows the world to be a passing dream, makes no bones about concealing his actions.

"The average man dresses decently, and pretends to forget that his mind is seething with primitive urges and that his body has functions that are humiliating – and what he calls euphemistically self-respect is, for the most part, vanity.

"A mast is utterly without vanity, and like a child, he allows his body to function in its own way, remaining himself consummately indifferent to it. Nor is he an eccentric exhibitionist, for his behaviour bears no relationship to the presence or absence of an audience."[32]

Unlike almost all other masts that came into Baba's fold, Karim was never bathed, although Baba fed him and sat with him several times a day.

At the end of June, William was called back to Meherabad. He left his colleagues at the Bangalore hospital and made his way to Baba's headquarters on the outskirts of Ahmednagar. His diary reflects his delight with the change:

"It is real good to be back in this ramshackle old hole after being so bored in Bangalore. The place on the hill [women's quarters at Upper Meherabad] is relatively grand compared to this place for we male mandali, but I love this place."

William went on to describe the crooked roof, which harboured scorpions and snakes.

"Wind-blown and crude as all is, it is a lovely place. Although it is no home really, I feel at home here. I suppose its deep link with Baba makes it so wonderful to be here."

William's joy at settling in at Meherabad was short-lived, however. By July 3, he, other followers, and the masts were off to Ranchi to the newly established mast outpost. Shortly after he arrived, William summed up his feelings about the new base of operations:

"I was really getting fed up with Ranchi a few days ago, with the filthily bad weather, the people, and even with Baba."

An incident prompting Baba to give William and Dr. Nilu a blast when the two were 20 minutes late returning from the post office may have prompted the discouragement.

"Baba gave Nilu and me a hell of a dressing-down. He told me if I did the same thing again I would have to leave, and he told Nilu to pack off tomorrow. I was so peeved that [I decided] I'd go too as it was as much my fault as Nilu's."

True to form, Baba made his own argument:

"[Baba] talking of relevant and irrelevant things ... brought us both to the verge of tears."

Baba quickly forgave the pair.

"We felt rather depressed till next day. But since then I've felt considerably better; and whatever else the row was for, it at least released the tension of my disgust for this place."

While at Ranchi, William harked back to his brief, but enjoyable, stopover at Meherabad:

"I enjoyed the last week in Meherabad very much indeed, going for walks, sleeping in Baba's [former] room, hobnobbing with everyone, and generally messing about the place for a week."

In a short time William gave his own opinion of the newest mast, Karim Baba:

"A big, black, surly-looking man. He had not spoken for 10 years in Calcutta.... He never washes, has long hair, and long nails; since Baba has been feeding him he has started talking a sort of hack Hindi poetry, and has been getting rather aggressive. I suppose he is regaining consciousness of the world again, and doesn't like it."

Tensions and tempers were running high at Ranchi, for Williams's diary entry of July 17 indicates on one occasion Baba talked to his followers about backbiting.

"Baba ... says he knows none of us will obey that order – which is on the year's order-list – which is quite true, none will. He says we must be on guard every day for a year against these enemies in ourselves." No backbiting was one of many orders Baba wanted his lovers to follow. In less than two weeks William and other mandali would be facing an additional strict list of behaviour orders from Baba.

The ashram at Ranchi was closed at the end of July and Karim Baba and the other mast inmates were then brought to Meherabad. On leaving Ranchi, the mandali again encountered an uproar with mast Chatti Baba. At one point en route Chatti would not re-board the train. William and two other mandali had to stay with him while Baba and the others went ahead.

"Next morning with the help of the police shouting at him we got him into the train; very tedious. All day he tried to get out of the train at every station. He looked very sad," William said of the continuing ordeal.

In Meherabad a special bamboo cage was built for the Calcutta mast Karim. Baba occupied an adjacent room and would go and sit with the mast many times each day and attend personally to his needs.

After only two weeks, Baba announced that his work with Karim was over and the mast was returned to Calcutta. Arrangements were made for his care with a doctor living in the city. Baba paid the doctor to feed Karim twice a day.

Although Baba returned to Calcutta at least twice after 1940 to feed the poor and contact other advanced souls there, Karim Baba would never again meet Meher Baba.

Settling in again at Meherabad, Baba told William to remain there until he was "called up" to report for wartime duty with the Indian Medical Service.

At this time, Baba gave William and the other men and women mandali special orders they were to follow for one year – from August 1, 1940, to July 31, 1941.

In addition to the men followers, a group of Eastern and Western women mandali were living a separate existence in the ashram.

Included in the group of women mandali at Meherabad was Mehera, whom Baba described as the "purest soul in the universe," saying that she "loved him as he ought to be loved." Another mandali was Baba's younger sister Mani, who had

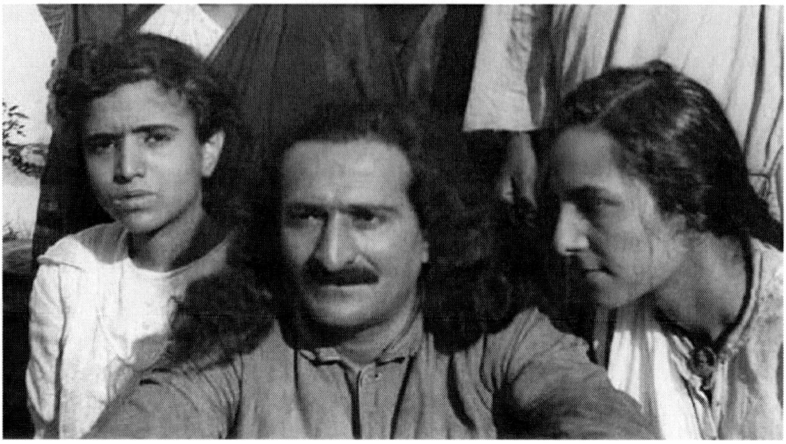

MSI Collection India

This early photo shows Mehera J. Irani, right, and Mani S. Irani with Baba. They were Meher Baba's closest woman disciples. Mehera, his chief woman disciple, joined the ashram at age 17 in 1924; and his sister Mani joined the ashram at age 14 in 1933.

joined Baba at the age of 14 in 1933 despite protests from their mother. Western women followers living at the ashram in 1940 included Kitty, Norina, Elizabeth, Rano, Irene Billo*, Nadine Tolstoy**, and Margaret.

The year-long orders that Baba issued emphasized the strictness of ashram life. A dozen of them include

> Do not indulge in tobacco smoking in any form.
> Do not drink alcoholic beverages of whatever kind.
> Do not eat meat.
> Do not eat fish.
> Do not eat eggs.

---

* Irene Billo, from Switzerland, met Meher Baba through her parents in 1938 in India. She spent eight years with him, which included much travel in India and life in the ashram at Meherabad.

** Nadia Tolstoy (nicknamed Nadine by Baba) was the daughter-in-law of Count Leo Tolstoy, the Russian author of *War and Peace*. She and her husband were spiritual seekers who met Baba in New York in 1931, where they were friends of American Baba followers Malcolm Schloss and Jean Adriel.

Perform no lustful action whatever, even with your lawful wife or husband.

[For men] Do not touch (even without a thought of lust) any woman over six years of age. [A list of exceptions to this order included nursing the sick and saving a woman's life or honour. A formal handshake between sexes was acceptable.]

[For women] The same rules as above pertaining to the opposite sex.

Do not tell lies.

Do not steal.

Do not criticize, scandalize, or speak ill of others.

Do not go to any cinema performance.

The final order on attending the cinema was relaxed only when Baba accompanied the group. Newly released movies of the day that Baba and others attended included *The Wizard of Oz* and *Gulliver's Travels*. Baba was also fond of Laurel and Hardy and Charlie Chaplin movies.

On one occasion while William was working in the hospital in Bangalore, a June 3, 1940, letter from Baba reminded him of the strict code of behaviour expected of him:

"I don't mind your giving lectures on eye surgery to sisters as long as your eye looks upon women as sisters. I trust you fully and hold you very dear."

There were 31 orders in all that William was to adhere to. Other orders dealt with avoiding outside influences such as theatre, magazines, and books, although he was allowed to read newspapers.

Rules on fasting were also issued and participants were ordered to meditate either upon the impersonal God or upon Baba. They were also to perform "conscientiously the prayers customary to your religion."

The issuing of the orders coincided with a period of Baba's seclusion on the hill at Upper Meherabad. Throughout his life Baba observed periods of seclusion – sometimes for days and other times for months. This particular seclusion would last a year with occasional lapses for travel.

At the end of August, William was ordered to go to Ankai Mountain.* Five of Baba's mandali were staying there in seclusion and William was to check on their condition and find out whether they wanted to continue their stay.

"They are in a man-made cave up there – a fine view about 900 feet above the plain and a sheer cliff all around," William noted in his diary.

Ankai was a spiritual site, and the day that William arrived there was a day of pilgrimage. He describes the crowded conditions on the single stairway up the mountain.

"I fought my way up with great difficulty. It took me a half hour or more what would take 10 minutes when the stairway was empty.... To get up I touched literally hundreds of women, although I am not allowed to do so by Baba's order."

Many of Baba's orders were difficult to follow or given with the idea that the order would be carried out sometime in the future when conditions were right.

One of William's orders stated that he was to observe silence for a full year. Another said he must beg for food for a full year and not accept any money offered. Often Baba would be pleased if a disciple tried his or her utmost to obey his order even if the person was unsuccessful.

When William told Baba the next day about touching the women on the Ankai Mountain stairway he was not annoyed, but told him that "to wipe this matter off" William was to fast the next day on milk only.

Although Baba was in seclusion, he did break his solitude once a week to visit the women mandali. Very often after these visits, William and Dr. Nilu would receive taunting messages from Baba asking why they were not treating certain of his followers better.

With the start of September, rumours started to circulate from the women mandali that Baba was talking about going to Honolulu and California in November. The men mandali were happy to hear this because it indicated that Baba's seclusion would end in November.

---

* Ankai is one of twin hills near Manmad that has Buddhist and Hindu caves and sculptures and ruins of a fort from Shivaji's time.

Although it appeared Baba was favouring the women mandali, the men still managed occasional sightings of his coming and going weekly at the women's quarters. An earlier explanation from Baba about his varying treatment of disciples argues that apparent benefits do not have lasting good effects. He outlined how some of the followers of Sai Baba – one of his Perfect Masters – appeared to have benefited from donated funds early in their lives only to suffer materially immensely in their later years.

"Baba one day told the mandali that they must never question Baba when he treats one man well and another badly.... He explained, however he treats one or the other disciple, never worry or enquire; he has very good reasons for pampering one, and cursing another."

Baba relayed on more than one occasion that "all suffering was a gift of God," and going through various trials helped address an individual's sanskaras (impressions), helping to pave the way to God-realization.

Because of Baba's seclusion, the men mandali were being deprived of his company and his explanations when they were needed. This must have made following his orders and dealing with one another without the Master's help especially difficult.

While William was anxious to have increased contact with Meher Baba, for the most part he had little time to dwell on the absence. In mid-September he again went to Ankai Mountain to convey Baba's orders that the mandali staying there should return to Meherabad.

"They were all glad at the order to return.... I think the last two weeks have been difficult for them.... The next day I saw Baba for the second time since his seclusion began to report results of the Ankai expedition. He seemed fit and in a good mood."

About this time Baba received a famous visitor. Swiss explorer Ella Maillart* arrived at Meherabad asking if she could see him. Maillart was turned down and went away without gaining an audience with Baba. No reason was given for the decision.

* Ella Maillart (1903–1997) was a Swiss adventurer and journalist who stayed with Countess Tolstoy in Moscow in 1930 and spent most of the war years (1939–1945) living south of Madras near the ashram of Ramana Maharshi.

Late in September, William had already shifted a certain amount of his attention to working at the hospital in Nagar (Ahmednagar), where he was giving anaesthetics and assisting operations. He expected his orders to report to the India Medical Service for wartime duty would arrive any day. When the Honolulu/California tour suddenly changed to a November tour of Ceylon* instead, Baba told William not to write to the authorities, but to wait to be asked up and then go, thus prolonging his time under Baba's influence.

"He wants me to obey the special [Baba] orders as long as possible."

The draft notice finally came in October, but on Baba's order William was able to obtain two months' deferment so that he could accompany the others on the Ceylon tour.

Preparations for the trip to Ceylon instantly took over. Mandali member Chanji** went off to Colombo to find a suitable bungalow for the group. Doctors William and Nilu were to arrange vaccinations for the travellers. Forty-two people were involved, including the masts Mohammed and Chatti Baba.

At the time William and Nilu were also dealing with Baba's glycosuria (urine glucose), and William gave his thoughts about their advice to Baba:

"We told him what we thought, but he'll never listen. As a patient he is really no good at all. But I suppose that Avatars can do as they please."

This nonchalant response about medical treatments was a fact of life with Baba, who on many occasions refused medical treatments. In the two major auto accidents he was to experience he downplayed his serious injuries.

Although the party was to go by train to Ceylon, vehicles that included the big bus and a car for their use were also being transported to the island at a cost of 2,000 rupees.

After a great deal of difficulty, William managed to get permission from the military to stay in Ceylon until January 1, 1941:

---

* Ceylon (now Sri Lanka) is the tropical island country to the south of India in the Indian Ocean.

** Chanji (Framroz Dadachanji) was Baba's first secretary and brought his large extended family to become Baba-lovers.

"I had to phone Delhi twice to get that result through.... No doubt it was only because of his [Baba's] will that the permit was given as now doctors are being called due to war spreading."

Baba and his followers continually tracked the war news. Although some of Baba's predictions were off the mark from a worldly point of view, others were accurate. William conveyed the gist of Baba's remarks in his November 1, 1940, entry:

"Britain will be crushed, but won't give in, and won't lose. Germany and Italy will be crushed and lose.

"England would have been wiped out except for Churchill. He is real clever, and if old Chamberlain had been prime minister, England would have been finished. Churchill has saved England."

At this time Baba was negotiating the purchase of another piece of land on the other side of Ahmednagar. This property would eventually become Meherazad and serve as Meher Baba's intimate home away from the busier pilgrimage centre of Meherabad about 20 kilometres away.

Once the caravan landed in Ceylon, they created quite a bit of interest in their travels on the island "what with Baba, Chatti Baba, Europeans, Indians and all."

William was held up at the crossing from India to Ceylon because his military permit was not in order. Nilu came back to India the next day to retrieve 79 pieces of luggage that hadn't made it on the first crossing, so William crossed over with him.

There were problems with transporting the large bus on the boat and they also wondered whether the bus would be allowed to travel on the restricted roads in Ceylon.

Chanji and William were dispatched to Kandy* to find a suitable bungalow for the stay. Baba went to see the bungalow along with William, Western women Kitty Davy and Rano Gayley, Eastern mandali Chanji, and two others. Baba approved of the residence and they then settled in at the tea plantation called Primrose Hill Estate.

---

* Kandy is one of the most scenic cities in Sri Lanka, in the midst of the hills in the Kandy Valley, which crosses an area of tropical plantations – mainly tea – in the central province of the island.

"A beautiful place, very fine view, and when weather is fine – very fine indeed. We drink fresh tea off the estate," William wrote.

Baba continued his partial seclusion in Ceylon, spending every second day in his hut. He was fasting on only one solid meal a day, while his followers were taking two. Shortly after their arrival in Ceylon, William was asked to make inquiries about the local weather. After learning it would be wet half the time they were there, Baba decided to cut their stay short to only 20 days, even though the bungalow had been rented for two months.

Chanji was quickly sent back to the Indian mainland to find suitable quarters for everyone at Cochin and Calicut*.

Departure day from Ceylon was December 5. Baba's party spent two weeks in Calicut before moving on to Rajputana** in Western India.

The constant travel and changes of plans created nagging tensions among followers. Flat tires, stuck vehicles, and mechanical breakdowns were the norm and such mishaps often occurred in the dead of night. Personality clashes and feuds with officials along the way happened so often they got to be routine.

"I had a nice row with the customs people ... and the station master – both foolish men. Station master, a first-class horror," said William of one confrontation.

"At Ramnad,*** Baba gave all the ladies a lecture saying they were hopeless and started Norina [Matchabelli] weeping, which she seldom does."[33]

William also appeared at the end of his patience as a diary entry of the same day indicates, "Baba slept with us men. He

* Cochin (now called Kochi) is one of India's principal seaports, located on the northern end of a peninsula on the southwest coast of India in the state of Kerala. It is bounded by the Arabian Sea on the west and estuaries to the east. Calicut (now called Kozhikode) is on the Arabian Sea coast of Kerala. It has beautiful beaches and a deep network of lakes, canals, estuaries, and wetlands running through the city.

** Rajputana (now the state of Rajasthan) is a large area northwest of the Aravalli Range that includes part of the Great Indian (Thar) Desert. It is the hill and plateau country between the north Indian plains and the main plateau of peninsular India.

*** Ramnad (Ramanathapuram) is a city and district in the southeast Indian state of Tamil Nadu that contains the Indian portion of Rama's Bridge, an east-west chain of low islands and shallow reefs that extend between India and Sri Lanka.

teases me a bit because I don't get up promptly ... and saying we're a hopeless lot. I try not to get annoyed – as that's all he's really trying to do – to get me to lose my temper. So mostly I keep quiet, though pretty glumly, as I am never at my brightest at 4:30 in the morning – and Baba ... an incurable early riser, capable of teasing anyone at their weakest moments."

The trip to Ceylon was not an official mast tour and Baba's followers might have thought they were off to enjoy a holiday rather than a collective ego-thrashing. Baba of course always alternated between loving and stern measures, and whenever he dressed someone down he was quick to forgive, embrace, and bring the person happily back into his circle. He also frowned on foul moods, insisting that whatever one was feeling inside, one must remain outwardly cheerful.

"Don't be garlic faced," Baba would often tell his followers, including William.

Calicut soon began to wear thin even on Baba:

"Baba dislikes this place. It is too hot, and we shall all be glad to leave.... I take the ladies at 6 a.m. in the bus to the beach for a bath," writes William.

The 1,800-mile trip north to Jaipur, Rajputana, passed with relatively few mishaps. The cooler weather was reflected in better moods all around – including Baba's.

"Baba very jaunty and humorous here, teasing us all in a good-natured way.... Baba put his cold hands on our warm stomachs in the cold morning. Makes us pull our shirts up to do it – it's like an electric shock. He teases Chanji; good-naturedly too – to the amusement of all."[34]

Life for William was about to change drastically. Shortly after their arrival in Jaipur, he received his notice to report directly to military medical duty in Poona on March 1, 1941.

"Baba says I am to go this time. So at last this calling up business has borne fruit. Baba seems pleased about it.... For me a new phase will be beginning shortly – where it will begin, I suppose, only Baba knows."[35]

Although this tour was not for contacting masts, Baba never turned away from meeting with them when good masts were found. In Jaipur a mast was brought to the compound, and

Baba also travelled to nearby Jodhpur with mandali members Gustadji and Eruch, where Baba fed "three very good masts."

Baba described one of the masts as having "practically no body consciousness at all." Baba went to this mast seven times with food and made Eruch and Gustadji take their turns of having darshan (blessing) from the mast first and last.

Baba also contacted an older female mast (mastani) in Jodhpur, whom Baba went to and fed three times, ordering the two mandali members to take darshan from her all three times.

Before William officially joined the military, Meher Baba started a publishing venture that would distribute his messages, including an explanation of the seven realities of Baba's teachings. He asked William to put the seven points into good English.

"This I did to the best of my ability, and now a new propaganda push has been ordered by Baba and the seven points are to be distributed all over India – about a million copies in all languages. Norina may go to the USA in June to carry on propaganda there before Baba goes to the West."

Later in the month William was given a Gujarati arti (prayer from the heart) of Baba's. Translated into English it reads:

> Oh God, command that the fire of ignorance
> be extinguished!
> Bestow upon Your lovers the light of faith
> for which they long.
> Oh Master Meher Baba!
> We lay our heads at Your feet.
> Oh Meher Baba! You are the One who knows
> the original state of God.
> You are the Lord of Truth!
> You are the lover and Beloved in one.
> You are the torrent of Infinite Knowledge
> and the Ocean of Oneness.
> Oh Beloved, bestow upon us seekers
> the knowledge of Ezad.
> For You, Paramatma, are omniscient,
> Divine Knowledge Itself!
> Intoxicate us by making us

drink from the cup of love divine.
Oh Saki, promise us a cup of wine!
We offer our lives in sacrifice to You.
Our ship founders in mid-ocean;
only if You steer can we remain afloat.
Oh Meher Baba! You are our captain and protector!

Baba was again anxious to get underway and was planning to go northward from Jaipur to Quetta* near the Afghanistan border. The 1,500-mile trip started on Baba's birthday and would take 15 days.

While Baba wanted William to accompany the group to Quetta, he realized that William would have to honour his military commitment. Baba felt it necessary to amend the long list of orders William was adhering to. He was ruthless, or perhaps kind, in easing the strictness because of the pressure William would face in doing wartime service. In the end William was given only three orders to follow, which he entered in his diary:

"No fasting or anything – but no lustful action;

"Communication with Baba twice a month giving address; and

"When things reach a climax and Baba writes me or wires me to come, I must come at once, without permission of authorities if necessary."

Previous orders of not to smoke, not to drink alcohol, and to abstain from eating meat, fish, or eggs were dropped once he joined the military.

Before William embarked on his wartime years of work in the Indian Medical Service, the reflections that this English doctor made of the mast ashrams and their elusive purpose are revealing. The breathless description of the seven main ashrams reflects William's own unanswered questions:

"Those things that matter most, such as the spiritual reality behind these centres for God-intoxicated souls; the ultimate reasons why Baba has done all this work; the invisible interplay

* Quetta (part of Pakistan after partition) consists of valleys which act as a natural fort surrounded by imposing hills on all sides. It is known as the "Fruit Garden of Pakistan" because of its diverse flora and fauna.

between the utterly perfect being of the Master, and the subordinate spiritual capacities of the masts – all of these things ... escape the power of words, and their explanation cannot, therefore, be found between the covers of this book."[36]

William continues striving in *The Wayfarers* to explain the one-on-one intimacy in the countless Baba/mast relationships. In the end his own heart cannot be contained and completes the telling task:

"But such secrets are, surely, Baba's affair and the mast's affair, and I suspect that, if Baba were to give an intellectual explanation of them, we should be intrinsically none the wiser, for these arcana must be experienced in a way that transcends the intellect before we can even begin to understand them.

"It is better, therefore, that we take a leaf from the book of a God-intoxicated soul, and seek to be overpowered by Divine Love, or like a God-absorbed soul, fly fast and straight across the measureless skies to the great homeland of the Infinite, rather than fritter away our intellectual and spiritual substance in profitless conceits."

Although William would not pen these words until a few years later when he began writing *The Wayfarers*, it's a fair guess that they capture his mood as he prepared to enter military service. His feelings about and ties to his Spiritual Master were also given in the early pages of the book:

"A subtle quintessence of love ... pervades everything that Baba does. His physical presence and the brilliance of his leadership have that impossible quality of the philosopher's stone, that by their magic touch, they transmute the base metal of the most commonplace routine into a treasure of loving service.

"This is perhaps an ornate way of describing something that is at once so real that one might think it easy to describe quite simply, and so transcendental that the spirit of it eludes the grasp of words.

"But this magic, this imponderable something, weaves itself like a golden thread into the fabric of everything that Baba does, and when the factual details of a phase of Baba's life are buried so deep in the ashes of one's mind to be almost forgotten, the memory of this splendid thing is still there."

6

War Years, Indian Medical Service

To say that William had a strong love for Meher Baba at this time would be accurate. One also gets a sense that no matter how lofty William's description of Baba and events surrounding him, one had to be there and live the life to fully absorb the experience.

Baba's expectation that William would drive the bus on the mast-hunting trip to Quetta was short-circuited when the 29-year-old Brit was told to report for military service at Poona on March 1, 1941.

William's diary suddenly became dormant. His next entry on May 19 was written from Bangalore, where he had been stationed administering to the needs of Italian prisoners of war (POWs)* in the 160-bed hospital there.

While with the Indian Medical Service (IMS) during the World War II, William served as a doctor at hospitals in Bangalore and Secunderabad**. He spoke 13 languages, and because he knew Italian, one of his medical duties was to treat the Italian POWs in the Bangalore Hospital. During the war years William served in Poona as well as Secunderabad and Bangalore.

William was able to visit Baba many times while on military leave from his medical duties. While his close proximity

* By 1945 there were about 100,000 Italian POWs in India spread over 28 locations. The British chose to incarcerate them in India rather than transport them to England.

** Secunderabad is just north of its twin city Hyderabad in Andhra state. Its people follow a mixture of religions and it is home to many famous temples and churches.

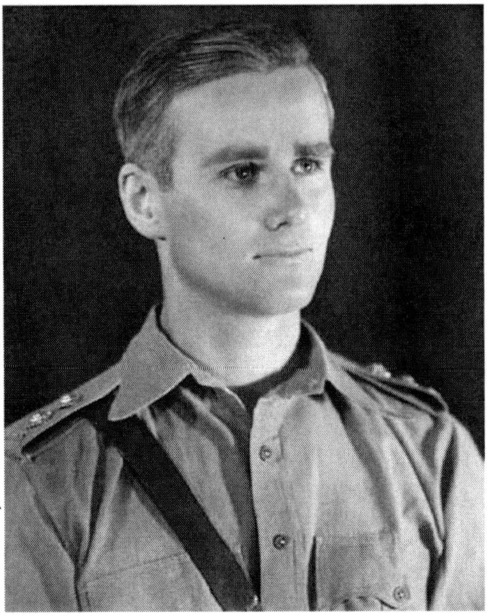

Donkin Family

William served as a doctor in the Indian Medical Service during World War II. He spoke a dozen languages. Because of his command of Italian, he was stationed for a period in the hospital in Bangalore that treated wounded Italian POWs.

to Baba in the war years might suggest divine intervention, one should realize that Baba's power and influence in practical matters was enormous. In short, he had contacts everywhere – many in important authoritative positions. Baba also explained that he does his work through his close ones, so no doubt William was also contributing toward this in some unknown way.

While William served in the hospital at Bangalore, on occasion mandali members would also pass through the city and bring messages from Baba to William.

Ironically, the mast ashram that Baba set up in Bangalore shortly after William's 1939 arrival in India had been gradually phased out and moved, on a smaller scale, to Meherabad. It was closed completely in the autumn of 1940. Six years would pass before Baba established another mast ashram in Mahabaleshwar in 1946. During that period he still continued his mast-hunting tours.

Baba's habit of initiating constant, ever-changing activity did not let up during the war.

In May 1941, Baba instructed Adi Sr., who was later to be his long-time secretary, to visit Upasni Maharaj, the Perfect Master with whom Baba had lived for many years.

"Adi [was] very overcome meeting Upasni, weeping a lot. Upasni said that suffering with a Master brings spiritual fruit.... He also said he was like a husk, all empty and lifeless; and his spirituality had been given to Baba."[37]

William complained in his diary that he did not "like this army job at all. Too much red tape and all...." However, he said that his Italian had improved as a result of working with the POWs in the hospital.

Four months passed from William's entry into the IMS before he saw Baba again. He was granted leave from Bangalore in late July 1941.

"Ghani*, Eruch, and I went off to Ahmednagar, leaving here on Sunday morning, reaching Nagar on Monday morning.

"As soon as we got to Meherabad and had a bit of breakfast, Baba called me up the hill.

"It was good to see Baba after so long. A couple of hours with him after four months absence is a real treat."[38]

William's military leave at Meherabad coincided with a meeting of the mandali with Baba, who outlined his upcoming six-month seclusion. It was to be in two parts. The first and strictest was to start August 1 and run two and a half months to mid-October at Meherabad. During this time only one mandali, Vishnu, would see Baba. Vishnu would receive orders to convey to other mandali. The second part of the seclusion would be carried out at Panchgani, another of Baba's favourite haunts.

Baba's periods of seclusion were strict, involving only one watchman to ensure Baba was not disturbed.

Baba also delivered a discourse to the mandali during this meeting. William conveys the gist of the message in his diary:

"Behind all our actions is egoism, mind, emotions, etc. Behind Baba's actions is the Infinite Truth. Both actions outwardly

---

* Dr. Abdul Ghani Munsiff was a school friend of Meher Baba and one of his early mandali. Ghani enjoyed a unique relationship with Baba because of their long and close friendship.

appear the same – eating, sleeping, getting angry, etc. But there is this great difference, of God behind Baba's actions – egoism behind ours."

Baba assigned William several minor duties while he was on leave. He was also reminded to write two letters to Baba before August 1.

On leaving Baba after his leave ended, William wrote, "Adi, Eruch, and I left Meherabad on Monday night. Ghani went on to Poona, and I got back to Bangalore this morning. Feeling rather depressed but it's been wonderful seeing Baba anyhow."

Another four months passed before William would again turn to his diary. The entry came after he heard that Baba was to stop in Bangalore after visiting the mast Chatti Baba in Negapatam. Other mandali were called from communities close to Bangalore for Baba's visit, and Baba delivered extensive discourses to those gathered. Baba spoke of darkness and light. Where, he asked the group, did darkness go when light appeared?

"Light was knowledge which made all things appear clear in the consciousness. Darkness was ignorance," wrote William.

Baba also gave those assembled a detailed description of the seven planes that humans pass through on their involution to God-realization and the period of darkness that appears on the fourth plane of this journey.

In his November 18, 1941, diary entry, William conveys Baba's message further:

"Spiritually darkness is the fourth plane, and all Avatars when they speak of darkness mean this fourth plane."

Baba then explained the journey to God on the planes:

"The first three steps are the first three planes, which lead us up to the House of God. The fourth plane is the threshold of the House of God, and it is in complete darkness. Here we are very easily misled, and if we fail, we tumble back down the three steps of the three planes and have to start up again."

Baba went on to say that if we are able to cross the threshold and make that transition under the safe guidance of a Spiritual Master, then we suddenly reach light and the fifth plane when one actually feels God.

"Then we go further into the House of God and see God [sixth plane]; and then we go up to God and become one with Him on the seventh plane."

William points out that Baba said all individuals are in reality God, but their levels of consciousness are not high enough to realize this.

"When a man is realized, his consciousness is that he is God, and when he returns – if he has to for duty [and this is the highest spiritual state] – his bliss remains the same always, and so his consciousness of God – but his suffering increases as he descends."[39]

One suspects that Baba is describing himself in this paragraph. His role as the Avatar meant that he had returned in response to his duty to mankind. His mention of suffering increasing as he descended no doubt referred to the experience coming from the Perfect Master Babajan in a God-realized state to be brought down over a seven-year period by another Perfect Master – Upasni Maharaj.

Baba would make a number of predictions about breaking his silence over the years. He vowed to speak the word of words that would have a profound effect on mankind – particularly on those who were at the right stage spiritually to receive the word.

Again in 1941 Baba said he "had already begun to speak to himself alone," and this would increase.

"Baba said he will never tell us when he is to speak. Does an earthquake announce its coming, he said. Nor would he announce his date of speaking," wrote William. "But when he spoke all would feel it – some a lot, some a little. People would know Christ had come, by feeling something really had happened."

Although many of Baba's followers were already accepting him as the Avatar or personification of God, Baba himself would not formally announce this until February 1954 in Meherasthan – a small village in the Hamirpur district – when he was nearly 60 years old.

The despair that gripped much of the world in the forties continued to make Baba's messages ring true for the small hodgepodge of people from various countries around the world who were his followers.

Before he would finally speak, he said, "Hate and destruction will grow and spread 'till all is chaos." After he spoke, he said, hate would be all gone, and there would be understanding and love and a world of friendly nations.

In the meantime Baba continued to work his magic on his followers:

"Baba flattered me a lot. It's like a deep drink of celestial wine to see Baba. He gives so much in these wonderful meetings," William wrote at the time.

On Boxing Day 1941, those in the ashram learned that the Perfect Master Upasni Maharaj had died on December 24. "So what! Baba has always said that when Upasni dies, He comes into His full power," wrote William in his diary on Boxing Day.

In a letter on May 26, 1942, William wrote to Baba from St. Martha's Hospital in Bangalore that he was very interested in the fracture work he was doing in treating the Italian POWs.

In a July 5 letter, Adi Sr. wrote to William, "Baba keeps kicking me about from place to place like 'a ball gathering no moss.' If I could steady myself for a minute even in the rolling, I shall be informing you of Baba's teasing and pranks with the mandali."[40]

A full eight months would pass before William turned to his diary in August 1942, again marking another personal meeting with Baba. Taking leave from his medical work at the Bangalore hospital, William was able to join Baba and the mandali at Dehra Dun in northern India. Apparently this generous leave was made possible through Baba, who had sent a telegram to someone on William's behalf. Baba told William at the time that the world was going to turn chaotic and that Germany and Japan would advance toward India.

"Baba also told me to smoke only one cigar daily, not more. Baba is looking very fit indeed, active and in a good mood. I am to stay here [Dehra Dun] ten days, and in Meherabad four days, and visit Hardwar, Rishikesh, and Mussoorie while here."[41]

Enjoying his leave, William began making more frequent entries in his diary.

"Baba talks about the war and the India situation. He agrees that non-violence is good and that India must be free, but he says the inconsistency of Gandhi and others is confusing and misleading, and will lead to chaos," William wrote on August 9, 1942.

Baba appeared to be in good spirits in Dehra Dun, calling everyone by odd nicknames. Donkin was mysteriously dubbed "the son of an ostrich."

Baba was also hinting at the time that within two and half months William would be free of his military service and "be with him and working for him."

"How he doesn't say – so we shall see.... Although I am very sceptical about Baba's promises; I naturally live in hope," wrote William.

William appears to have enjoyed this leave and even had "a good gossip with Kitty [Davy], Margaret [Craske], and Rano [Gayley]," three of the Western women who were also staying in Dehra Dun.

By August 21, William had travelled south to Nasik and Meherabad, where he was waiting to return to his military doctor post in Bangalore the next day. William wrote very little about his work with the Italian POWs in the Bangalore Hospital or what he did in his off time during his many months away from Meher Baba. However, during his off-duty times in Bangalore he was involved in Baba-related chores. He took on the job of getting enlarged photographs of Meher Baba made and also made visits to the Byramangala Spiritual Centre on occasion to carry out work.

William told Baba in a September 1942 letter that he had been promoted to captain and that his retroactive pay for the new rank would date back to November 1941.

An October 14 letter he writes to Will and Mary Backett in England echoes his yearnings to be with Baba:

"I don't see much of Baba these days except whenever I can get leave every few months, and I was in Dehra Dun for three weeks in August seeing Baba every day."

William describes the joy he experienced when Baba sent him off to Rishikesh and Hardwar during the visit:

"You would have loved these famous Hindu pilgrim centers, at Rishikesh, where the Ganges comes sweeping out of the Himalayas ... Hardwar, or 'God's door,' is 15 miles below

Rishikesh. The Ganges passes through a small cut in a line of hills there ... a fascinating place."

That Baba was often thinking of William is reflected in a call he received in October to meet his Spiritual Master at midnight between Bangalore and Madras* when Baba was returning from Negapatam for his meeting there with the mast Chatti Baba. Adi Sr. wrote to William about the meeting on October 16, 1942, "Since your writing to Baba longing deeply to see him ... Baba has decided to see you at Jolarpet. This trip has been arranged expressly to see this very loving doctor as he has put it."

"I met him at Jolarpet Station** at midnight and was with him until 2 a.m. Baba made the deviation off his route specially to meet me.

"He said that we must die for God, while others die for their country. Baba was in an excellent mood and we strolled about the station in the moonlight together.... Such occasional meetings with Baba are really very satisfying indeed – a sort of deep thirst is assuaged." [42]

William's yearning to be permanently in Baba's presence is reflected in his October 11, 1942, letter to Adi Sr. from St. Martha's Hospital about the possibility of seeing Baba again soon:

"If it were a real call which must be obeyed, I would come without permission and damn the consequences."

On working and living in Bangalore, William added, "In this war everyone is on jobs and in places they would prefer not to be. So even if I stay here, my heart at least is with Baba always.... I long for the time of reunion with Baba, and envy you fellows with him very much...."[43]

The job with the Italian POWs at the Bangalore Hospital ended in January 1943 when William was transferred to a new field ambulance job in Secunderabad.

---

* Madras (now Chennai, capital of Tamil Nadu), on the southeast coastal plain, was originally a fishing village. It was selected as the first permanent British settlement in India and has some Victorian architectural influences. During World War II, it was attacked by German U-boats.

** Jolarpet is an important railway junction in Tamil Nadu in southern India. It is a mostly flat area, but not far from the Yelagiri Hills, which are surrounded by orchards, rose-gardens and green valleys.

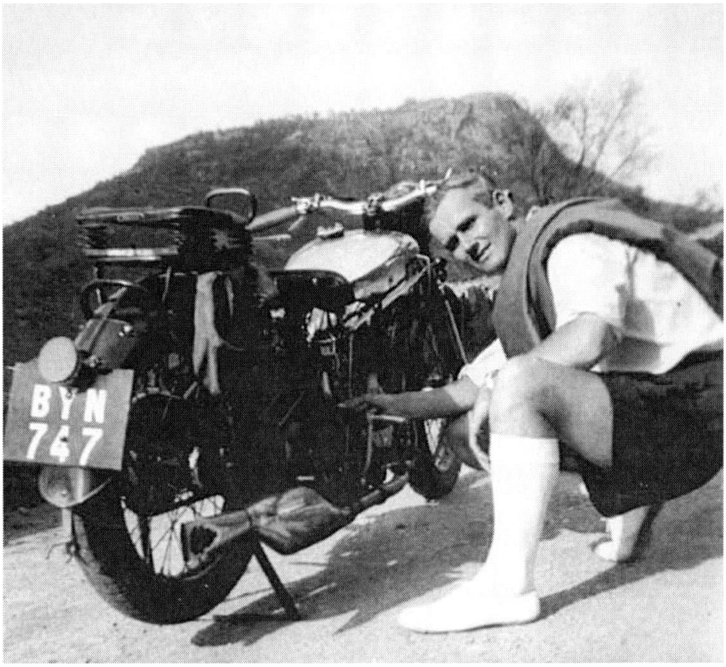

MN Publications

William, shown in 1941, had a motorcycle for many of the years he stayed in India. He was meticulous in maintaining such machines, often stripping them down, cleaning all the parts, and putting them back together again.

Before taking up this new job, he was called to a one-day meeting in Meherabad involving 100 followers of Meher Baba. After returning from the meeting, William received several written orders which were not to be opened until February 1, 1943. Although the orders were to be carried out "at the cost of life if necessary," William chose not to detail them in his diary.

At Secunderabad William was much closer to Meherabad but that didn't seem to counter his uneasiness over his medical duties: "This field ambulance job, I am loathing it, and writing grumbling letters to Baba every few days."

When April came, William was told that he would be spending May 14 until June 15 in other parts of India with Baba and other members of the mandali.

Shireen, Baba's mother, passed away on February 25, 1943. Baba had travelled from Mahabaleshwar by car, arriving a half-hour before his mother died. She had apparently suffered a stroke and was in Sassoon Hospital (Baba's birthplace) in Poona for a few days. She had gone home from the hospital and died a few days later.

Pendu*, one of the mandali, was preparing a grave for her next to Nonny Gayley's grave on Meherabad Hill.

At the end of February, William was moved from Secunderabad to Wah**, just beyond Rawalpindi. At this point, William seemed to realize that his medical duties would not take him outside of India, and he was pleased:

"The thing is that I don't want to leave India, because Baba is here and I want to come closer and closer to him."

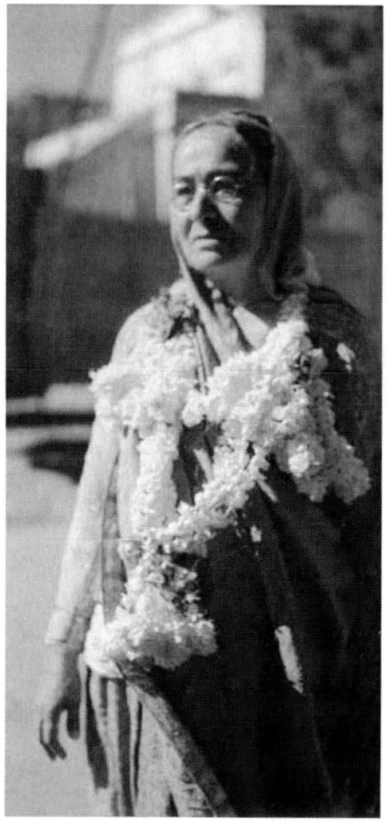

MSI Collection India

Meher Baba's mother Shireen Sheriar Irani died in Poona at age 65 on February 25, 1943, her son's birthday.

The next diary entry in April 1943 noted a brief meeting with Baba as William was travelling to Poona on army business. Baba assured him again he would be spending May 14 to June 15 with Baba, through special leave from the medical service.

* Pendu (Aspandiar R. Irani, 1903–1986) was Baba's maternal cousin and one of the earliest members of the mandali.

** Wah is a city in the Punjab near Rawalpindi, now part of Pakistan. Legend says that a Mughal Emperor, possibly Akbar, after drinking from a spring there on a journey to Kashmir, exclaimed "Wah" which translates as "Wow," giving the city its name.

Throughout the war years, William continued to manage to get days off here and there so he could make his way to Baba and the mandali wherever they happened to be in India.

"Last weekend I went up to Panchgani to spend a day with Baba. I was allowed to hob-nob with Margaret, Kitty, and Rano for 20 minutes."[44]

These three Western women were to spend long periods with Meher Baba in India during the thirties and forties. Margaret Craske would stay seven years; Kitty Davy, fifteen years; and Rano Gayley, for the rest of her life. (She died in 1986.)

William undoubtedly talked about the war with these women, but they also would catch up with news related to other Baba followers.

"They told me that Baba had said that Norina's present publicity lectures in the USA were not his way of working, but that it did ... help his work," William wrote in April. At this time Norina Matchabelli was giving high-profile lectures in the US, claiming that Meher Baba was speaking directly through her or channelling his messages in what she called "spiritual thought transmissions."

Although Baba did not allow prophesying and often chose to travel incognito, he sometimes let his followers pursue their own directions in relaying his messages to the world. Norina, who had a strong theatrical background, chose for a period of time to relay his message in this flamboyant manner.

During William's short Panchgani stay, Baba put a figure on the number of male mandali he considered close: "He says that ... he is happy to have his 24 chief male disciples. They are jewels he says – in spite of their obvious faults," William wrote.

Although Baba's followers were expected to work hard on extinguishing their egos, a direct comment about William Donkin's service that Baba made at this time, recorded in Bhau Kalchuri's* *Lord Meher* series, might have proved difficult for William to forget.

---

* Bhau (Vir Singh) Kalchuri joined Baba in 1953. He was Baba's night watchman. On Baba's instruction he wrote ghazals (poetry) and a biography of Baba in Hindi *(Meher Prabhu)* and English *(Lord Meher)* and other works, and served for many years as Chairman of the Avatar Meher Baba Trust.

"I am extremely happy when I see men like Don [William]. What a spirit of self-sacrifice, everyone so near and dear [his family], and while serving the government dedicating all to me. What sacrifice and service could be greater? This is what makes me happy with my men mandali. They are men [heroes] in the real sense of the word."[45]

The month-long furlough William was to receive in mid-May was in part to allow him to attend a major meeting of 120 of Baba's followers. The program was to last four or five days during which a diagram or chart outlining evolution of the species and involution of the soul through the planes of consciousness was to be unveiled. Women mandali member and artist Rano Gayley drew the chart under Baba's direction.

Those assembled were asked to meditate on the chart for three and a half hours, which for William was quite a chore.

"We all meditated from 7 a.m. to 10:30 a.m. on the chart sitting about in places shown by Baba. I was in the main hall at Meherabad opposite the clock, and so could see how slowly the hours passed," says William in his diary. He said Baba wanted the group to experience and allow strange thoughts to come in, but he "wanted us to fight them," while meditating on the chart.

Throughout his lifetime, Baba made only minor references to meditation, stating that physical contact with him and being in his presence were much more important. He did, however, cover the topic of specific levels of meditation in his published work *Discourses*.*

On the day following the chart meditation experience, the mandali were asked to bathe and feed the poor. Each one of the mandali looked after one man, whom they were to consider as Baba at the time.

William gave his own interpretation of the four-day meeting and chart meditation, stating that it was beyond the group to decipher Baba's spiritual intent:

"I rather feel that apart from Baba's spiritual working; about which we can know nothing, that the meeting was a

* *Discourses* is a book of Meher Baba's talks on a variety of mostly spiritual topics, as recorded by his disciples and close followers. It has been published in seven editions, in five volumes, three volumes, and a single volume.

chance for all to see a lot of Baba, and that the program was just a way of filling in time, and keeping all happy. The thing that really matters is contact with Baba."[46]

During William's month with Baba, he and various other mandali were going back and forth between Panchgani, Meherabad, and Poona. On some of these trips, William again found himself driving the old Blue Bus. On one stay in Panchgani, William drove Baba to the Hindu High School for Boys there, and he relayed the scene at the school:

"He [Baba] really looked as fresh and simple as a child as he sat there. For all His 49 years – mischief monger as He is nevertheless."

An episode between Baba and William during this month-long leave typified Baba's persnickety approach and the frustration his followers sometimes experienced. A trunk of William's personal possessions was being kept in Baba's room at Meherabad while he was away in the army. During his leave, William took the trunk from Baba's room to rearrange his possessions.

"When Baba came and found it was gone, he was very fed up and gave me a dressing down accordingly."

Later, Baba told William he had ordered the trunk kept in his room on William's absence as "a link with me."

"I didn't of course know about this special order of Baba's – that it should not be touched."

William was ordered to fast, taking two meals a day only and also to again meditate on the evolution chart that Rano had created. "I didn't like the fast – too fond of eating to enjoy fasting – but the meditation business was not very arduous." Knowing William's ability to creatively adapt to myriad situations, the tongue-in-cheek comment may well have meant he spent some of his meditative time catching up on sleep.

Baba appeared to want to interact with his mandali most naturally during this time. A certain amount of the day was spent discussing the war, but there were also sessions for more light-hearted pursuits such as card-playing, in which Baba took part.

Shortly after William returned to his medical duties, Baba informed him that he wanted to meet him for a day between

July 4 and 14 at Lahore* in northern India.

Even during the war years Meher Baba and his followers did not ignore sudden national emergencies. In October 1943, Baba and a large number of disciples visited Calcutta during the terrible famine**, when millions died of hunger. Baba fed about 1,000 people, organized the distribution of about 10,000 chapattis (an Indian flatbread) and distributed 2,000 vests to children.

"A number of middle-class people who were invited to the feast could not ask for charitable relief because of their social position.

"When all were seated in the school building where the feast was given, some of the orthodox Hindus were disconcerted at being served by a non-Hindu [Baba], whose identity was kept secret. However, the social workers of Calcutta who had helped organize the gathering explained to the guests that Baba and his disciples had come all the way from Bombay to serve them, and that they should be grateful.

"Nearly all accepted his generosity and were even struck by the fact that the originator of the charity had himself come to serve them and supervise the work. When the feast was over, Baba personally gave each person clothes and money."[47]

Another five months passed before William again put pen to pages in his diary. In mid-November, he visited Baba in Lahore, having seen him only briefly in Rawalpindi in August and in Lahore in June before that. There are no details on this meeting between the two.

Baba and the other mandali left Lahore on November 25, 1943, to return to Meherabad after spending almost five months in northern India.

William continued his usual pattern of fulfilling his medical duties and when on leave scurrying off to see Baba wherever he was in India. Five months after William's Lahore visit,

---

* Lahore is a major city in the Punjab region, now in Pakistan, which has a rich Mughal heritage and many British colonial structures that combined Gothic, Victorian, and Mughal building styles.

** The 1943 Famine in India claimed the lives of about 3.5 million people. It is considered to have been entirely man made, as the British did not store any of the grain grown in the area, and they were exporting wheat from India and did no rationing of the rice that was available.

the two travelled toward each other to meet halfway at Jhansi* in Uttar Pradesh.

"We all had a meal. Rice, dal, and two sorts of vegetables, then fruit and tea. We sat talking – Baba of course by signs – until about midnight, and then off to bed."[48]

After William complained to Baba the next morning about his medical duties in the army, Baba proposed that "all this would be OK" if he could locate seven masts in Jhansi. William and the other mandali were successful in finding seven masts and were able to locate another seven in a side trip to Gwalior.** William relates an amusing incident which occurred on the train trip to Gwalior, which helped alleviate any tension or overtiredness the group was feeling:

"While in the train, Chanji had been drying Baba's pyjamas out of the train window. In the scramble to get out at Gwalior, Chanji lost these night clothes and discovered the loss at the hotel. Baba pretended to be annoyed, and Chanji was quite cut up about it, but I think Baba was rather amused."

William saw Baba only briefly (an hour in Bombay in July) during the next six-month period. At that time Baba told William he would soon obtain more interesting work in the military.

"And I have! On September 16 [1944] I reached Secunderabad, being posted to ... permanent surgical duties; and am a trainee for grading in orthopaedic surgery, and very happy too."[49]

At this time William received word from Adi Sr. that Chanji (Baba's secretary and a long-time mandali) had died in Baba's presence.

"Dear old Chanji, teased by Baba most of all. I have seen Baba throw things at Chanji when he was very obstinate, absent-minded, muddled-headed, teased by all of the mandali. But he loved Baba and worked for Him; travelled all over the world with Him.

"Dear old Chanji – we loved him for all his shortcomings."

---

* Jhansi is a city that grew up around the stone fort strategically built on a hill rising out of the plain. It is a major rail and road junction.

** Gwalior is a city and fortress in Madhya Pradesh. It is known for many palaces in the Hindu style of architecture and the Jai Vilas Palace, patterned on the French palace of Versailles.

On his next leave, William joined Baba in Aurangabad.* "[Baba] made me give a pretty full account of myself."

Baba told William he was to write down a number of points related to the next seven months. William's points in brief:

1) To remain at the hospital in Secunderabad until March 1, 1945.
2) To come see Baba for a day or two in January.
3) To spend a month with Baba in April 1945.
4) At the start of May to go to work in another big hospital – possibly Poona; where I would be physically nearer to Baba, and would do more surgery.

Baba also told William to look after his health and stay out of the sun.

In a conversation about the war, Baba said although the Allies – the United States and England – were going to win the war, they might lose the peace, because Russia would dominate peace negotiations.

The mandali, including William, accompanied Baba on a visit to the Ellora Caves.** Passing through Khuldabad,*** Baba said he liked the spiritual atmosphere there and mentioned that Sai Baba, one of his Perfect Masters, had stayed there for a long time.

During this period, William was trying to learn the Persian language. Baba instructed him to spend a half hour studying each day. Baba mentioned Hafiz,**** one of his favourite Persian poets, and spelled out some couplets of Hafiz on his alphabet board.

---

* Aurangabad, a city in Maharashtra, is known for its many gates and historical monuments, including the Ajanta Caves and Ellora Caves. It is also home to Bibi Ka Maqbara, the "mini-Taj," a small building that is a replica of the Taj Mahal.

** Ellora Caves are 34 rock-cut caves containing carved-rock sculptures that were carved between the fifth and tenth centuries. The caves were carved in a hillside and used as temples for Buddhists and Jains.

*** Khuldabad (Heavenly Abode) is a walled town considered the holy shrine of Deccan Muslims. Among the many historical figures buried there is Aurangzeb, the last major Mughal emperor.

**** Hafiz is the most beloved Persian Sufi poet. He expressed the spiritual experiences of a mystic in the words of the lover for his Beloved.

"He said if he was speaking now, he would teach me Persian very quickly," William said in his diary on October 29, 1944, in Secunderabad.

William's "day or two" with Baba early in 1945 occurred in February rather than January. On this occasion, Baba reiterated his thoughts about Russia and the peace negotiations. He also brought up the search for an ideal site for a spiritual centre in the United States and hinted that William might eventually work there. Baba had just approved a site in Myrtle Beach, South Carolina.

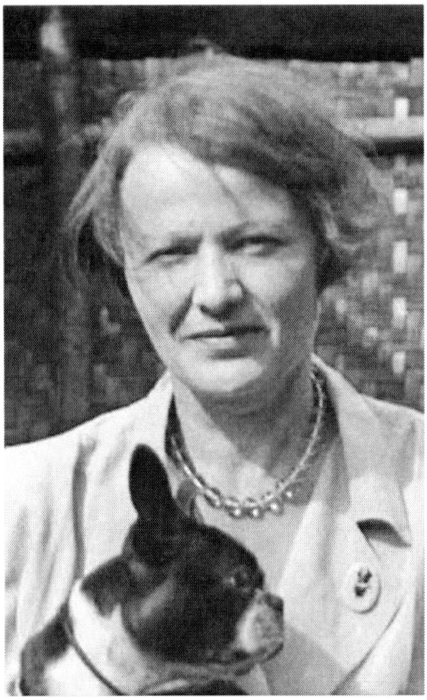

Elizabeth Chapin Patterson Photo Archives

Elizabeth Patterson

"It appears Elizabeth [Patterson's] ... father has left a lot of land and money, and a centre is being planned there. It sounds ... interesting."[50]

In the same diary entry, William indicated that Baba was spoiling him on the brief three-day visit:

"Baba ... told me that I was the luckiest of all the Westerners, having seen so much of Him during the past years; and that this was due to past connections with Him."

William also enjoyed a chat with Margaret Craske during the visit. On his departure, Baba asked William to find a suitable bungalow for the group in Secunderabad or Hyderabad.*

Mandali member Bal Natu** wrote in Volume 8 of *Glimpses of the Godman,* a series about Meher Baba, about the rigmarole involved in finding adequate accommodations for the party.

---

* Hyderabad is the twin city of Secunderabad in Andhra in south India.

** Bal Natu, a schoolteacher from Kurduwadi, became a close follower of Meher Baba and would spend long periods of time with him in the 1950s and -60s. He joined the mandali in Meherazad in 1977 when he retired.

"Baba wished to make Hyderabad His headquarters for contacting masts in southern India.... Dr. Donkin selected two or three bungalows and wrote to Baba about them. Baba sent Pendu with certain instructions to finalize this matter."

Based on Baba's assessment criteria, William's choices for bungalows did not measure up. In an area called Jubilee Hills, a new villa was nearing completion with a well-kept garden and small swimming pool – both items that Baba had stipulated.

"Pendu made inquiries of the owner who was a prominent lawyer in Hyderabad.... Baba personally visited ... liked the bungalow and asked Pendu and Donkin to lease it."[51]

The bungalow saga had many logistical tentacles connected with it. The owner was so busy that William and Pendu could only see him late at night. They talked about the rent, and the lawyer instructed his clerk to draft a compliance agreement concerning the facilities in the villa and the advance money to be paid.

Despite the late hour, when William and Pendu returned to their hotel, Baba wanted to know the full details of the agreement. Unfortunately it was written in Urdu. Pendu was dispatched to find someone in the hotel who could translate the letter, and the only person available was an inebriated partygoer.

"Pendu requested him to visit the room of his 'elder brother.' Though drunk, the man seemed sober enough to read out to Baba the agreement drawn in Urdu. While listening, Baba gave certain instructions to Pendu, regarding changes to be made in the draft. Thus, even a tipsy man was of timely help. This account is given to convey how particular Baba was in selecting His residences as He moved from place to place."[52]

Not to dwell on this particular bungalow search – but it is telling in that it shows that Baba used even seemingly simple chores to wear down the egos of his followers to get them to the point where they couldn't care less what stress they created and what other people thought of them.

A sidebar description of acquiring Jubilee Hills is given by David Fenster in his book *Mehera-Meher*, Volume II:

"The owner had wanted to complete construction on the house before renting it, but Baba was anxious and sent William and Rano to persuade him.

"'Only the lampshades are left,' [to do] the owner told them in a beseeching tone.

"'We don't want them,' they replied.

"'But what about the locks? At least let me have the locks installed before you move in.'"

The locks were put on, but when Baba and the women mandali moved in they had to see with the harsh light of naked light bulbs rather than the softer light that lampshades would have provided.

"The washbasins had no faucets and work remained to be done on the windows. But there was a thick red Persian carpet in the hallway, and the house was partially furnished – though they had to supply their own beds."

While it might appear to the reader that Baba was always looking for luxury accommodations, he was primarily thinking of the needs of his followers – particularly of Mehera and the other women mandali. Also, the accounts of the intense mast-hunting excursions conducted over the years indicated that Baba himself spent little idle time in the accommodations he chose.

To visit Baba and the other mandali, William often cycled eight miles from the hospital in Secunderabad to Hyderabad. "I usually got there rather hot and sweaty ... a shower, and change a shirt and cool off, and then go down to Baba's bungalow."

On May 1, William was ordered to fast and also to inform those in Ahmednagar and Meherabad to do the same.

"There are about 400 on the fast, so I have had as much food as I could stuff in before seven this morning in preparation for the day's fast."[53]

While the larger group fasted for only one day, Meher Baba chose to fast for at least 11 days (longer if his strength held up) on glucose and lime juice. William monitored Baba's condition on his daily visits.

At about this time, the ashram received word that one of Baba's women mandali – Nadine Tolstoy, daughter-in-law of author Leo Tolstoy – had been diagnosed with amyotrophic lateral sclerosis (Lou Gehrig's Disease), and was not expected to live more than a year or two.

Baba continued to butter William up in front of the other mandali, saying he was his best Western follower.

"Of course it's nice to be smarmed up, but I know that in such times Baba doesn't praise one because of any genuine goodness on one's part. In fact, the better the disciple, the more he maligns and teases usually."

William' astuteness in assessing Baba's methods was growing with time. He saw Baba's praise as a "prelude to trouble." But he did admit that his Spiritual Master was usually diplomatic in slipping the stiletto in:

"I think to a certain extent he likes to magnify and draw out and nourish one's faults until one becomes aware of them, and gets them off the chest. Instead of suppressing them – after all what's bad in one is best out.

"Anyhow with Baba, from whom one can't hide anything really, he always digs it out, even if one did not know it was there."

William was predicting that Baba and the mandali would stay in Hyderabad another two months "since the ladies like the bungalow ... that usually has a big influence on Baba's moves."

William's diary entry of May 14, 1945, mentions victory in Europe, and indications that his Indian Medical Service duties would soon be winding down.

When William describes the "orgy of drunkenness" that accompanied the victory night celebrations, Baba expressed disappointment at the behaviour.

"He was a bit disgusted.... He says to take a little liquor occasionally and be cheerful is good, but to drink mainly to get drunk is silly."[54]

William's next diary entry as the war is ending indicates he is seriously thinking about his relationship with Meher Baba and his life in India:

"There's no doubt Baba makes a mess of one's life. One's old life that is, though of course I met him at the beginning of it. Though it is a strain nevertheless, changing one's values and having the bees in the bonnet taken out.

"I often wonder if I am genuinely and intrinsically better in the eyes of God than before I met Baba. I feel I am; somehow cleaner and freer inside. I am sure something is happening, bit by bit inside for the better."

His questioning and uncertain mood continued in another diary entry at the time:

"I went up the other evening after a foul day in a rotten mood, fed up with work, myself, Baba, and everything. Baba at once began asking after my health, and mood, and I told him [my] mood was so-so. As usual he asked why, and in front of the others I gave a few of the reasons."

Baba then chose to read William's "fate," by opening a page of the work of the Persian poet Hafiz.

"Muslims seem to do this, and Baba often does it half in fun. I don't remember the couplet except that it fit my mood, and was about the numbers of my enemies, with only You for a friend. And how I am restless day and night to be united to You. In Hafiz 'You' means God."

Throughout Baba's life he often told his followers that yearning to be with him both physically and in Divine Love was as important as or even more important than being with him.

"Well that was one of my reasons for [the] bad mood. Difficulties in work, enemies in self, and annoyance with Baba. All this fooling around – why can't we be one with what he really is. I've known Baba now for 13 years. Anyhow he bucked me up eventually."[55]

Baba left on a 10-day mast tour at this time, and William did not go. At the time Baba again reiterated his feelings about William to the other mandali, as noted in *Lord Meher,* Volume 8:

"Donkin's deep love for me, unshakable faith in me, and unparalleled service for me are beyond praise. Don comes from a wealthy family. His faith and love for me are unique. He serves in the army for me alone, saves money for me, and always gives me help."

Baba also indicated to William that he was fitting in nicely with his Eastern followers, during a discussion about Baba's health, which had taken a turn for the worse because of the rigours of the mast tours:

"He [Baba] told me the other day when we were discussing the steps to be taken about getting him fitter that I was like all his intimate Eastern disciples and not like his intimate Western disciples. [That is] I believed him to be all powerful, and that he can make himself fit as and when he pleases. And this is more or less true, because as a patient he is impossible."

From the outset Baba had told his followers that the Eastern countries, particularly India, were more spiritual than Western nations. He said masts could be found only in the East, although he did have "agents" in the West. One agent meeting in the United States occurred in Albuquerque, New Mexico, in December 1934, and is described in William's book *The Wayfarers*:

"In 1934, when Baba and a few of his disciples were on their way to California, the train stopped at Albuquerque for a short time. Baba spelt out the word 'Indian' on the palm of his hand. And went with Ruano away from the station into a small street nearby. At a street corner they noticed two American Indians; one was selling bows and arrows, and he walked away as soon as Baba approached. The other, a tall, impressive figure with a red band tied around his head, stayed where he was, and for a few moments Baba and he stood facing one another, each looking intently into the other's eyes. Baba then abruptly walked back to the station."

In addition to discussing spiritual matters, the gatherings at the Jubilee Hills bungalow in Hyderabad included ongoing talk about the global conflict that was coming to a close. Baba also spoke of India's push to independence, and predicted that a Hindu-Muslim civil war was approaching.

There seemed little let-up in the onslaught of spiritual discipline; even small, innocent events could lead to a rap on the knuckles. On one occasion, William had escorted Rano Gayley to an optometrist, and on their way home he bought some toffees for the mandali. While Rano refused to take any toffees, she eventually gave in, knowing Margaret Craske was fond of them.

When Baba later learned that Rano had given sweets to Margaret, he asked, "Why not me first?" Baba chastised William for giving sweets to the mandali, telling him, "I want them as thin as air."[56]

William's own version of the event perhaps reflects that he was indeed becoming attuned to Baba's ways of working:

"I got a moderate ticking off for giving some toffees to Rano ... and she was made to return them to me – but Baba teased me quite nicely really."[57]

A story related in Bhau Kalchuri's multi-volume *Lord Meher* series shows that humour was still an essential part of ashram life:

"During this period, Donkin was serving in the military hospital at Secunderabad, and would cycle ... over to the mandali's or Baba's bungalow to be with them during their stay at Hyderabad.

"Baba had given ... two black bull terrier puppies to Donkin to look after, named Raja [king] and Rani [queen], and had told Donkin to bring them with him whenever he came.

"Margaret Craske came down with a case of dysentery, and Dr. Donkin began coming more often to check on her. He would carry the puppies in a basket on his bike, but on the ride, they always seemed to find some way to jump out. Donkin had to stop, get off his bike and catch them, and his exertions proved amusing entertainment for passers-by."[58]

Meher Baba and various followers stayed in Hyderabad from March 10 to September 6, 1945. He contacted masts all over Hyderabad state. Figures show that he contacted more masts in Hyderabad city than in any other city in India.

The war was finally ending, which gave William the opportunity to accompany Baba and his band on a mast tour late in July. The party of five took a train from Hyderabad to Madras on the coast. William saw the city as "a horrible place, with a horrible climate, and a very dull, poor and dispirited population."

Despite the depressing description, mast-hunting in the area was successful.

"During the two days in Madras, Baba contacted nineteen masts, of which five were really good. One was ... naked;

the second best one, called Punjabi, used to walk about with button-less trousers, holding them up with his hands."[59]

However, the travels took a toll on Baba, who, walking with his followers from noon until 10 p.m. each day, developed sores on his feet from wearing his chappals (sandals).

The group then travelled north back up to Raichur.* The party's condition attracted the attention of a policeman who entered the names of everyone on the "suspicious strangers roll," recalls William in his diary.

William was quickly immersed in a street event at Raichur, where Baba washed and gave money to a group of 40 poor people. According to William's diary, "Baba washed their feet, and I dried them. Baidul and Eruch lifting water about. Afterwards Baba gave 3 rupees to each one, mostly miserable beggars, and many blind."

Baba, it seems, saw the divine appeal in the masts he came across no matter the circumstances in which they were found.

"Baba contacted one really good mast ... a great drunkard. We found him in a toddy shop, well pickled when we got there; a long beard and a charming face; always smiling. Baba was frightfully pleased at contacting him."

The travellers later headed back to Hyderabad on the train. At this time Baba gave a talk about meat-eating and sanskaras (impressions). After, William's diary indicated the spiritual objection to meat-eating, according to Baba:

"He said that the sanskaras of an animal hang onto the body for three days after its death, and that on the fourth day the animal takes on a new body.

"A human being takes on a new body on the fourth day, or any time later, say even up to 400 years. When one eats fresh meat one consumes animal sanskaras, which are a hindrance."

Never one to leave a subject unexplored, William asked Baba whether frozen meat that had been dead for months posed the same sanskara problem. Baba said that this was like eating dead germs to feed live germs – "germs" meaning sanskaras.

---

* Raichur in the middle of Karnataka state and on the banks of the Tungabhadra River, is known for its imposing fort, which has inscriptions in Arabic and Persian on its bastions and gateways.

7

Global Reach, *The Wayfarers*, and Sufism Reoriented

Baba was still commenting about participating countries in the war at this time, and said Russia is the world's one brigand left.

"But she will eventually make a mess of things trying to swallow too much, and there will be a popular reaction against her, but not a war."

World War II officially ended on September 2, 1945, and Baba and his followers made plans to leave Hyderabad on September 6 to move westward to Panchgani and Wai.*

Although William makes no formal mention of mustering out of the Indian Medical Service, he did so after the war ended.

In October 1945, Adi Sr., Meher Baba's secretary, published a small book of his Master's discourses titled *Messages*. William wrote the foreword for the book, providing his own insight into the war's aftermath:

"We, the human race, stand before two problems: one, the world as it is today, and the other, the world as it should be in the years that lie ahead. What it should be, and how to make it so is the preoccupation, not only of the world's leaders, but of every man and woman alive.

"Behind the veil of a demi-peace and an unfinished war is a background of terrible suffering which must be relieved.

* Wai is a beautiful town located on the banks of the Krishna River in Satara District, Maharashtra. Wai is famous for its temples as well as seven Ghats (broad flight of steps leading to the river).

There have been hitherto, so many answers that even the leaders at the world's conference tables have found it difficult to draft decisions, because they find themselves confronted by the protagonists of opposing ideas.

"Between the covers of this book is an answer. The reader may consider that he has heard such an answer before. But there are, I think, differences. First and foremost, the advice is grounded on direct Spiritual Knowledge. Secondly, there is, in some of these pages a warning that to camouflage weakness and material advantage with our ethical veneer is dangerous and solves nothing. Thirdly, there is an assertion that if our life is centred in a search for God, everything will go well; that there is no need to evade the applications of science or the differences inherent in life, because the search for God unites everyone and everything and is the root of the meaning of life...."[60]

In October and November 1945, Baba and his followers stayed in motion searching for masts. Although Wai, near Panchgani, was their home base, they travelled constantly. They went as far east as Calcutta and north to Muttra*, visiting close to 20 communities.

Baba, for his own reasons, always travelled incognito and, as stated earlier, asked to be described by other members of the party as their "older or elder brother."

Even though the war had ended, the pressure on 34-year-old William continued. His release from the Indian Medical Service and the horrors he had witnessed in wartime hospitals did not mean Baba thought he now deserved a holiday.

Living with Meher Baba was an ongoing whirl at the best of times. In addition to being immediately thrown into a number of mast tours, William was expected to respond to the health needs of other mandali, other followers of Baba, and their extended families.

Because his detailed diary ended in mid-1945, it's a fair guess that he was beginning to keep some kind of written record

---

* Muttra is on the right bank of the Jumna (Yamuna) River, 30 miles north of Agra. It is an important railway junction and an agricultural trade centre. Historically it is important to Buddhists and Jains and is considered to be Krishna's birthplace.

of the various masts Baba was contacting at the time. Baba also complicated matters by spending much of the last half of 1945 in seclusion doing what he termed his "universal work." For the most part he was available only to those staying with him.

Added to the travels in India were two significant new developments – one in India and the other in the United States in South Carolina. In 1944, development of the 500-acre Meher Spiritual Center in Myrtle Beach, South Carolina, and Meher Baba's new personal residence at Meherazad, a short distance from Ahmednagar, were proceeding simultaneously. William would be an active participant in both projects – living for a time at Meherazad and within a year travelling to the United States to visit South Carolina and report back to Baba on the status of the new spiritual centre.

Baba had for some time been looking for a spot "near Ahmednagar for a quiet stay and work." When he was informed that a piece of property near Pimpalgaon was to be auctioned off, he visited the site and liked it.

Through the generosity of his followers, the land was acquired in February 1944, just four months prior to the inauguration of the Meher Spiritual Center in Myrtle Beach, South Carolina.

Bal Natu, in his *Glimpses* series on the life of Meher Baba, describes Baba's shift from Meherabad to Meherazad:

"That Baba was preferring to no longer stay permanently at Meherabad is reflected in the report that he accepted the offer [earlier in the year] of accommodation in Ahmednagar from January 31 to March 9, 1945, from one of his followers [Rusi Irani]. This follower's daughter – Dr. Goher Irani – would later join Baba's ashram in 1947 and become a mandali member and Baba's personal physician.

While life was vigorously progressing for Baba and his followers, life was changing and ending for a number of Western devotees. Irene Billo returned to her home in Switzerland in March 1946 after a seven-year stay with Baba in India. William played an important part in getting Irene safely back to Switzerland, but Irene and William's behaviour in the process did not win favour with Baba.

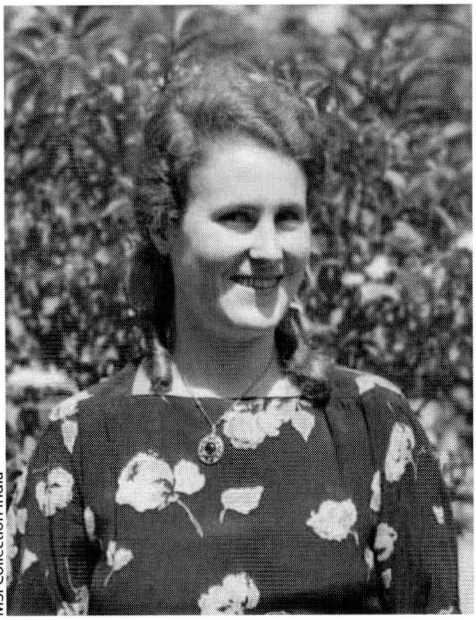

Irene Billo, who grew up in Switzerland, joined the ashram in 1938 at 21. Irene had learned about Baba from her parents, who were followers.

"Around March 26, Irene was sent to Bombay with Don [William] for the day to arrange boat passage home. Usually, during the tours, when travelling in India by train, Irene was ill and travelled first class with someone, while others in the ashram went second or third class.

"Don [William] was a major in the army, so he always sat in a first-class military compartment. For this trip, he listed himself as 'Major Donkin and his wife,' so that Irene could travel with him. But Don wanted Irene not to mention this in the ashram when they returned. After the boat tickets were purchased they also went to see a movie."[61]

When the pair returned to Meherabad, Baba inquired about their activities in Bombay. After he pushed for details, Irene finally admitted that they had gone to see a movie.

Baba immediately scolded her: "As soon as you're on the loose, you take advantage! You shouldn't have gone to the cinema without my permission, when you know that others here don't get to go. You shouldn't have taken liberties, others don't have."

Later, Irene noted, "After being so strict in the ashram, one felt happy to be a bit free, to walk around, to do as one liked. It was natural. But afterwards, we felt so bad."[62]

Baba was undoubtedly trying to keep the lid on any personal interaction, particularly flirtatious behaviour, between female and male members of the ashram. People are only human and Baba knew that there would less likely be such behaviour if he had sanctioned certain small freedoms and knew exactly what was happening. Those involved would feel Baba's nazar (gaze) on them and would be more inclined to behave properly. That a similar ebb and flow of human emotions still occurs today worldwide between Baba followers trying to comply with his wishes is not surprising.

On April 16, 1946, less than a month after the incident with Irene, William found himself travelling with three women mandali, and again used his military influence for the occasion.

"Kitty, Rano, and Margaret did not even know where they were going, when they were sent ahead with Don [William]. In Delhi, they were to wait for Baba and proceed with him to a 'place of seclusion.'

"On the train, Don passed the women off as his relatives so that they could occupy a military compartment with him, as Irene had. The three women were wearing their solar topees [pith helmets], but before entering an army rest house along the way, Don said to them, 'For God's sake, take off those topees, before we go inside. You look like a bunch of missionaries.'"[63]

Again, one can speculate on William's inner train of thought and consider whether looking "like a bunch of missionaries" might have been better for decorum' in an army rest house.

In May 1946, another Western woman – Margaret Craske – who had spent eight years in India with Baba, left to return to England. Another close mandali member, Nadine Tolstoy, passed away at age 62 on April 14, 1946. Nadine, who had married Count Ilya, son of Leo Tolstoy, the great Russian novelist, had met Meher Baba in 1931.

"Countess Tolstoy met Baba during his first visit to America in 1931. A Russian, she attended the University of Petrograd, studying psychology, logic, and philosophy. Afterwards she

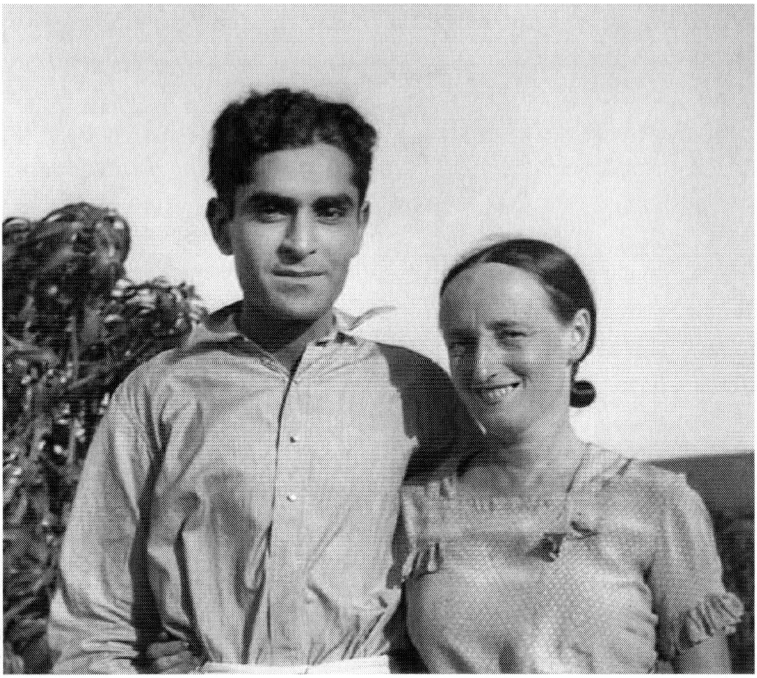
MSI Collection India

Ballerina Margaret Craske, shown here with Baba's youngest brother Adi Jr., became a well-known ballet instructor in London and New York. She lived at the ashram in India in the 1930s and -40s.

continued her studies at Lausanne University in Switzerland and also studied piano, later entering the Moscow Conservatory."[64]

"Nadine met Count Ilya, Leo's oldest son, and they both left Russia in 1917 to live permanently in the United States, where they were married.

"Count Ilya also met Baba in New York and remarked, 'It is the first time in my life that I met a man who has Divine Love.'"[65]

Nadine had spent a number of years in India with Baba. Adele Wolkin*, a long-time Baba lover – who has played a significant role in the New York, Los Angeles, and Myrtle Beach

* Adele Wolkin (with her friend Filis Frederick) first heard of Baba from Norina Matchabelli and Elizabeth Patterson in New York. After a glimpse of Baba stolen as Baba boarded the train for South Carolina, she finally met him on May 10, 1952. She has spent the rest of her life in service to Meher Baba.

Baba communities – looked after Nadine in New York in the final months before her death from Lou Gehrig's disease in 1946.

"Nadine was very maternal and I felt very close to her. When I first met her she asked me to sit on her knee," says Adele of their first meeting at the East 67th Street home of Elizabeth Patterson. Later Baba asked Adele to care for Nadine in her final months.

"I could spend a whole evening talking with Nadine," recalls Adele. "This is the first time I ever witnessed death or anyone dying. She died with ease, so beautifully, although she suffered from a debilitating disease. People could not console her because she was so cheerful, so bright, so able to talk about spiritual subjects. They would be just captured by the atmosphere around her, which was anything but morbid."[66]

Mast travels took on a new intensity in April 1946, and Baba continued to insist that his lovers in India and around the world should not try to contact him directly.

Again, William was put to good use on the India travels. Meher Baba's sister Mani recalls one side trip that four mandali women were on with Baba to Kullu Valley* at the foot of the Himalayas.

"It was a privately hired bus. Don was with us, arranging everything for the trip....[67]

The usual routine of putting up a sheet between the women and men mandali in the bus was observed so the women could not see the men, but they could hear them.

"Don was lying down in front, since it was a long journey. When we came to a [British] post, where we had to show the permit or license to go on, Kaka shouted, 'Donkin!'

"Don sat up, so the Indian official could see the British face and wave us on. Then Don would lie down again."[68]

On this particular trip the group stayed in Kullu Valley for some time. Although horses had to bring in provisions, William, through his own ingenuity, was able to offer an array of expensive jams, honey, and cheese to the party.

---

* Kullu Valley, by the banks of the river Beas, was once known as "the end of the habitable world," beyond which rose the forbidding heights of the Himalayas. It first became accessible by car after independence in 1947.

Rano got hepatitis during the trip, and was isolated in a room over the stables. William, who diagnosed and treated her, advised Rano to eat some of the appetizing things that were available, but Baba did not agree with William's recommendation.

"He [Baba] fed her with his own hands, remarking, 'I brought you here to look after my requirements, but now I have to look after yours.'

"'It's my bad luck,' Rano replied.

"'Not bad luck,' Baba corrected. 'It's your good luck.'

"With Baba's treatment, Rano improved quickly."[69]

William was reminded on another occasion of the contradictory life with Baba. Horses were hired so that the women mandali could have a ride in the mountains.

"The first day, the horseman was told to bring the horses at 4:30 p.m., but he came an hour late. Baba was not pleased and told Don to scold him. Don began shouting at the gorewala [horseman], telling him to leave. The man removed his turban and laid it at Don's feet, begging forgiveness, but Don kept up his tirade, as he thought this is what Baba wanted. But Baba, who was watching, tapped Don on the shoulder, asked him why he was so upset, and forgave the man."[70]

It was at about this time that William's duties and orders took an even more bizarre twist, when the "Boja Fund" was created, taking William to England and the United States.

Dr. Ghani Munsiff, a friend of Baba's since childhood and long-time mandali, had been falsely accused of murder in 1940. Ghani faced debts from legal costs, and Baba decided William should visit London and the United States to collect enough money to pay off these debts. Any vestige of pride still lingering in William would have been tested by this begging-bowl errand.

Records indicate that William was away in London and the US for much of August and September 1946. In addition to collecting for the Boja (Burden) Fund, William was also directed to pass a message along to Margaret Craske in England that she should "accept any temporary work."

Margaret, who had left India earlier in 1946, later wrote two books, *Dancing With Love* and *Still Dancing With Love*, about her life with Meher Baba. She describes her take on

William's trip to the UK and US and their meeting in London in her second book:

"This was at the time when I was in London making every effort on Baba's orders to get to America myself. My difficulties, however, did not prevent Baba from sending me an order to get a round-trip ticket for Donkin to go to that country." Margaret confronted obstacles in obtaining a ticket facing "firm refusals, rudeness, and downright snubs" by every travel agent she approached.

"One afternoon, feeling most baffled by a rude refusal, I was turning to leave the counter when a clerk – not the one who had crushed me – wrote something on a piece of paper, put it under a blotter, pushed the whole thing toward me, signed to me to take the paper and clear out quickly. I took the paper and found on it the address of a small agency located in a nearby unimportant street.

"I at once went to the address and at once was given a ticket. No trouble at all."

Margaret goes on to describe her meeting with William later at the corner of Oxford Street and Tottenham Court Road:

"He was full of dry British humour and shook hands with me saying, 'Dr. Livingston, I presume.' After this piece of idiocy – enjoyed by both of us – he seemed delighted to receive his ticket, and to hear about the seeming miracle that had produced it."

Baba also had asked his dispatched English disciple to "inform and impress Elizabeth and Norina [in Myrtle Beach, South Carolina] that my coming [to the West] depends on my return from the Himalayas," which could postpone his coming by a month or two.

William brought back news on the progress of the spiritual centre in Myrtle Beach. Shortly after he returned to Meherabad, William was to embark on the major literary project *(The Wayfarers)* that would involve much of his time for two to three years.

William's diary entries, begun in 1939, ended in 1946. It's not surprising, however, as the mammoth task of collecting material and writing *The Wayfarers* soon consumed him. It's certain that William had not thought his simple observation and suggestion to Baba in the fall of 1946 about someone doing a written account of the God-intoxicated would result in a project falling completely into his lap.

The birth of the book began innocently enough on William's part. Bhau Kalchuri describes the naive start of the project in *Lord Meher,* Volume 9:

"Donkin had always been profoundly impressed by Baba's work with the masts – the way Baba selflessly kept himself occupied day and night travelling under most difficult conditions, at times without food and water, hunting for the great souls. After his return from England (and the US) in the fall of 1946, Donkin began thinking, 'In the history of past advents of the Avatars, never has such work been recorded. It is something quite new for both the people of the East and the West. What Baba is doing in this age is unprecedented and unparalleled. If any of the past Avatars have done such work, history has not recorded it.'

"One day ... while in Dehra Dun, he voiced these thoughts to Baba:

"'Your work with the masts is so important, fascinating, and significant, yet there is no record of it. If an account were compiled and written down, it would be most useful and interesting to future generations.'"

"Baba told William that he would think about it. Two days later he came to the hut where Donkin, Nilu, and Vishnu were resting. Baba remarked to Donkin, 'Your suggestion about a book on masts is excellent. Why don't you write it?'

"Donkin had not expected this.

"'Me? I'm no writer. I've never written a book. I'm not fit to write it.'

"But Baba assured him, 'You are the proper person to write it. I will help you.'

Bhau Kalchuri says in *Lord Meher* that William was encouraged and the seed for *The Wayfarers* took hold.

"Baba began giving William explanations, detailing the various types of masts, and explaining about them in general. Dr. Donkin wrote studiously and with devoted labour and attention to detail, collaborating with those who went on the mast tours with Baba.

"On one occasion Donkin [said] about the book, 'So I did it. My aim being only to make a faithful record of Baba's work with masts and others – his external and visible work, that is. His real inner work he would not tell us about – but then why should he?'"[71]

When *The Wayfarers* was finally published in 1948, Baba was critical of the book, saying William's account of the masts was "too dry."

While Baba did review the entire manuscript before the book was published, William, because of Baba's hectic schedule, often had difficulty getting Baba to spend time with him on individual aspects of the research.

William, as a bright and inquisitive man, undoubtedly would have pressed Baba about his specific reasons for contacting hundreds of these people. In the end, however, he had to accept his Spiritual Master's lack of detailed explanation.

A reader of *The Wayfarers* quite naturally recognizes that while the "who, what, when, and where" are covered in precise detail, the "why" remains an unanswered mystery. If this shortcoming results in readers asking "What's the point?" it's a responsibility that Meher Baba himself may have to share with William for not at least trying to explain the "why," even though William's own words exonerated him for not doing so.

There are, however, a few tiny trickle-down moments and snippets in the pages of *The Wayfarers* from Baba on the nature of his inner work with the masts. One brief explanation of Baba's is found early in the book. William's long, breathless, sentence style reads, "When a mast gets walled-in by his own self-sufficiency and desirelessness, only the Master can draw him out of the isolation of his choice; by awakening within him an expansive love that breaks through all limitations, and prepares him for shouldering the important responsibilities of rendering true service to others who are in need of spiritual help.

"Because of his being stationed on the inner planes, which are free from the limitations and handicaps of the gross world, a mast can be, and often is in contact with a far greater number of souls than is possible for an ordinary person.... A mast can therefore be a more effective agent for spiritual work than the most able persons of the gross world....

"In a thousand ways, the Master makes an irresistible appeal to the innermost being of masts, and awakens in them the undying spring of creative action."[72]

This explanation in the foreword of *The Wayfarers* may indeed be a paramount clue in interpreting Meher Baba's work with the masts. That they could serve as a contact to multiple human souls throughout the world after their contact with Baba may justify the years of hard work that went into mast-hunting and working with them.

The remainder of the late forties was spent on more mast tours, but these were always interspersed with other adventures, some as respites from the vigorous mast-chasing ordeals. On one occasion when Baba wanted a change, William suggested the group travel to Vengurla* "for its beauty and privacy."

A quiet beach resort on the west coast of India, Vengurla is reached by travelling down hairpin curves through forest until one reaches the sea. The group going there included Baba, William, Mehera, Mani, Meheru, and Kitty. The women enjoyed the place, and they stayed there for four days at a dak bungalow, a government rest house.

"Vengurla was a nice, seaside town," Mehera said. "It was an old type of village, not very modern. A small out-of-the-way place not frequented by tourists, so Baba could relax and not be recognized."[73]

On one walk along the beach, William sculpted Baba's face in the sand and Baba called the women over to see it. During another outing they collected seashells and walked through a thick cashew forest, past a cashew nut factory.

"It was lovely there," said Mehera. "Moonlight on the ocean, watching the fishermen in their little boats going out to fish, the early morning sunrises. Very, very quiet. No people around."[74]

---

* Vengurla is a town just north of Goa in Maharashtra, India. It is surrounded on the north, east, and south by a range of hills with lush green foliage of mainly cashew, mango, coconut, and different kinds of berry trees. The Arabian Sea is located west of the town.

Elizabeth Patterson and Norina Matchabelli arrived in India from the US in July 1947 for a stay at Satara.* The two women had worked hard launching the Meher Spiritual Center in South Carolina. Norina had been ill with a heart condition and would spend the next two years in India with Baba. She was immediately ordered to spend her first six months in India observing strict silence. This was undoubtedly a tough order for Norina, who had frequently spoken publicly about Baba during her years in America.

Shortly before the two women arrived, William, after eight months of research and information-gathering, began the actual writing of *The Wayfarers* while in Satara.

The stay at Satara, recorded as an actual mast ashram, was brief, lasting only through June and July. A number of other locations were used for short-term mast quarters throughout 1947, but Meherabad remained the main base of operations.

William's work on the mast book continued as 1947 drew to a close. Baba's sister Mani helped William by typing his handwritten account into clean copy. Baba had indicated that he wanted the book completed by the end of July. William worked on *The Wayfarers* six hours a day and contacted Baba's secretary Adi Sr. frequently, seeking help in finding photographs for the book.

In one letter to Adi Sr., William specifically asked him to locate photos of a bullock cart and tonga. William said photographs were necessary because Westerners would not be able to understand what these Indian means of transportation were without photos. He also asked Adi Sr. for a photograph of a crowded Indian train and a picture of Mohammed the mast for the book.[75]

William pursued other initiatives in 1947, including designing and clearing a path up Seclusion Hill, which overlooks Meherazad (Baba's new residential compound outside of Ahmednagar). William personally worked on the project for six months as a surprise for his spiritual master. The hill was to be an important site for Baba's future seclusion work.

---

* Satara is a town in Maharashtra on the Deccan Plain that is surrounded by seven ("sat") hills ("tara"). It is the site of Baba's December 2, 1956, car accident.

The sense of dedication within William was reflected in another incident at the time. A close Baba follower, Savak Kotwal, was living with his wife, two daughters, and son in Meherabad. The son, eight-year-old Adi, became ill with typhoid and pneumonia, and it was thought that he would not survive. The oldest daughter Najoo recalls William's role in her book, *He Gives the Ocean,* which is an account of the family's life with Baba:

"Since there were no medicines at that time for typhoid fever, Dr. Donkin and Dr. Nilu concentrated on treating Adi's pneumonia with penicillin injections and his typhoid with diet therapy. A penicillin factory had started in Poona, but only a doctor could get the medication, and it had to be kept refrigerated. Since we did not have a real refrigerator, Dr. Donkin made several trips on his motorbike to Poona, where he would buy two ampules at a time and immediately bring them back to the cottage. These trips took many hours. He would give Adi one injection when he returned, and the second he kept in Mummy's improvised refrigerator made from earthen pots until it was needed."

Adi recovered from his illness.

An event early in 1948 brought more worldwide exposure to Meher Baba, when an American woman, Ivy Duce, and her teenage daughter Charmian came to stay with Baba at his new residential quarters in Meherazad. Ivy was not just another fan of Baba's. She would be a pivotal person in his widening global circle.

A few years earlier, Ivy had met Murshida Rabia (Ada) Martin, head of the Sufi Order in the United States. Martin had told her about Meher Baba, expressing the belief that he was a genuine Spiritual Master.

Murshida Martin had headed the Sufi Order in America since the 1927 death of Hazrat Inayat Khan of Baroda. Inayat Khan had brought the Sufi message to the West in 1910.

Although Murshida Martin became convinced of Meher Baba's divinity after meeting Norina Matchabelli and corresponding with Baba's disciple Dr. Abdul Ghani Munsiff, she passed away in 1947 and did not have the chance to meet Baba. Before her death, Martin appointed Ivy Duce as her successor.

At Christmas 1946, Ivy and her daughter met Norina Matchabelli in New York. During the meeting Ivy had a strong emotional experience, and like her predecessor, she soon embraced Baba as a genuine Spiritual Master.

Later in July 1947, when one of Baba's close Eastern disciples, Meherjee Karkaria,* came to New York, Ivy and a group of other Sufis invited him to lunch.

"While we were lunching, I kept wondering how this man could look so young, as I knew he was at least 40.

"Finally I asked him. 'Don't you ever worry?'

"He looked astonished and replied, 'Why no! The Master forbids it!'

"It was the turn of the luncheon group to look astonished. In fact, it sounded so absurd that we could hardly refrain from laughter."[76]

On another occasion Meherjee joined the Duces for lunch. On this occasion when Meherjee saw a photo of Baba that Ivy kept beside a vase of flowers he almost burst into tears himself.

When they later parted, Meherjee said to Ivy, "I'll see you soon in India, Mrs. Duce."

In October of the same year, Ivy's husband Terry, an oil company executive, suggested Ivy and their daughter accompany him on a trip to Saudi Arabia. A side trip to India for mother and daughter developed after permission to visit Meher Baba came from Meherazad. The two arrived at Baba's residential compound on January 7, 1948.

Both women dissolved in tears when Baba said to them, "Oh, you two have been with me since ages."

The only Western disciples living in India at the time were Elizabeth Patterson, Norina Matchabelli, Kitty Davy, Rano Gayley, and William.

From Ivy's account in her 1975 book *How a Master Works,* she had a number of conversations with William during her stay at Meherazad. Her description of him probably aptly sizes up William and his frame of mind after nearly nine years in India:

---

* Meherjee Karkaria first met Baba in 1927 when he accompanied Chanji one weekend to visit Meherabad. He was a teacher in the Meher Ashram School and later was a successful businessman with a factory in Poona.

Sufism Reoriented

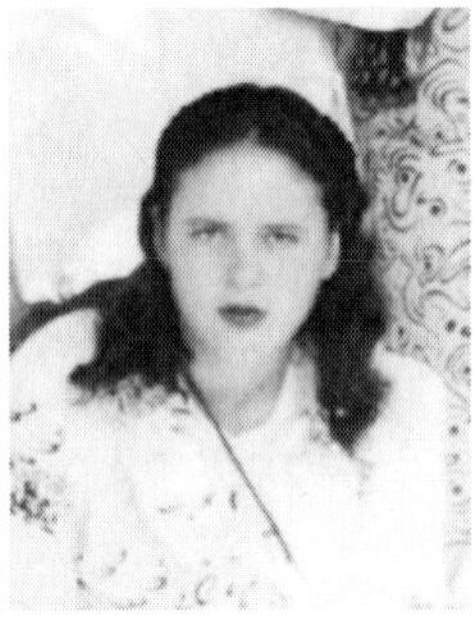

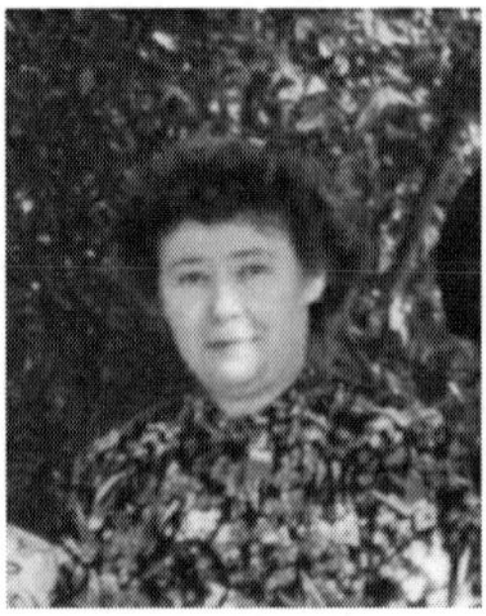

Ivy Duce, right, and her daughter Charmian visited Meher Baba at Meherazad in January 1948. The two women became lifelong followers. Ivy served as Murshida of the California-based Sufism Reoriented for nearly 30 years.

"Dr. William Donkin was typically British – a fine-looking chap with deep blue eyes, tall and slender. He had met Baba in England while studying medicine, and when asked his reaction to Baba he exclaimed, 'Well, you know, he just bowls you over!'

"Of all Baba's close disciples, I would imagine the hard life privations might have been peculiarly difficult for him. Not that he has any lack of physical stamina, for he had been a great mountain climber and had served five years as a doctor in the British [Indian Medical Service] army. But there was no other man from the Western world to offer camaraderie, and Baba used him to accomplish what seemed the impossible in many a mission. He always fitted in well with the others, however, having a dry sense of humour and a native modesty."[77]

While Ivy and Charmian's five-day stay at Meherazad did not seem to be marked with any high emotional drama, there were some timely reminders to the two Western women about rules of behaviour. Ivy describes one occasion when a group of five, including herself and William, were talking about the "war and the Russians," when another of the mandali dropped in on them and said, "Baba says you must have forgotten the instructions he gave you last night."

Baba on many occasions would instruct his followers not to discuss politics.

Ivy, who was a bit of a fashion diva, described two instances where she appeared to be competing with Baba and his own sense of style. Ivy loved hats and wore "a lacy hat with a single pink rose on my head and carried a cocktail hat of pure magenta feathers." Shortly after the "photo op" capturing this moment, Baba appeared in a doorway in a magenta jacket, and literally started preening himself in front of Ivy, William, and Dr. Ghani.

"We admired it," said Ivy. "It was the exact colour of my hat – and then he disappeared. Dr. Donkin stared at Dr. Ghani and asked, 'Where did he get that one?'

"Ghani replied, 'Damned if I know, I never saw it on him before.'"[78]

Baba later slipped the group a typed note, given to them for their own interpretation, of the fashion competition. Ivy relays the message in her book:

"Perfection has both the human and divine qualities in full, and expresses itself in high and low alike. A perfect man has infinite love, inviolable spirituality and [the] greatest sense of humour. He comes down to the level of the devotee and yet is all the time the master."

Baba had a good reason for asking Dr. Ghani to join the group at Meherazad when the Duces were there. Ghani was the leader of the Sufis in Poona, and after Ivy returned to the US, he served as her link to Baba through written correspondence.

Ivy describes Ghani's story about his meeting with Baba many years before:

"I asked him about his relationship to Baba, and he told me that he went to Deccan College with Baba and eventually became a doctor.

"He opened a dispensary, and one day, after hearing a knock, he went to the door and was horrified to see his old friend, Merwan, standing there in a white robe.

"'For heaven's sake,' Ghani exclaimed. 'You were the brightest one in our school. What in the world are you doing running around in a white robe. Is this the only way you can make a living?'"[79]

"On that same day after meeting with Baba, Ghani decided to close his clinic and begin his new life with his old friend. He did admit to Ivy that it would be some time before he embraced Baba fully.

"'How long did it take you, Dr. Ghani,' I asked, 'to accept Baba's ideas?'

"He looked at me rather shamefully and said, 'I'm ashamed to tell you Mrs. Duce, but it took about seven years. I was so hard-headed.'"

Dr. Ghani, who had known Hazrat Inayat Khan personally, asked Ivy to mail all of Murshid Khan's books from the United States to him in India. Ivy recalls his response in her book:

"I later learned that when he went over them he remarked in exasperation to Dr. Donkin, 'For heaven's sake, is this all the knowledge that Inayat Khan gave to the West? He knew far more'; to which Donkin retorted, 'Well, probably that was all they could take!'"[80]

William's sense of humour served him well in his life with Meher Baba, for many years later he would reveal his own take on "how a master works" to Ivy, which she relates:

"On a later visit to the United States, he told me that Baba's two chief methods – one could almost call them weapons – for whittling down the false ego of aspirants were humiliation and exhaustion.

"Now a quarter century later, I can appreciate this, for when you have been pulverized you no longer care anymore what happens to you and you are then fit for the state known as 'becoming dust at the feet of the Master.'"

Ivy and daughter Charmian left India on January 16 and later flew from Arabia home to New York.

8

Discipline Intensifies, Mast Travels, Seclusions

Baba's work with the masts continued as January 1948 unfolded. On one occasion Baba was using William's room at Meherazad for seclusion with one of the masts. This may have interrupted William's work on *The Wayfarers,* although he probably found an alternate writing perch nearby.

On January 30, 1948, Baba and the ashram received the shocking news of the assassination of Mahatma Gandhi. Baba and Gandhi had met on the steamer *Rajputana* in 1931, when Gandhi was on his way to the Indian Round Table Conference in London and Baba was making his first trip to the West. Baba had always praised Gandhi's sincerity and honesty in life.

Later, in February, the mandali and Baba got together to look over published articles on Gandhi's life. Baba seized the occasion to question the mandali on their feelings:

"'People regard Gandhi as a mahatma. What do you take me to be? And do you wish to hold on to me till the very end?

"He also added, 'If any of you really feels confused or disappointed [over my status], he should be rendering me a great service by leaving me. I want you to be honest to yourself and to me. I am what I am, what I really was, and will ever be. So once and for all, think well before you decide.'

"He instructed each of the mandali to give Him a written and signed reply."[81]

Replies received from four of the Western women mandali indicate their loyalty:

"Norina: 'In You ... I believe. For You, I am ready to live and die.'

"Elizabeth: 'One thing I know; if you had not come into my life there would have been no other Master for me. Having come, there is no other way for me.'

"Kitty: 'Your love brought me to you, your love has kept me with you, and your love will bind me to you till the end.'

"Rano: 'The one certainty in my life is you, beloved Meher Baba. I am yours and always will be yours.'"[82]

The *Glimpses* account also gives positive comments from a dozen other Eastern male mandali members. A reply from William Donkin was not published in the account.

Throughout February 1948 Baba made numerous overland journeys, washing the feet of the poor, making cash donations to villages, and passing out grain bundles.

Contacting masts continued to take a lot of Baba's time, and when William was not writing *The Wayfarers,* he would accompany him on these trips. William picked up more information for his book on such journeys, as evidenced by one of his entries in the published work:

"A person of inquiring mind may wonder whether masts may be found in other parts of the world, and if they are not, then why it is that India alone is gifted with such souls.

"Baba, in explaining this paradox to his disciples, told them once that India was nearest to the 'creation point,' and was therefore, the most significant country in the world in the realm of spirituality.

"It was for this reason, he explained, that there were very few masts outside of India, and none in Europe or the Americas; although there were mystics, saints, and God-lovers there.

"It is therefore not surprising that in the Western world, there are, as far as I am aware, no traditions about these God-intoxicated souls, and that when a Westerner is confronted for the first time by eccentric characteristics of a mast, his reaction is, quite possibly, one of incredulity and abhorrence."[83]

Earlier in 1948, Baba asked followers to adhere to five orders from February 1–25:

To take one meal a day and tea or coffee only twice.
To observe silence.
To feed every day, one poor person with one's own hands, a different person each day.
To abstain absolutely from any sexual relations whatsoever.
To meditate one hour each day.

Followers, even those in the West, were asked to return the signed list of orders and indicate which ones they were to fulfil. In many instances a back-and-forth correspondence ensued on particular interpretations of the orders. Baba was pleased if participants were sincerely trying to observe the orders he gave.

Mast tours to the Bombay and Calcutta regions continued throughout March. Baba had a great love for animals, and one of the masts he found, called Maharaj, shared this devotion to animals. According to William, one bullock was very attracted to the mast:

"There was one spirited brown and white bullock that would lick him all over with his tongue. The mast would screw up his eyes when his face was being licked, or would lie supine between the forelegs of the bullock, while the front of his body was licked from head to foot."

By the time March 1948 came, William's 400-page manuscript about the masts was already in the hands of the printers. But the work did not go smoothly. In the book *Mehera-Meher: A Divine Romance,* the difficulty is described:

"While Baba was away, the women occupied themselves with helping Donkin on his book, *The Wayfarers.* Mani met with Don privately in a separate room, where she pronounced the Urdu names in his account, so he could spell them correctly. Don had also drawn a colour map of India to accompany the book, but it came back from the printers full of misprints. Mani, Mehera, and Meheru took on the job of correcting them."

Mehera recalled the painstaking task that was taking place at Meherazad while Baba was searching for masts in Calcutta and Rishikesh:

"Don was very particular. We were told to do the corrections so perfectly, that no one could tell that they had been corrected. We were given razor blades, erasers, and black ink. In one place we had to put a *B* instead of a *P;* in another an *o* instead of an *e.* We did it every morning, sitting near the door, where there was more light; a certain number every day. It was painstaking work, but I liked doing it."

Because Baba's work with the masts continued, William felt obligated to continue tracking the activity. He did so until August 1, 1949, and this material, while first published as a separate pamphlet, eventually found itself into *The Wayfarers* as two supplements totalling 70 pages. The added sections covered two separate mast-hunting periods – mid-March 1948 to mid-May 1948 and June 8, 1948, to August 1, 1949.

Again, the mast travels could not be billed as a picnic. The first half of April 1948 was spent in the Himalayas of northern India, specifically in the village of Uttar Kashi*. William describes the area as a series of rivers and estuaries where the sacred Ganges is born.

"About halfway between the source of the Bhagirathi [as the Ganges is called here] and the confluence of Devaprayag is the village of Uttar Kashi, famous as a centre for spiritual aspirants, yogis, and advanced souls. Uttar Kashi is the focal point ... for it was to this little village that Baba went in April 1948. Uttar Kashi is not high by Himalayan standards, for it lies less than 4,000 feet above sea level; but to get there the traveller must ride or walk along the stony track from Tehri Garhwal**, a distance of some 40 miles."[84]

William, perhaps harkening back to his Sahara experience and his mountaineering exploits, appeared to relish such Baba-initiated adventures.

Again the trek he described was no casual stroll. Wheeled traffic of any kind was unable to move on the rough roads, and

---

* Uttar Kashi is a holy city with many ashrams and temples in a hilly area. The region has many small and large rivers and is known for its excellent trekking.

** Tehri Garhwal is an agrarian district where people farm on the hillsides. It runs from the Himalayas to the foothills at Rishikesh. Recently the river was dammed and a lake submerged the town, which was rebuilt 15 miles away.

even depending on mules and ponies was a nuisance in such rugged terrain.

"Most travellers ... find pack animals tiresome and unreliable, and the backbone of Himalayan transport [in India] is the back of the Nepalese or the Dhotiyal porter. These tough little men will carry up to 60 pounds over the roughest sort of country, and I have seen them walk barefoot on hard snow for several hours, without complaints."[85]

William again took time to reflect on Baba's work with masts in the first of the *Wayfarers* supplements:

"My impression is that his work is either so personal that its nature and meaning are none of our business, or that the ins

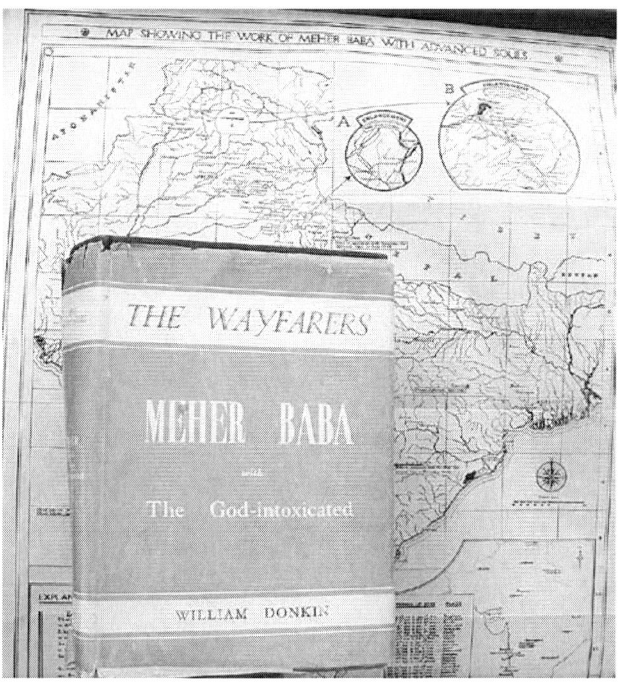

S of L

The Wayfarers was first published in 1948. The book was a major undertaking for William Donkin. At least two mandali members say William became mast-like himself after finishing the book, which details Baba's work with the God-intoxicated of India.

and outs of it are so intricate and obscure that even a detailed explanation would be quite beyond our grasp."

The trip to the Himalayas certainly was not preceded by a lengthy rest or build-up of strength for the followers. The party had just come off of mast journeys to Bombay and Calcutta. It was Baba's fourth visit to Calcutta, with other trips made in 1940, 1943, and 1945. From Calcutta, the group had taken a train to Hardwar, and then travelled by bus to Rishikesh. Here coolies were hired to transport the luggage to Uttar Kashi.

Baba and the group then took another bus from Rishikesh to Tehri Garhwal, where they rested a day before starting their 40-mile walk.

William's book provides embellished details of the journey:

"Think, then, of this little town of Tehri buried in a hot and steamy valley, with the murky torrent of the Bhagirathi [River] thundering along its centre, swollen by the melting snow from the great heights that are 70 or 80 miles away.

"See, in your mind's eye, the terraced fields cut into the mountain sides above you like giants' staircases, interrupted only by irregular patches of forests, by deep-cut gullies, or by outcrops of sheer rock."

The foot journey would last three full days and the toll was felt by all:

"The final day the scenery was impressive and the track full of peasants moving up to the high pastures for the summer with their goats, sheep, cows, dogs, and tents. The path however was rough, and Baba's feet and the feet of those with him were painfully blistered by the time they reached Uttar Kashi."

Although Baba seemed to prefer contact with masts on the higher planes of consciousness, he would not miss the opportunity to interact with a seeker on his journeys, particularly when the person appeared sincere. William relates one such incident in Hardwar, not far from Uttar Kashi.

Two of Baba's disciples approached an old man in rags sitting upon a wooden platform at the side of the street. The pair was to ask the old man about masts and advanced souls in the city of Hardwar. Soon after this contact, the old man began following them through the streets.

"Since the tenacity of his pursuit seems not to be relaxed, Baba ordered Eruch [his close disciple] to ask why he was following them."

The old man said he was seeking a guru, and quoted Kabir* that there could be no realization without the help of a guru.

"Finally he addressed Baba directly and said, 'I find you to be the right man to guide me.'

Baba in reply told the man to love God more and more so that his love became like that of a fish out of the ocean whose only desire is to return to the ocean.

Baba met the man again later on the street and ordered three oranges bought and given to the man with his blessings.

"Baba told him to seek God within himself with an ever-increasing love; and said that if he did so, he would soon see God," wrote William. Baba's identity was never divulged to the man.

During Baba's stay in Uttar Kashi, a total of 25 sadhus** were contacted.

At this point William was approaching his tenth year in India with Meher Baba. Although on many occasions he bemoaned the secrecy that surrounded Baba's contact with the God-advanced, William continued on occasion to offer his personal feelings on the worth of these peculiar personalities.

"Were you to ask a disciple of Baba's why such and such a man was a mast and not a madman, he would probably simply reply, 'because Baba says so.'

"In other words, the average man or the average disciple is not in a position to judge these people because his only measure is to assess them by their external actions."[86]

During William's two years writing *The Wayfarers*, his insights into the world of the masts opened up, especially with the additional clarifications he received from Baba.

---

* Kabir is considered one of the world's greatest poets. He was one of Baba's favourites and is widely quoted in India. Baba said Kabir was a Perfect Master.

** Sadhus are renunciates, who have left behind all material and sexual attachments and live in caves, forests, and temples all over India and Nepal.

"There is, however, one quality in masts – in those, at any rate, who have had much contact with Baba – and this is that, however strange they may behave, they make one feel unmistakably happy in their company.

"They do not exhale any of that subtle antipathy that seems to emanate from the insane, but actually kindle a sense of harmony in one's self, a harmony of which one may not be immediately aware, but which becomes eventually a real and obvious thing.

"Thus if you were to ask the men at Meherabad whether they liked or disliked Mohammed and Ali Shah, you would find, I believe, that everyone felt spontaneously attracted to them."[87]

William's final addition to *The Wayfarers,* which he completed in September 1949, includes Baba's work with the masts from mid-May 1948 to August 1, 1949. The book was published in September 1949 – just a month before Baba would initiate a major upset in the lives of his followers worldwide.

William's approach to this final addition to *The Wayfarers* appears to have been vetted by Baba, who had criticized the original volume as "too dry." One can also see William's stabs at providing colourful description in some of his accounts, perhaps his own effort at "wetting down" previous accounts that Baba had criticized. His description of Ahmedabad* in June 1948 might go a bit overboard in this desire to please:

"This city is a pasticcio of a place, a hotchpotch of ancient monuments, rococo villas, cotton mills, and thousands of hutches so squalid that they beggar description."

In the introduction to the final addition, William wrote, "As soon as work was started on this small volume, it became obvious that to present the full story in diary form, so that no details were left out, would be to make an admirable record of Baba's work – but a quite unreadable one."

---

* Ahmedabad, the largest city in the state of Gujarat, is bifurcated by the river Sabarmati. The eastern side is the older part of the city, with crowded bazaars, temples, jam-packed buildings, railway station, post office, and buildings from the British era. Gandhi had two ashrams in the Ahmedabad area.

It is also important to note that William depended on the accounts of disciples Eruch and Baidul* for this addition, indicating that he did not accompany Baba on these trips.

In 1949 Meher Baba's major work with the masts of India ended, although he would often house various masts at his headquarters at Meherabad, including Mohammed, who lived out his life there. In William's description of these final months, Baba apparently took a greater interest in his writing and would provide "occasional notes on the spiritual state or stage of masts."

The final year of mast-hunting did not turn up any outstanding masts other than when Baba and his party reconnected with a favourite mast from the earlier years.

Baba also widened his net in 1948–49 to include sadhus, and his visit to Ahmedabad was specifically to contact a large number of them. William's interpretation of the sadhu as seen through the local community's eyes provides insight into their standing throughout India:

"The Western reader should understand that sadhus as a class have a mixed reputation in India, in much the same way and for much the same reasons that the monks and friars of medieval Europe had a similar reputation."

William went on to point out the lofty misconceptions often evident in categorizing sadhus.

"Although, ostensibly every sadhu is presumed to have renounced the world, most Indian householders condemn nine out of ten of them as wasters. There are, indeed, exceptions – jewels of the finest water – but there seems little doubt that the average sadhu is a petty parasite on the body of a country already emaciated by poverty.

"In any case, whether sadhus as a class are worthy or not, there are times when Baba contacts sadhus ... without reference to their spiritual status or merits."

Again Baba's identity was always kept from the sadhus, and his disciples were not allowed to witness his work with them. Baba always gave each sadhu five rupees at the time of contact.

---

* Baidul was one of Baba's earliest mandali and was known as the "mast-hunter" because he was able to "sniff" out masts for Baba to work with.

That the group was still coming across interesting characters is depicted in one of William's descriptions:

"Baitullah Shah is an advanced pilgrim ... who lives in a suburb of Ahmedabad, and he has a woman disciple who wears a gown of patches. He reads the Quran [Koran] aloud from 11 o'clock every Thursday night to 3 o'clock the following afternoon, and during these 16 hours he neither eats, drinks, nor sleeps."

Baba and his disciples later travelled to Madras on the southeast coast of India. The masts he visited and met with there were often those he had previously contacted. On a number of occasions the masts would give Baba gifts of food and special keepsakes, indicating that these were "last contacts." Baba always cherished these gifts, devouring the food items given and often planting the seeds from the fruit on the land surrounding Meherabad or Meherazad upon his return.

Part of Baba's intention in going to Madras was to go further south to Tiruvalar, which was close to Negapatam and the home of Chatti Baba, who was one of his five favourite masts.

Sixth-plane mast Chatti Baba maintained a nomadic lifestyle in the area, but he was so well known that the locals usually always knew where he could be found.

The group was disappointed by Chatti Baba's condition when they found him, however, "for he, once known for his pleasing smile, was now emaciated and looked sad and old, and they felt that he had not long to live."

William said that while Baba "will stint neither time, nor trouble, nor expense, in promoting their [wellbeing] very often the general population will ignore these eccentrics."

"If a Perfect Master shows that a faultless patience is indispensable when working with masts it is hardly surprising that ordinary people, even though they may respect a mast, will seldom go to the trouble and expense of housing and feeding him for long – and this explains, perhaps, why Chatti Baba is not well cared for."[88]

While travelling along the southeastern coast of India, an incident occurred that involved a theft, showing Baba's approach to such thieves. The youth involved had a palsied hand and had tried to steal a 10-rupee note from one of the mandalis' pockets. When the youth was caught, the mandali member he robbed wanted to call the police immediately, but Baba said no, and forgave the would-be thief on the spot. He punished him only by twisting his ear gently and admonishing him never to steal again.

William's interpretation of how Baba dealt with the youth provides insight into the Spiritual Master as the strategist:

"The most obvious feature is bound up with the question of why people do anti-social acts. Psychologists and others are beginning to insist that delinquency is a symptom of a psychic disease that is not necessarily the fault of those who suffer from it, and they say that we should seek to heal delinquents rather than punish them."[89]

William's take on how Baba handled the situation was that he had responded in the same manner that contemporary psychologists would have. He says further in his free-flow narrative:

"The final feature is a spiritual one, and is bound up with the fact that Baba, because he is a Perfect Master, is one with the Divine Ground of all living beings. He therefore knows the *fons et origo* [source and origin] of this man's palsied arm and the full course of his psychic malady, and he feels his torment as he stands exposed as a thief. But though he feels this torment, he is its master also, and having allowed the youth to suffer this first vicious cut to his self-conceit, he now catches him off his guard and gives him a more than human absolution, and a draught of Divine Love that he will remember for the rest of his days. Baba's mandali are well acquainted with this technique, for it is one that Baba has used on each of them."

The human caravan kept moving, leaving southern India and travelling to the northwest coast to Junagadh* near the Pakistan border.

The city is famous as a place of pilgrimage. The hill of Datar is a climb of many thousand steps. Datar is named after Bapuzamil Shah Datar, a God-realized being of ancient times. It

* Junagadh is an ancient city of temples, museums, palaces, and caves on the northern fringes of the Gir forest. It features many hills, a fort, and a flora and fauna nature reserve. It is one of the few places where Asiatic lions still roam free.

is said that Datar disappeared in a cave near the summit of the hill never to be seen again. Today, pilgrims still come to the cave to pay homage to the saint.

Baba wanted to spend two days in seclusion on the hill fasting on water only. Baba had contacted a mast in Junagarh with whom he wished to spend the two days.

After this seclusion period ended, Baba and his men climbed one of the peaks of the nearby Girnar Hills, which are steeped in spiritual folklore. In ancient times anyone could legally throw himself to death from the cliffs.

"[The act] however, was not prompted by any personal disaster, but was undertaken it seems, by those who aspired to pass on to a better and higher posthumous existence," writes William in *The Wayfarers*.

The next stop on the adventure was Delhi and then onto Ajmer*, one of Baba's favourite mast haunts. From there they travelled south again to Baroda, where they reconnected with Chambu Shah, one of Baba's old mast contacts. Chambu Shah was given new clothes, and Baba later wore the mast's old ones for a period of time.

William focused on this meeting to point out some common interpretations of the strange contacts:

"Those who dismiss as arrant nonsense the notion that so-called masts are anything more than madmen or eccentrics may look upon Chambu Shah with opprobrium [extreme scorn], or may condemn him as hypocritical and a possible lecherous eccentric who trades on the credulity of dupes.... It is worth recording that most of those who go with Baba on these tours can be as cynical as any of you incisive intellectuals, and as worldly-wise as the most hard-headed Yorkshireman."[90]

From Baroda, the group again went westward to the coastal area and Morvi**. After that they moved onto Ahmeda-

* Ajmer, surrounded by the Aravalli Mountains, is a place of pilgrimage to tombs of saints as well as a centre of culture and education. It has a seventh-century fort and to the north is an artificial lake made in the twelfth century.

** Morvi on the Macchu River is a prosperous city-state in Gujerat. It is famous for its architecture and buildings. Known as the Paris of India, Morvi has the Green Tower, inspired by the Eiffel Tower.

bad and then headed back home to Meherabad and Meherazad.

"You may imagine, then, that Baba's men, when they left Ahmedabad for home, were dreaming of four heavenly blessings only; a lavish bath, the touch of spotless linen, the taste of a solid meal, and the bliss of sleep on a clean bed for a thousand years," says William of the mood at the time.

William did not go on all the mast tours and accounts indicate he was often staying at Meherazad, Baba's newly opened residential compound. Meherazad is situated nine miles north of Ahmednagar and Meherabad, the larger centre, is six miles south of the city.

Living with Baba changed with the move to Meherazad. Baba's English disciple Kitty Davy, who lived there until 1952, describes the altered atmosphere in her book *Love Alone Prevails*:

"There was a big change in Meherazad. Things were never quite the same after Baba moved there. There was much more laxity. Baba's training must have been complete....

"Only a few were called to live at Meherazad – those who were less moody, who needed less pampering, who knew how to stand on their own feet more, who didn't worry Baba with their little worries and troubles...."

Kitty described Meherazad as more like a family home, one that had been established with his chief woman disciple Mehera in mind.

"I felt it was different. It was Mehera's home. Baba had trained Mehera up until then absolutely strictly. Then she became free. [In Urdu] Mehera-azad means 'Mehera free or relaxed.'" Kitty points out that Baba was now more attentive to Mehera and that she needed this move now that she was older.

Another account describes a homey scene at Meherazad:

"We began reading aloud. We sat together in the evenings and had jokes. Mehera began to be a little bit free.

"Margaret [Craske] says Baba had taken them [Easterners] to the spiritual heights, and now he had to bring them down again – slowly, slowly – into the material world. He had taken them out of the physical world; they couldn't have any contact whatsoever. Then when we [Westerners] came on the scene, we felt that gradually, a tiny, tiny bit [Baba did it so

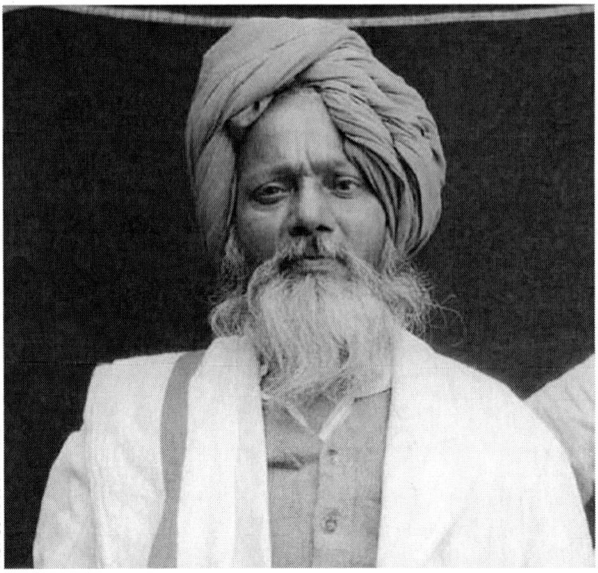

Ali Shah was one of Baba's five favourite masts. Baba spent considerable time with the fifth-plane mast at Meherabad and Meherazad in the 1940s.

slowly]; he brought them a little bit back in touch with the physical, material world."[91]

It is apparent that as William wrote the two supplementary pamphlets that would be published in a subsequent printing of *The Wayfarers,* he was studying the mast/Spiritual Master connection more closely.

Ali Shah, one of Meher Baba's favourite masts, spent considerable time at Meherabad and Meherazad. While in previous descriptions of Baba's contact with the mast, Baba appeared to be doing all the work, William noticed that a two-way street existed with Ali Shah when he was taken from Meherabad to Meherazad to spend a month with Baba in January 1949.

"Baba fed him and sat with him every day. I have brought this possibly unexciting detail into the main text in order to fill in an omission in *The Wayfarers* and also to record a small personal observation."

William said the omission was that Ali Shah is generally known in Meherabad and elsewhere as Bapji, and this name has now almost eclipsed his earlier name of Ali Shah.

"The personal observation may be thought unimportant, but it adds weight to the surmise that one of the reasons, if not the chief reason, for Baba's contact with the God-intoxicated, is to give them work. The observation in question is simply whenever Bapji returns to Meherabad after a period of contact with Baba; he spends almost the entire day in the privacy of his little room for a week or 10 days and seems to resent any intrusion. If you peep in at him he appears to be making more gestures than usual with his hands, and the impression is that he is concentrating on some kind of special task. After a week or 10 days, however, he comes out again from his room and mixes freely with the mandali, as if he now had leisure to do as he pleased."[92]

Just what work Bapji (aka Ali Shah) was engaged in is a mystery, but his popularity with Baba is beyond question. Earlier in *The Wayfarers*, William pointed out that Baba contacted Bapji on 20 different occasions between 1943 and 1947.

William's flowery description of Mount Abu*, Baba's next stopping off point, reflects his ongoing efforts at spicing up the prose in his book on the masts. Mount Abu has an important place in the histories of both Jains** and Hindus, and William points out, "It is said of Abu that if you fast there but one day all your sins are forgiven you and that if you live there but one year you will become the preceptor of all mankind."

Baba decided to use this northwestern India site as his headquarters for three months. Meheru*** rememberd the stay in the area:

---

* Mount Abu is the highest peak in the Aravalli mountain range in Rajasthan. The town is a popular hill station with carved marble Jain temples, Hindu temples carved out of rock, the beautiful Nakki Lake, and a fort.

** Jainism is an Indian religion that prescribes a path of non-violence toward all living beings. Its philosophy and practice emphasize the necessity of self-effort to move the soul toward divine consciousness and liberation.

*** Meheru was Mehera's niece (daughter of Mehera's sister Freiny and Adi K. Irani's brother Rustom). She joined Baba's mandali as a young woman and was one of only four women mandali accompanying Baba on the New Life.

"The house we stayed in was very comfortable. Right near the bazaar," Meheru recalls. "The men in the town would be drunk and noisy however and Don [William] was permitted to sleep at our place on the front veranda."[93]

While little happened at Abu to record, William described some side trips. On one occasion, Baba travelled to Ajmer where he contacted Chacha, one of his five favourite masts. On this occasion Baba also gave five rupees each to forty-four widows in the area.

While Baba occasionally contacted groups of the poor, it was unusual for him to actually give alms to widows. These meetings were usually behind closed doors, and William offers his own interpretation of the event:

"I think ... that we are justified in the assumption that the gift itself, whether it be money or cloth or grain or anything else, is a kind of catalyst by which Baba is able to bring about a certain spiritual reaction. Baba, we know, often gives charity to individual people, with apparently no other aim than to lessen the burden of their material cares, but these gifts are of quite another kind and involved no contact."

William went on to describe an arduous and comical journey by bullock cart to track down a mast, during which Eruch lost 700 rupees from his shirt pocket. When Baba was informed of the loss, he told the mandali that it was more important to concentrate on finding the mast than worrying about lost money.

Ironically enough, after a successful meeting with the mast, the money was found and recovered on the trip back along with a single shoe of Eruch's* that had been lost on the same adventure.

William continues his descriptive narrative, covering a number of mast expeditions from the Mount Abu headquarters. He indicates that difficulties are a natural part of life with a Spiritual Master and occur for specific reasons:

---

* Eruch Jessawala (1916–2001) joined Meher Baba in 1938. He served as Baba's attendant and main interpreter, in both the English-language alphabet board and later Baba's sign language. Eruch took dictation from the alphabet board for Meher Baba's book *God Speaks,* wrote the ninth chapter of that book under Baba's direct supervision, and wrote the book's conclusion. Eruch's stories of his life with Meher Baba were also published in a few books.

"Baba has explained many times that resistance of one kind or another is necessary for his work. If we take this as our starting point, it is surely justifiable to surmise that when resistance is not forthcoming of its own accord, a Perfect Master may deliberately invite it by walking with open eyes into a situation that he knows will bring difficulties and perhaps even disasters upon him."[94]

William's explanations as the final supplement to *The Wayfarers* took shape indicate that he reached new conclusions that were not to be found in the original manuscript.

He said it was natural for the reader to question the "Perfection" of a Perfect Master who often allows himself to be humiliated or obstructed to the point of absurdity.

"It would be impossible, for me at least, to define what I really know nothing about," says William. "But in this context we can certainly ask ourselves, whether, if we accept that Christ was spiritually perfect, He was only the less Perfect because He deliberately allowed Himself to be nailed to a cross like a common criminal."

While William admits it may seem unfair to compare the agony of crucifixion with a night of petty annoyances on the road with Meher Baba, "It seems to me that the principle common to both is that a Perfect Master deliberately allows himself to suffer in a way, and at a time, that answers to the needs of his work."

"The particular reason for enduring a particular difficulty or disaster may be beyond our understanding, but I am certain of one thing at least that all such voluntary sufferings, whether great or small, are borne by those Realized Beings for salvation of mankind."[95]

Later in this section Baba elaborates further on why masts often are found in filthy surroundings. Some even chose to live surrounded by their own bodily wastes.

As a lead-up to his explanation about masts and their often filthy hovels, Baba, through notes that William borrowed from Dr. Ghani, says, "'I like two things – masts and children. I like masts for their strength and children for their helplessness. The fire of love is terrible indeed, and masts present a challenge – of this terrible fire of love – to God, the Beloved.'

"Baba goes on to say, dictating on his [alphabet] board, 'Because of the terrible fire of their love, [they] present a challenge to the Beloved, and this challenge – that the Beloved should manifest Himself – is always accompanied by heroic efforts to achieve total self-elimination or egoless-ness; efforts that may take many forms.

"To live in dirty surroundings, such as in or near a latrine or a urinal, is one way of utterly forgetting one's bodily existence. And the beauty of it is that when the body is utterly neglected or forgotten – because the consciousness is afire only of love for the Divine Beloved – it does not deteriorate but takes care of itself automatically. The minds of ordinary people are constantly looking after their bodies, but they find that in spite of taking every kind of precaution and care, deterioration can never be avoided altogether.'"

Baba went on to point out how difficult becoming a lover of God could be:

"It is not given to everybody to be a lover of God. Such lovers are so consumed in the fire of love that they are not conscious of their stage of spiritual progress and they do not have any thought of union with God. They simply 'enjoy' the torture of love, and long for more and more of it.

"These lovers do not have any thought about their separation from the Beloved, or as I have already told you, any thoughts of union with Him. They are resigned to the state in which they find themselves, and, when their resignation reaches its climax; it is the Beloved who seeks union with them."[96]

In the early months of 1949, Baba made another trip with the women mandali and Eruch, Adi Sr., and William to the seaside village of Vengurla.

William travelled ahead to make reservations at the same cliff-side government rest house where they had stayed previously. Female mandali member Dr. Goher recalled the experience:

"It was a beautiful trip, a complete holiday for Baba. We went on walks with him, waded in the water. Sometimes, Baba went ahead with Eruch or Don, while we swam. There was a nice cook, who cooked well."[97]

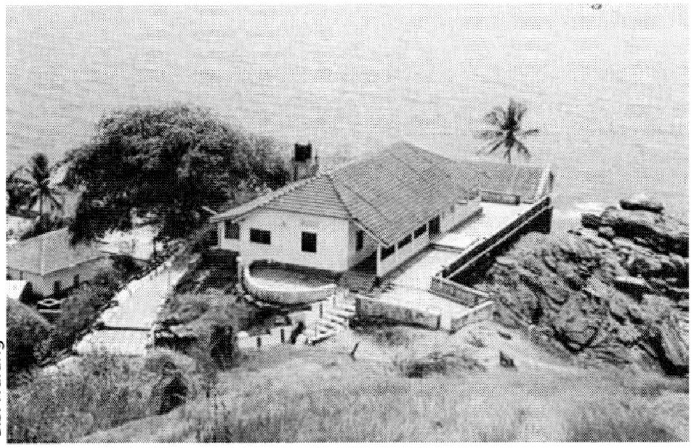

B.S. Warang

Baba, several of the woman mandali, and William first stayed in this seaside Government Rest House in Vengurla on India's west coast in 1947. Male mandali members Eruch and Adi Sr. accompanied Baba and the same group on a follow-up visit in 1949. The two visits were mainly holidays.

The trip was not without the usual humorous mishaps and controversy. On one occasion, Dr. Goher got stuck in a broken chair that she had warned others not to sit on. Baba, Mehera, Mani, and Meheru, who witnessed the incident, laughed heartily.

On another occasion William's meticulous nature got under Goher's skin. He had been too thorough in tying up the bed rolls, and Goher scolded him when she had trouble untying hers at bedtime. Bedbugs were also a problem at one stopover on the trip to the point that William asked everyone to turn in their mattresses, which he promptly set afire to get rid of the problem.

Other than this brief holiday, working side trips from Baba's new home base at Meherazad were the norm.

A surprising gift was delivered to the new residential compound that year. William's father Sydney Bryan paid for a gas generator which was to be installed there to provide electric lights. Meherwan, Eruch Jessawala's younger brother, recalls the generator's short life at Meherazad:

"It was installed and lit up the colony only once. At 10 o'clock that night Baba said 'shut it off'. He referred to it as a 'petrol-driven monster'."

Meherwan says the generator, which only ran for three hours, was a big piece of machinery that took up an entire room at Meherazad. It was soon moved to the larger Meherabad colony and used there.[98]

In April 1949 Baba and his followers travelled from Abu to Benares,* the city that overlooks the wide waters of the Ganges.** A memorable mast contact was made in Benares. Of Batwa Shah,*** Baba says, "When I sat near Batwa Shah I felt as if I was sitting near Chacha." Chacha had been described earlier in *The Wayfarers* as a God-realized being or majzoob of the seventh plane.

Batwa Shah was prone to phases of irritability, but also had a fondness for children. The mast had a distinctive habit of carrying sheets of paper wherever he went and whenever he sat down, he took out a peculiar long pencil and covered sheet after sheet with writing. Although reluctant at first to meet with Baba, Batwa Shah shared his food with Baba and also asked Baba to scratch him, which Baba did for about an hour.

William admits, as this final section of *The Wayfarers* supplement comes to an end, that the mandali could at times be frustrated with the mast-chasing exploits:

"In striving to do justice to this work of Meher Baba with advanced souls and others, I find myself jostled by the horns of a dilemma...."

William says that in the beginning, the tours had a "morning freshness" about them, which stimulated the mandali to "vital enthusiasm" for the work, but the years took their toll on this keenness.

---

* Benares (now Varanasi) is in the state of Uttar Pradesh. It is regarded as a holy city by Hindus, Buddhists, and Jains.

** The Ganges is one of the major rivers in India, starting in the western Himalayas and flowing through Bangladesh into the Bay of Bengal. It is holy to the Hindus and has been declared India's National River.

*** Batwa Shah was a well-known mast in Benares who had come from a wealthy family but who was found living in a filthy state.

"These labours have now gone on for so many years that the men who go with Baba on these tours have begun to show symptoms of languor of the spirit. One of the results of this is that their descriptions of all except the most exceptional contacts are inclined to be perfunctory, or worse still, to consist of a mere inventory of physical peculiarities."

William, who admitted his own enthusiasm was low, voices his frustration at trying to extract second-hand information from those accompanying Baba on the tours.

"And then, of course, it is clear that no one, except Baba himself, knows the real meaning of these contacts.... This ... is only half the dilemma, and the other half is an almost neurotic obsession in my own mind, that all this work of Meher Baba with advanced souls, sadhus, and the mad, and poor, must be put on record with a faithful attention to detail."[99]

In the last section of William's second pamphlet and thus the final pages of *The Wayfarers*, he deals with Meher Baba's 40-day seclusion from June 22 to July 31, 1949.

Oddly enough, Baba chose the body of the old Blue Bus as his seclusion sanctuary. The bus, which William often drove and Baba had used in his travels in the pre-war days, had been disassembled. The body had to be retrieved from a garage yard and resurrected at Meherazad.

During Baba's seclusion in the refurbished bus, which William described as the "sweetest and gayest little cabin," Baba would contact twenty-one poor people, the fifth-plane mast Ali Shah, and seven mad people. The forty-day seclusion was divided into five distinct phases.

Baba spent the first and last phases of the seclusion working almost entirely with the mast Ali Shah in the confines of the bus cabin. Between these two periods, in a surprising turnabout, Baba left the bus and travelled to Poona for nine days."The phase that was spent in Poona was [one is bound to admit], really no seclusion at all. In this context one remembers a dig that Baba once made at himself: 'I am consistent,' he said, 'in inconsistency.'"

Most of the Poona days were spent contacting masts. While the reader may interpret Baba's break from his seclusion as a sign of "spinelessness" or even "wilful dishonesty," William held firm on the point that because of Baba's elevated existence, he did not have to justify his actions to anyone or continue his seclusion for "spiritual profit."

"We know that there never has been and never will be any question of the slightest spiritual profit for Baba himself. Because he is spiritually Perfect. He has no personal axe to grind, and to carry through this thankless job he has extended his consciousness from the Shoreless Ocean of Infinite Power, Knowledge, and Bliss, to the choking smog of this wretched yet lovable earth of ours."

As William approaches the final 10 pages of his writing, he very openly praises Meher Baba, but admits he is butting up against forces afoot within his own psyche.

"When it comes to a Great Being – who knows and is one with the uttermost secrets of the universe; who is the Master of masters and the Genius of geniuses; who is, as the old prayer goes, King of kings, Lord of lords, and the only Ruler of princes – we hide our ears and tail under the cap and gown of an egregious self-complacency, and bray at him how he should or should not do his job."

William goes on to describe his own mental gymnastics in dealing with Baba's trip to Poona in the midst of his 40-day seclusion:

"You may suspect all this to be an acute attack of grandiloquence, and it should, therefore, be made clear that the antecedent paragraphs constitute a puja* – emotional rather than logical – directed *imprimis* from one department of my own mind to another department of it."

Baba chose a house on a hill overlooking his birthplace city of Poona for his nine-day stay. Although he left Meherazad with the mast Ali Shah and two other mandali, he was soon joined at the house by three other mandali. William gives a brief description of the five mandali members and Ali Shah, weaving a humorous hodgepodge of the inhabitants.

---

* Puja is a religious ritual performed by Hindus as an offering to a deity, distinguished person, or special guest with the idea of receiving their blessing.

While Baba described the Poona adventure as a period of relaxation, his work with Ali Shah and the mandali's efforts at contacting more masts was relentless. William describes one mast contacted as being very boisterous and a great source of humour for Meher Baba and the party. Another mast who lived in a public urinal was both "a public and revered figure in Poona." While Baba has already given "spiritual reasons" why these God-intoxicated people choose to live in filthy surroundings, William, perhaps predicting his book would be read by people outside of India, again tried his best to explain masts' habitat preferences:

"Spiritual explanations, however, are not quite the cup of tea of the average modern Westerner, although he is ready at any time to play fast and loose with specimens of jargon from normal and morbid psychology."

William goes on to predict that most Westerners might think the "so-called masts that live in latrines and urinals are nothing more than perverts."

The Wayfarers author says the adult population of India is as discerning as any adult population in any part of the world, and their reverence for many of these beings proves their worth, even if the basis of this conviction remains a mystery:

"Since we can neither prove that masts are spiritually advanced, nor disprove that they are psychotics or psychoneurotics, we may as well ... keep an open mind on the subject. For my own part, in any case, I accept what Baba tells us about these great souls, in the same way as I would accept, for example, what Niels Bohr* might tell us about nuclear fission."

In the final page of *The Wayfarers,* William describes Keshav, the urinal-inhabiting mast, and the efforts Baba made to bathe him. Eventually Baba was allowed to pour water on Keshav's feet as he sat in a jeep. After this, Keshav bowed to Baba's will, allowing him to feed and spoil and have contact with him before he was sent back to his urinal home.

---

* Niels Bohr was a Nobel Prize winner in physics who worked on understanding atomic structure and was part of the Manhattan Project, which did the research for developing the first atomic bomb for the US.

Bhau Kalchuri, in his multi-volume *Lord Meher* series, would later laud William's book, but Kalchuri also added, "It was said that Donkin was never the same after he finished *The Wayfarers.*"

If William felt taxed by this undertaking, it is certain that he, along with the entire global community of Baba followers, would soon feel the extra pressures of life with the God-man. Before 1949 came to a close, Baba would launch a program of "hopelessness and helplessness," which would affect everyone in his fold. Some were hit more directly than others, with William on the very front line of the experiment.

9

The New Life, Doctor's Clinic

Hints of the "New Life," which was to run from mid-October 1949 until February 1952, were given as early as 1931 according to Baba's close disciple and interpreter Eruch Jessawala. Eruch said Baba used the term "new life" on a visit to the West in 1931, when a young woman came before him and admitted she was so distraught she felt that suicide was her only escape.

"Baba looked at her very solemnly, and said, 'Then why don't you commit suicide?'

"And saying that, He pressed her head to His feet and again said, 'Commit suicide!'

"A few moments later, Baba raised her head and told her, 'Now you are no longer yourself, begin to live the new life. Think of Me, remember Me, and love Me.'"[100]

A few paragraphs later in the book, Eruch says of the New Life that it was an intense period of incognito travel, which Baba was to initiate 18 years later in 1949.

"Meher Baba's New Life was a blueprint for our life for we can find examples in it to help us in every incident; to be cheerful under all circumstances, to try to curb anger and never to worry about the future but to depend solely on the Lord's Will."[101]

Eruch's brother Meherwan, who was in his late teens at the time, says Baba "exploded an atom bomb" when he came out of seclusion for a day on June 21, 1949, to announce the New Life. "He wanted to dispose of everything – cars, property, everything. He said 'let them collect things – I will dispose of all.'"

Eruch and William would both have an all-encompassing direct involvement in the New Life. Baba carefully chose the four women and sixteen men who would accompany him on the New Life travels.

Meher Baba's followers worldwide were informed of the New Life plan early and invited to join the process in some capacity at a meeting that Baba called in India. The sacrifices for most followers were not insignificant, and for the group chosen to go with Baba, they were overwhelming.

At the outset Baba said all ashrams would be completely disassembled. Throughout his life Baba warned his followers about the institutions, window dressings, and trappings of world religions, which he said interfered with true spirituality. He may have thought that the colonies of his followers at both Meherabad and Meherazad needed to feel some upheaval. He always insisted that true spirituality would not be found by hiding away or secluding oneself from life's trials. He may even have felt that his followers were not truly living in the spirit of renunciation. He was determined to place them as much as possible in situations where renunciation would have to be fully confronted.

While tearing down ashrams and divesting himself of properties showed his determination to upset the status quo, he also outlined major changes and choices that his followers would have to consider.

The 21 who accompanied him were for the most part the only people in contact with him for three or four months, and those who were left behind were expected to assume new lives away from their previous patterns in the ashrams.

Long-time Western disciple Kitty Davy, who would have to leave the home base of Meherabad after 12 years, went to teach school in Bombay for the New Life period. She explains how the New Life "bombshell" affected the mandali directly:

"All at Meherabad were called to Meherazad to a big meeting.... In brief, Baba had decided to close all ashrams, dispose of all their contents, and relinquish all properties in India, except the Meherabad Hill premises.

"The majority of those living with Baba at the time were to be sent back into the world to live and work.

"A few disciples would form His 'chosen companions to accompany Him in the New Life....' Those agreeing to the severe conditions of the New Life [hence called 'yeswallas'*] had to be prepared to look upon themselves as dead, in the sense that the dead have no desires, concerns, attachments, questions or provisions for the morrow."[102]

William was immediately involved in New Life preparations. While still in seclusion in the Blue Bus body, Baba asked those representing the various religions to read passages from the Bible, Koran, Zend-Avesta, and Bhagavad Gita as part of the lead-up to the start of the New Life. William read the Sermon on the Mount, one of Baba's favourite Bible passages. William also helped draw up the circular outlining New Life rules.

Kitty Davy relates Baba's comments related to the circular:

"I want you all to go through this circular word by word most carefully before you decide.... Although your faith, love and service for Me have been greater than Mine would have been for My own Master, yet these conditions might prove your undoing. So unless you are ready to live the life of complete satyanashi [self-annihilation and/or hopelessness] and absolute obedience, it would be better to stay behind and obey instructions that will be given to you.... The decision is entirely to be made by you and you alone. May God give you the required strength."[103]

Specifically, Baba gave the women four alternatives:

1) Stay in the Meherabad Hill quarters if a family member can provide financial help;
2) Work for a living and contribute anything that could be spared for families that had so far been depending on Baba;
3) Do what they liked and have nothing more to do with Baba; or
4) Leave everything to Baba and do exactly as He said, accepting with full faith whatever decision He made....

---

* "Walla" (in "yeswalla") is a Hindi word that literally means 'connected or pertaining to' and refers to someone's particular job, responsibility, or activity.

While Kitty wanted very much to accompany Baba as a female companion on the New Life, in the end Baba chose only four Eastern women disciples. He believed that taking Western women disciples on a foot journey through India might attract unwanted attention and questions from Indian authorities.

In the group of 16 men who were finally chosen, William was the only Western disciple to join Baba in the New Life.

When different mandali members read out passages from the various holy books, Baba would follow with explanations on their meaning.

When William read from the Sermon on the Mount "Be ye therefore perfect, even as your Father, which in heaven is perfect," Baba explained that Jesus used to tell people that God-realization is the goal of each individual and that everyone is potentially God.

He added that few people at the time of Jesus were ready to hear such truths directly.[104]

At the close of William's reading of the Sermon, Baba spelled out on his alphabet board, "This is my favourite section[105] of the Bible."

In Bal Natu's *Glimpses of the Godman,* Volume II, the author says that William received word in July from Baba that he was to mark out important passages in some books on Christian mysticism and then forward the books to Meherazad.

"He was specially asked to send the books of Friar Juniper.* The other books were *The Little Flower's Life, Mirror of Saint Francis, Classics of the Inner Life,* and *The Cloud of Unknowing.*"

William carried out other Christian readings as the months passed in preparation for the New Life. At one point he read out the Crucifixion of Jesus from the Gospel of St. Matthew.

At another meeting on August 9, 1949, Baba had a message read out in four languages. Part of the message in English that William read was,

> May God, whom the Muslims call Allah,
> whom the Zoroastrians call Ahuramazda,

* Friar Juniper was one of the brothers who lived and worked with Saint Francis of Assisi.

whom the Hindus call Ishwar Paramatma,
and whom many others call by many other names,

May He whose union lovers seek in self-annihilation,
whom the seers see as the only Reality,
and whom the knowers know as their own real Self,

May this Supreme Conscious Being,
this conscious Soul of souls, who eternally manifests
as Avatar and Perfect Masters,

May He through His all-merciful act
bestow on us His grace....[106]

Baba also asked William and Dr. Ghani to prepare the final draft of the New Life conditions. They were to have the job finished by August 21, and Baba stressed the "seriousness and finality of these conditions."

Although the conditions were sent out to more than 1,000 Baba lovers, Baba finally selected only 32 men who would be given the choice of accompanying him on the New Life. The 32 names were finally reduced to 16 who would take on the arduous travels.

A few days after the men were asked to decide on taking part in the New Life, Baba met with the women mandali. After this session, Baba chose only four women to accompany him – Mehera, Mani, Meheru, and Goher.

During preparations for the October 16 start of the New Life, Baba continuously emphasized the importance of the holy books of different world religions. In addition to reading Bible passages, William was also given the job of reading out the conditions of the New Life in English to his fellow companions at a final meeting on August 31.

When he finished reading these conditions a deep silence prevailed among those gathered.

Those who were to travel directly with Baba were going to have a completely different relationship with him than in the past. Although they were to obey him implicitly, the orders they followed were all preordained according to the conditions in writing they agreed to and signed prior to the start of the New Life journeys. Baba insisted that on the actual travels he would only be a companion to the other members of the group and was not to be treated as their Master. As per his usual instructions, his identity would be kept from anyone they came in contact with.

The earlier description which Baba had given about the New Life being one of "hopelessness and helplessness" was indeed apt in that the companions were to exist only on what they could acquire through begging.

Ivy Duce, in her book *How a Master Works,* describes the group's departure on the New Life: "The first day of walking was a long trek of 17 miles and was tiring especially for the elderly ones, notably Dr. Ghani, who led a sedentary life.

"The men companions walked in front, and a short distance behind, Baba and the women followed."

Sore and battered feet were regular ailments for companions, including Baba.

"On the journey Baba's feet became sore due to a new pair of sandals. Mehera offered Him her broken-in sandals which fit Baba comfortably. Dr. Donkin applied gauze and adhesive tape to Baba's blistered feet...."[107]

At one point "[Dr.] Ghani complained to the other men, 'Dr. Donkin and Dr. Nilu totally led me astray. They were saying that Baba's health was such that he would not be able to walk more than four or five miles a day.'

"He was humorously suggesting that he wanted another rest, but Baba just smiled and they all pushed on."[108]

Dr. Ghani suffered a mild heart attack just a couple of days into the journey, and William and Dr. Nilu attended him.

"Baba gestured for him to sit under a roadside tree in the shade for 15 minutes. He was then given water to sip and one of the companions splashed water over his face. Due to this help Ghani was able to cool down."[109]

Ghani recovered enough to keep travelling after they took rest in a government rest house. Ivy says the companions also adopted a sort of uniform at the beginning of their journeys.

Baba and the men wore white kafnis* and green turbans. William was excused from wearing the turban because he could not balance it on his head Instead he wore a makeshift Arab head covering**.

"The first day out on the journey, the women companions wore cotton saris of the same colour – slate blue. Afterwards they wore clothes that were more practical and did not interfere with the walking – long pants or trousers with a frock over them."[110]

Their first destination was Sarnath, said to be where Buddha delivered his first sermon. Buddhist monuments abound there as well as many monasteries. The ancient ruins in Sarnath are the most expansive on the Buddhist trail, and their haunting beauty at certain times of the day reflects the deep spiritual history there.

The travellers' procession became even more theatrical when they moved on to Benares. Here the group acquired several animals to take on their journeys, including a white horse.

Ivy describes the bizarre parade that was a result of the added menagerie:

"The scene was like a pageant being enacted before us. First came Dr. Donkin wearing an Arab-like head-dress and a white kafni, leading the beautiful white horse....Then followed the camel cart and bullock carts. Hanging from the neck of the stately camel was a Persian bell which sounded melodiously. Some of the companions were driving the carts, the rest coming on foot. Last came the caravan drawn by two bullocks, and tied to the caravan were two donkeys who were not used to being led like horses and resisted this treatment all the way."

Although comical to envision, the life of the companions was tough at the best of times. Each member of the group, including Baba, had a bhiksha (begging) bowl and a couple of companions at a time were dispatched to beg at dwellings for food and other necessities.

---

* A kafni is a knee-length shirt or lightweight coat.

** The Arab head covering may have been a keffiyah or ghutra – which is a folded cloth that is bound onto the head with a cloth band.

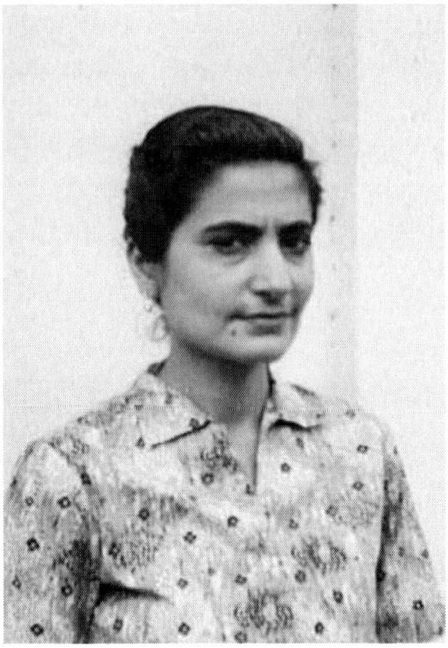

MSI Collection India

Meheru R. Irani, was a lifelong woman mandali of Meher Baba. She accompanied Baba on the New Life travels. Meheru was the daughter of Rustom K. Irani and Freiny Irani (Mehera's sister). Rustom was the first of Meher Baba's mandali to travel to countries of the West in 1928.

Being cheerful and calm was one of the conditions of the New Life. The members were also never to speak impatiently or get angry with anyone, even under provocation.

The party usually got underway at 4 a.m. in bitter cold conditions. They would walk all day then set up camp tired and footsore. Water would have to be fetched from a well and tents and bedding set up and arranged for the night.

In her book, Ivy relates William's description of his experience during the New Life, which he later conveyed to her in person:

"Will Donkin's facial expression was really comical as he described with wry humour how awful he felt when begging for food at someone's back door; and the housewife on looking him over noting his strong British body and healthy good looks would remark scathingly that he shouldn't be so lazy – he should go to work."

From the outset, William had trouble with the white horse put in his care. The animal overnight turned into a sort of demon, putting its ears back and baring its teeth. The horse would eat from a feed bag that William held. Before getting down to the last few munches, it would begin to turn around preparing to kick William.

Calamities facing the group finally spilled over into a full-fledged protest with William deep in the fray, recalls Eruch Jessawala in *Tales From the New Life.*

"Donkin ... flared up saying, 'Do you know how to handle this horse? He's not a horse, he's a devil.'"

William's comment came in the midst of a complaint session by a number of men companions, who thought they were bearing the brunt of the suffering in the journeys while Baba and the women companions were getting off relatively easy.

One issue brought up was tending all of the animals, including milking the cow each morning and even carrying newborn calves. They also cited the rough conditions for older members of the party and the difficulties they encountered with villagers along the way.

Eruch, who was head of the male companions, reminded them that when they took their grievances to Baba everyone was to maintain a cheerful face as per New Life orders. In the end, Dr. Ghani, an old school chum of Baba's, was chosen to relay the issues to Baba, but it had to be done without rancour or resentment.

There was a bit of cat-and-mouse activity between Baba and the other companions the next day before Ghani faced Baba. He apparently was quite obtuse in his explanation, telling Baba that the companions were a little put off that they were not being treated as well as the animals they were in charge of.

Whatever the tactic used, Baba appeared to have understood, the air was cleared, and the need for a repeat performance did not come up again in the New Life. Shortly after the companions' flare-up, Baba decided the group should take a week off from travelling and stay in one place.

"Let us rest, except we will still have to go out begging for our meals," Baba conveyed on the alphabet board.

Egos were certainly being hacked away rather than just whittled down in the New Life. But the blueprint for the New Life had been made clear in a declaration to all Baba-lovers worldwide before this phase began. Two circulars – one sent out in March 1950 and the other in September 1950 – together had laid out Baba's expectations clearly to everyone:

"This New Life is endless and even after my physical death, it will be kept alive by those who live the life of complete renunciation of falsehood, lies, hatred, anger, greed and lust; and who to accomplish all this do no lustful actions, do no harm to anyone, do no backbiting, do not seek material possessions or power, who accept no homage, neither covet honour, nor shun disgrace, and fear no one and nothing."

The two circulars continue, "By those who rely wholly and solely on God and who love God purely for the sake of loving, who believe in the lovers of God and in the reality of Manifestation, and yet do not expect any spiritual or material reward, who do not let go the hand of Truth, and who, without being upset by calamities, bravely and wholeheartedly face all hardships with 100 per cent cheerfulness, and give no importance to caste, creed, and religious ceremonies.

"This New Life will live by itself eternally, even if there is no one to live it."[111]

While most of Baba's followers worldwide were aware of the difficulties in adhering to these principles and perhaps compromised certain interpretations; the companions who actually travelled with him were under direct pressure to toe the line.

Though William felt the duress along with Baba's other direct companions, he was at times given duties that he felt were of value. For a period during the New Life, Baba asked William, on his behalf, to communicate with Elizabeth Patterson and Norina Matchabelli ["Elinora" as Baba referred to them], who were heavily involved in clearing land and establishing a small network of cabins at the new Meher Spiritual Center on the coast of South Carolina. Baba had indicated that he would soon visit the Center.

As the only Westerner travelling in the New Life, William stood out. There was also talk among Eastern members about incidents of favouritism bestowed on William. On one occasion Baba had blankets and sheets distributed to his companions, and William was the only individual to receive a mosquito net.

Baba, perhaps sensing the feelings of others, seized the occasion at the October 25 meeting to bring up William's courage in taking part in the New Life:

"In his case, the little consideration in giving him a mosquito net was not a concession of favouritism. Compared to the other men, he has suffered most and yet he does not grumble. On the contrary I find him keeping a very good and cheerful mood. His tastes in food, his habits of sitting, sleeping, toilet and bathing are altogether different. But without mulling over them, he keeps himself cheerful. Not to make a hard life harder, he has been shown some consideration which, in turn, is neither a concession nor partiality."[112]

Although eliminating the ego was one of Baba's major goals in working with his followers, he knew there was a limit to how much they could take at once. He would also often give them a boost, either verbally or through a pat on the back or embrace, cueing in to when the individual needed encouragement.

While all of the companions were equally slogging out the New Life under trying circumstances, there were times when William was undoubtedly overburdened.

He continued to tend the cantankerous white horse, which was later harnessed to a tonga (horse cart) with the hope that the job would settle it down. After one particularly nasty day tending to the whims of the animal, William collapsed exhausted in front of the campfire for the night, without even undoing his bedroll.

William would later relay in a letter his determination to follow Baba's rules:

"Moods due to illness, want of sleep, etc., were one thing and this Baba understood and it was not deemed a fault, but if rising out of anger and irritation because of putting up with hardships, etc., then they would be deemed faults not to be tolerated." And Baba warned them all that he had complete freedom to send any away or to keep them with him.

However, it was noticed that "throughout the New Life, [although] Baba was very strict, he was also very forgiving, and not without his jovial moods and eternal humour."[113]

After more than 10 years living directly with Meher Baba, William understood the Master/disciple relationship. Baba said more than once that his Western lovers "were hard nuts to crack" when it came to eliminating their egos – the major requirement for achieving a human state where divine love and God-realization were possible.

That his approach was accomplished very much on a one-on-one basis must have made the task difficult for Meher Baba. For while he would issue all kinds of rules and orders; they were almost always interpreted on an individual basis. If, as Baba said, that the East, particularly India, was more prone to spiritual matters than the materialistic West, this may have made compliance easier for those followers who were reared in his own country.

As November gave way to December, the companions were travelling northward in India from Benares to Hardwar.

"Baba ... asked Donkin to study a map to determine the most convenient road for the journey on foot from Benares to Hardwar. He said that he expected the New Life to become so difficult that 'not a single one from amongst you will remain with me.... I am expecting of you in this New Life something which is superhuman in some aspects. I, too, am in the soup along with you.'"[114] Though the Ganges does not lose its rapids completely, it nevertheless becomes quiet and calm in Hardwar, a major pilgrimage site. The water is clean and people prefer taking baths on the numerous ghats built on the river shores. It is said that taking a bath here purifies the soul and opens the way for the ultimate freedom – Nirvana.

As per Baba's usual procedure, his identity was kept secret wherever they went, and he was referred to as the "elder brother." Despite the secrecy, there were occasions where people would recognize Baba, and small crowds would form seeking his darshan.

At one point in Belgaum people "heard of Baba and his companions' presence in the local newspaper and came for darshan ... Baba addressed the companions about dealing with inquiries from people while on the New Life.

"'Now remember, there will be occasions when people will ask all sorts of questions and such occasions will often arise. Donkin should be the one to go and meet the Westerners, and either Ghani, Adi, Nilu, Eruch, Pendu, or Vishnu should explain matters to Indian questioners.'"[115]

William was instructed to tell any Westerners that a meeting or darshan was not possible, and the Indian mandali were to deal with the Easterners in the same manner. The extent and seriousness of this order is reflected in an incident which took place on November 10:

"Jal Rusi, Dr. Goher's younger brother ... made no attempt to see Baba or the companions. Although he was staying in Belgaum and Donkin had seen him several times on the road, both immediately turned their faces away."

Added to William's chores of caring for animals, looking after the health of fellow companions, and begging for meals, Baba asked him to be the "newspaper reader" for the group.

No task which Baba gave out was without an element of intrigue, and William's newspaper reading chore had its unique points. He was to keep 75 rupees with him, which Baba calculated would suffice to cover the purchase of a daily newspaper for two years.

Baba's directive regarding the newspaper process as relayed in Bhau Kalchuri's *Lord Meher,* Volume 10 states, "Donkin himself should go through the newspaper and cut out news items from it required for our purpose, in keeping with our New Life.

"You Donkin cut out such items and show them to me, and these after approval I shall give to the companions to read."

Baba expected William not to relay any political and world news to any of the other companions. Local items which may have borne on their travel plans were all that Baba was interested in conveying, according to the *Lord Meher* account:

"Donkin should cut out only news items relating to ... new laws, riots, curfews ... strikes, epidemics and so forth. Then forget what you have read and destroy the newspaper. This is Donkin's lifetime duty."

At one point during the journey, a discussion was held about possibly taking on camels to serve as pack animals. William admitted his experience with camels during his Sahara desert adventure before he met Baba. After this he ended up inheriting part of the care of these animals, although their stay was short when they proved too much of a nuisance.

The begging process for the companions in the morning followed a particular pattern. They usually got underway very early and would eventually notice smoke coming from the huts they passed, indicating the first meal of the day.

"On some such occasion Baba would send Eruch to those distant huts for bhiksha [charity] and then [ask him] to rejoin Him on the main road. Eruch's experiences of begging were pleasant and amusing too. He observed that those living in mansions were not large-hearted, but the village folk readily offered something from what they had."[116]

To meet expenses one day, Baba asked the companions for their watches so they could be sold.

"Every man took off his watch.... Baba, however, told Donkin [and two other companions] to keep theirs as they were often sent on outside work for which they would need their watches to be punctual."[117]

Baba always appeared to be trying to neutralize the sanskaras (impressions) that the companions were experiencing to keep inflated egos at bay. At one point after the group left Hardwar and were travelling to nearby Dehra Dun, Baba had occasion to admonish Adi Sr., his long-time mandali and secretary. Adi had arranged outside accommodations that were not to Baba's liking, and he had to accept the dressing down. In the course of the discussion, Adi described the food and railway fare arrangements he had made on behalf of the travellers, about which Baba expressed his gratitude.

Bal Natu offers his own take on this bit of psychology in his *Glimpses* series:

"Baba's sneering and cheering were equally significant. They were meant to free his dear ones from the binding snares of 'I did it.'"

The companions were undoubtedly learning as the New Life progressed and becoming more guarded in their responses to Baba's requests. Although they were following Baba's orders, they were also asked to treat him equally as just another companion. They soon got a chance to test this "equality" factor when Baba sought out a manager for the group to deal with the cooking of the food and other matters.

"Baba consulted Adi, Pendu, Eruch, Donkin, and Sadashiv, but each man declined ... convinced this innocent-looking dependence would in fact turn into a rope around his neck."[118]

William proposed the formation of a committee of managers, perhaps in an effort to keep the heat off any one individual. The idea was finally put aside when no one could come to an agreement. Baba must have felt that he was shouldering too much responsibility, for at the time he emphatically stated on his alphabet board, "You men fail to grasp that I really want to be free to look after other details for the New Life."

Despite the admonishment, Baba's sense of caring came through on many occasions, including on the road travelling toward Dehra Dun in early January 1950:

"During these long marches, Donkin tended to get very shaky after long periods without eating, but he never complained. Since the women always carried fruit and sweets ... one day when Donkin became so shaky he almost fainted, Baba went to the women and took an orange. He then walked all the way back to Donkin and gave it to him. Donkin immediately consumed it. Later he said it was a lifesaver."[119]

The group stay in Dehra Dun in a well-appointed bungalow owned by an English woman was not to be for long. Oddly enough, while at the bungalow, Baba, in another twist to routine, offered help to an English couple – the Angelos – who were having trouble getting out of India and returning to England. William provided financial help to the couple for their return home.

Baba, the women mandali, and at least two of the older mandali, including Dr. Abdul Ghani Munsiff, had made the last leg of the trip to Dehra Dun by train due to the strain of the New Life travels.

Other companions, including William, made the trip overland to get the various vehicles (bullock carts) and animals to Dehra Dun. The caravan encountered all types of difficulties, not to mention detours, in getting the vehicles and animals to the city. Mandali member Bhau Kalchuri's book *Meher Baba's New Life* outlines the problems encountered:

"Eight days after leaving Benares, Pendu, Donkin, Aloba, Baidul, and Sadashiv arrived ... with the carts and animals....

"The group was late ... because they took a shortcut. Caravan got stuck in the mud while crossing rivulet in a wild and secluded place.

"Then following Donkin's advice, they laid branches in front of the wheels to give the tires the same traction and the caravan eventually eased onto the road again, but now it was late evening."

Little did they know that on reaching their destination another surprise would come from Baba. A close follower, Bal Natu (author of the *Glimpses of the Godman* series and *Conversations with the Awakener* series), was not a companion, but offers a description of the New Life process and the hint of the major change that was coming for the companions:

"After reaching Dehra Dun, Baba thought of revising some of the conditions being followed by His companions in the New Life.

"They had passed through the phases of training, begging, and gypsy life. These phases had offered Baba's companions some objective lessons, which had helped them to understand their own weaknesses and merits. Everyone had enough experiences of the comforts and discomforts, the thrill and the fatigue of the New Life phase. This life had many surprises; some aggravating, some soothing. They had to pass through them all with considerable unconcern. Sometimes it was natural for them to feel depressed and dejected but they had to laugh it off soon – the sooner the better.[120]

The second phase of the New Life, enacted in Dehra Dun, brought yet another major shift in direction for most of the companions. Three new plans were introduced. In one, four of the companions were to return to their former homes. In the second plan (Plan No. 1-B), William and two older mandali were to settle in Dehra Dun, where William would open a medical dispensary and work as a doctor. The third group, which included eight Eastern disciples, would continue the New Life travels with Baba. All the original companions were to continue to live under New Life orders even if they were not physically accompanying Baba. The women companions would also no longer travel with Baba, and were to stay in accommodations near Dehra Dun.

On January 26, 1950, Baba spoke with Donkin about Plan 1-B. A bungalow had been located which would serve as a medical dispensary. Baba and the women were staying in a separate bungalow in the village of Manjri Mafi.

"Gustadji and Kaka, both in poor health, were eventually to stay with Donkin under his care. For the time being, however, they were at Manjri Mafi, and it was arranged that Donkin would pay 150 rupees a month for their food and lodging there.

"In this way, a provision was made in this plan to care for those who are elderly, ill, disabled, or destitute....

"In the late afternoon of the 26th, Baba, Eruch, Donkin, Nilu, and Vishnu went up to the open terrace of the roof of the ... bungalow to witness the magnificent view of the snow-covered peaks of the Mussorie Hills, lit by sunlight against a clear blue sky."[121]

Just after the late group's arrival, Baba again lauded William for how he had persevered on the eight-day journey bringing the caravan of vehicles and animals to Dehra Dun.

"Donkin showed the greatest courage, which brave-hearted men like Pendu and Baidul [Eastern mandali accompanying William] appreciated. Baba later stated that Donkin provided an example of love for Him in the New Life worthy of being followed."[122]

The shift in plans indicated that the journey to northern India had taken its toll on New Life companions. Of the women mandali, Mehera and Mani were not well, and Kaka and Gustadji, the two male mandali to be left in William's care, were unable to continue – one because of illness and the other because of old age.

It appeared that William was finally going to be able to practise medicine, and he was sent off on January 27 to Meherabad and Bombay to bring back supplies and purchase necessary medicines and equipment for the dispensary.

"Before stepping onto the Delhi Express, Donkin was instructed by Baba to carry out various other errands, which included going to Meherabad and Meherazad."[123]

An aside on William's frame of mind during the New Life is reflected in an observation made by Najoo Kotwal in her book:

"Baba ... informed Mummy that whenever Dr. Donkin came to Meherabad, she was to be in charge of his food. Mummy carried out Baba's orders religiously, taking great pains to cook three different items for each of Dr. Donkin's meals. But to Mummy's dismay, he would mix everything together in the plate before starting to eat. In those days he had a fiery temper, and I particularly remember one day when Mummy was five minutes late in sending his evening tea. When Hilloo [younger sister] and I delivered it to him, he took the mug, looked at his watch, and then flung the tea, mug and all, out the door. Frightened we ran to tell Mummy what had happened. Mummy did not seem disturbed; she just started to make more tea. And 10 minutes later, when Dr. Donkin came to her, she calmly said, 'Donkin, I have made your tea again, so please have it.'

"He started to sit, then gave a roaring laugh and hugged first Mummy, and then Hilloo and me before drinking his tea....

"Despite Donkin's temper, we found him very pleasant to talk to. Hilloo used to sit next to him when he had his meals and listen to all he said attentively, as he was very intelligent and interesting and often very amusing...."[124]

Others give similar descriptions of William's outbursts during much of his life in India. Such behaviour was certainly against New Life orders where one was expected to be cheerful and calm and to never speak impatiently or get angry with anyone. Perhaps William, being out of Baba's physical presence, was just letting off steam or his sense of decorum was falling by the wayside along with his ego.

Strangely enough, when William was away collecting supplies and doing errands, those remaining in Dehra Dun were not shy about discussing his welfare without him being present, and even talked about the viability of setting up the medical dispensary.

"Baba called all the companions in the hall at 6:30 a.m. to discuss the availability of Donkin's bungalow. Opinions of the companions were invited about sending a wire to Donkin to postpone or cancel buying medical equipment at Bombay on account of uncertainty of obtaining a suitable bungalow for Donkin to start his medical practice."[125]

After further discussion, it was decided to move quickly to find a suitable bungalow for William rather than sending him the wire saying the medical dispensary plan was off.

William returned to Dehra Dun on February 10 bringing woman disciple Naja from Meherabad to help look after Mehera and Mani as they recuperated from the New Life travels.

Common points in the various plans that the now disassembled companions were to continue to follow included not to touch any woman with lustful intention, not to discuss politics, not to create situations that would invite homage, and above all to remain cheerful.

In *Glimpses,* Bal Natu presses home the core ingredient of the New Life:

"In the New Life, Baba often stirred up the companions' emotions and then helped them to face their weaknesses. The plans and the many changes in the external aspect of the New Life were made by Baba to keep the spirit of the New Life [helplessness and hopelessness] intact.... "

Baba gave some timely advice at this time about remaining cheerful, which he said was a divine attribute that helped to make others happy.

"If you worry about yourself, God does not worry about you. And why should He? If you stop worrying, God has to begin to worry for you. Remember him wholeheartedly; leave your worrying to Him and be free to remain cheerful," Baba said through the alphabet board.

Years later in the 1960s, Baba's famous saying, "Don't Worry Be Happy," would adorn small cards and large posters and eventually inspire the popular Bobby McFerrin song. McFerrin would later say, "Whenever you see a poster of Meher Baba, it usually says 'Don't worry, be happy,' which is a pretty neat philosophy in four words, I think."

A cheerful disposition was certainly of major importance to Baba in regards to his followers, and in relation to the discomforts of grim and cold weather of the New Life, he said, "If you don't want to be old before your time, be cheerful in deed and word and in appearance – most of all in appearance. It is a divine art to look cheerful; it helps others."

William was taxed to the limit to remain cheerful when added to his other duties was the job of selling the menagerie of animals collected on the New Life to raise 5,000 rupees to help finance his new clinic. In the end, William was allowed to give away the cantankerous white horse.

Baba and the women New Life companions were settling into life at the Manjri Mafi bungalow not far from Dehra Dun. Naja, fresh from the outside world, became part of the household, but was ordered not to relay anything about her life in Bombay to the companions, in accordance with New Life orders.

William then turned his attention to setting up his dispensary. Again Baba seemed to relish the idea of heaping more responsibilities onto close mandali. Not only was William expected to look after the welfare of mandali members Kaka and Gustadji as leader of the Plan 1-B group, but all extra funds he earned at the dispensary were to be turned over to help support those living under the other plans, including the women disciples.

At one point William voiced his impatience and was "a bit peevish" about the slow progress in turning the bungalow into a medical clinic. Despite this glitch, great fanfare occurred on the day the clinic finally opened in late February, 1950. "Baba told all the companions to be ready by 2:30 p.m. to attend the opening ceremony of Dr. Donkin's consulting clinic in Dehra Dun.... Donkin invited Dr. Prakash, one of the leading physicians of Dehra Dun.... All helped Don in making the function a success.... Baba personally served sweets [rava, etc.] and tea."[126]

William was to be taught a lesson shortly after getting the clinic started. Another doctor and his office boy had a business up the street from William's dispensary, and the boy began dropping in on William at unusual hours to chat with him. One day, when William was told the boy was approaching, he said, "Tell him, I am out!"

"Almost instantaneously Baba seemed to appear from nowhere, and as he stood in the doorway, reprimanded

Dr. Donkin beginning with, 'Didn't I tell you that you had to be 100-percent honest?'

"Dr. Donkin defended himself by stating that this was only a little tiny white lie, as is often used in social circumstances. Baba insisted that there could be no white lies and Dr. Donkin must make up his mind whether he was 'in' or 'out' and act accordingly."[127]

Baba was in regular communication with Elizabeth Patterson in the West through letters he dictated through William, and at this point he was indicating he would make a trip to the West in the summer of 1950.

William also offered his own anecdotes in the correspondence on Baba's behalf with Elizabeth and Norina in South Carolina, as in this excerpt from his letter of March 10, 1950:

"As far as Baba's New Life goes not one of us companions can make head nor tail of it.... It is all a mystery, a mystery and again a mystery, and very difficult for those who are with Baba and those away from him.

"I went into Plan B [taking a temporary job] since that's what I felt Baba wanted me to do; but whether it is a frightful waste of money, I really do not know. Also I do not know, as you can realize, how long Baba will keep me at it, whether for a month, a year or a lifetime.... But as far as Baba himself goes, he is as adorable as ever....[128]

William had good reason to express apprehension about the viability of the medical dispensary. From the outset the clinic appeared to be run on a charitable basis. Baba followers in Dehra Dun were included in the patient list and Baba told William not to charge these devotees. On one occasion William treated an older woman, collecting only one quarter of the bill with the rest coming out of his own pocket.

Baba, however, did not appear concerned that William would turn a profit in running the clinic. One of his main concerns, according to a reference in the *Lord Meher* series, appears to be over the pressures that running the clinic put on William's own personal health.

"Don't worry in the least about earning money. If patients come well and good, and if they don't, don't be anxious about it. Don't economize regarding your food; eat well; and keep healthy and fit."

Bhau Kalchuri's account goes on to say that William had "wanted to help the companions financially and had originally thought of the idea of opening a dispensary for that purpose. But he experienced one disappointment after another. The sick would take advantage of his generosity and he continued to lose money."

Baba could still be a stickler for detail when it came to the clinic. There was to be an exchange of medical instruments – one in Baba's possession and one in William's – which did not occur to Baba's satisfaction. Baba pointed out that William had not kept his promise in this regard, but later forgave William and allowed him to keep both instruments. On the flip-side, Baba would continue to ask how William was feeling.

On one visit to Baba and the women mandali's residence, the toll the running of the clinic was taking on William was evident.

"After seeing the worried expression on Don's face, Baba observed that it was a sheer mistake on Don's part not to give up worrying about earning money through the practice, when he was repeatedly told by him that he should not worry about it in the least....

"In fact, it is quite true that Don has to practise his science with a meagre capital amidst unfavourable conditions. Being an Englishman; he is unknown to the people here and has no large circle of friends here to help him.

"Certain medical and personal requirements, urgently necessary, are not available to him. In spite of all these difficulties, Don has put his heart and soul into the work. When patients are wanting; he gets worried and restless. His one desire is to earn and help the New Life of Baba."[129]

Although William's clinic did show short spurts of success, its overall viability was failing as the weeks evolved. Positive reports in late March gave way to dismal reports by mid-April.

The overall ill health of the New Life companions had led to the adoption of the various new plans. Companions also noticed how Baba behaved differently from the Old Life, where he had always expressed concern over the slightest sickness of his followers; in the New Life he seemed unconcerned about their health.

Bal Natu's *Glimpses* series indicates that when the New Life evolved into the new series of plans, Baba took on a serious mood at the meeting to discuss the changes:

"Baba looked very solemn. He was curt in admonishing the companions for the slightest mistakes they had committed."

There was still strict adherence to certain New Life rules, especially the one which forbade the group from communicating with any Old Life followers or receiving any news from the Old Life.

The strictness of this particular edict was driven home when William received word that the mother (also a Baba follower) of one of the New Life companions had died in Poona. William conveyed the news to Baba and was chastised for doing so.

"Donkin ought not to have given me the news concerning people in the Old Life whom I have left behind," said Baba.[130]

The next day Baba cautioned William further, "From now on, do not give any news relating to anyone in the Old Life, even if someone has died. Do not inform me unless and until I ask you, if the occasion arises."

This rule would hit William directly less than a year later when his mother became very ill in England.

Changes were continuously afoot in Dehra Dun. It was decided to disband the colony and close the medical clinic. William, still determined to have a successful clinic so he could contribute funds to support other mandali, had proposed to Baba that it might be more prosperous to set up a clinic that he and Dr. Nilu would run in a more populated centre.

"Donkin ... suggested that if [Nilu] joined him as a doctor ... in a clinic on a large scale at Delhi, there seemed a good probability of maintaining the companions. Baba liked the suggestion and said that the idea would have to be kept pending till in future the companions had sufficient funds to establish such a clinic which would help to earn livelihood for maintenance of all."[131]

The Dehra Dun clinic was shut down on May 1, and it was decided that a medical clinic would be opened in Delhi starting May 10. In the meantime, Baba and the women mandali moved from the quarters they were occupying into William's abandoned medical clinic at 29 Lytton Road.

While William and Dr. Nilu were attempting to set up the Delhi medical clinic, Baba developed eye pains and the mumps, and both doctors were summoned back to Dehra Dun to tend to him.

At this time another curve ball suddenly appeared. Baba had borrowed 40,000 rupees from two followers with the assurance that another follower was selling two houses in Poona with 40,000 rupees from the sale destined to come into Baba's hands. Complications arose in this deal when the Baba follower who had offered the proceeds of his house to Baba changed his mind. Baba felt obligated to the two other followers who had fronted the 40,000 rupees. When the money did not come through, Baba decided to seek donations from Eastern and Western followers to pay off the loan.

It was suddenly decided William would travel to the West – England and the United States – in an effort to collect donations from Baba followers in those two countries. The amount Baba wanted raised was 50,000 rupees. The extra 10,000 rupees would go for work with the God-intoxicated, the mad, and the poor.

10

New Directions, Death of the Mind

Again, changes were made to the different New Life plans that the mandali were living under. William's Plan 1-B was scrapped altogether, but he was still to adhere to most of the disciplines in the plan. It is interesting to note that on several occasions throughout Baba's lifetime with the mandali, he gave them a no-strings option to leave him completely if they wished.

The latest change of plans indicated that Baba was making yet another effort to enact stringent New Life rules for a select smaller group, for he wanted to achieve more success with a smaller number of companions than he had in the initial 12-month New Life phase. Padri, one of Baba's long-time mandali, decided not to participate as a companion in the revamped New Life. Baba was disappointed at Padri's reluctance and also that the original New Life plan with the 16 men and four women had not held together. He seized the occasion to explain what he now saw as the evolving status of the New Life:

"I am trying my best to help you all as much as I can so that all of you may be able to stick to me till the end.

"There is absolutely no question of any tests and trials after all these years that you have been with me.

"It is a fact that the New Life is going to be difficult, hard, exacting, and in certain respects disastrous. It will be foolish on the part of anyone to presume that I will purposely create any situation or situations that will compel anyone to leave me.

"Why should I do that? For example, I could have easily asked Donkin to go to the West and do a particular duty to me there and he would have had no reason to be dissatisfied in doing that."[132]

It is notable that Baba not only appreciated but prompted humour throughout the serious tone of the New Life. The final words in the volume of New Life circulars were, "Appreciating the good humour and good cheer consistently displayed by the mandali, Baba once said, 'Thank God, we can still laugh.'"

The companion network was beginning to break up and leave Dehra Dun, and by the time July 1950 arrived, Baba had committed to spend a month in Satara in the middle of India, where he had had a mast ashram in mid-1947. Baba invited Kitty Davy and Rano Gayley to leave their teaching jobs and join him for a month in Satara.

A July 8 excerpt from Kitty's diary describes the reunion:

"Last evening Baba returned at 7:00 from Poona. We saw him for the first time in nine months. He was wearing a nice pink coat lined in white and looked so happy and lovely.... We all ate together that evening and Baba went early to bed. Naja and I cooked ... I read to Baba for an hour or so...."

The plan for William to start a medical clinic in Delhi gained little momentum. In fact, members of the group who had gone to Delhi suddenly embarked on a ghee (clarified butter) business. This business venture failed, however, and those involved were told to sell any equipment to help finance the colony that Baba was setting up in Satara.

Baba, like most New Life companions, was still suffering from ailments contracted during the demanding journeys. William was often needed to attend to these conditions. Kitty's August 1 diary entry gives further details on Baba's condition:

"Baba is not at all well. He is suffering from gastritis.... He is also much troubled with sinus, which affects Him and causes giddiness, and he is suffering from grittiness in both eyes. Evidently this year is a bad one for Baba's health."[133]

The topsy-turvy upheavals of the New Life continued when William was suddenly dispatched on his international begging trip to both London and the United States. The debt

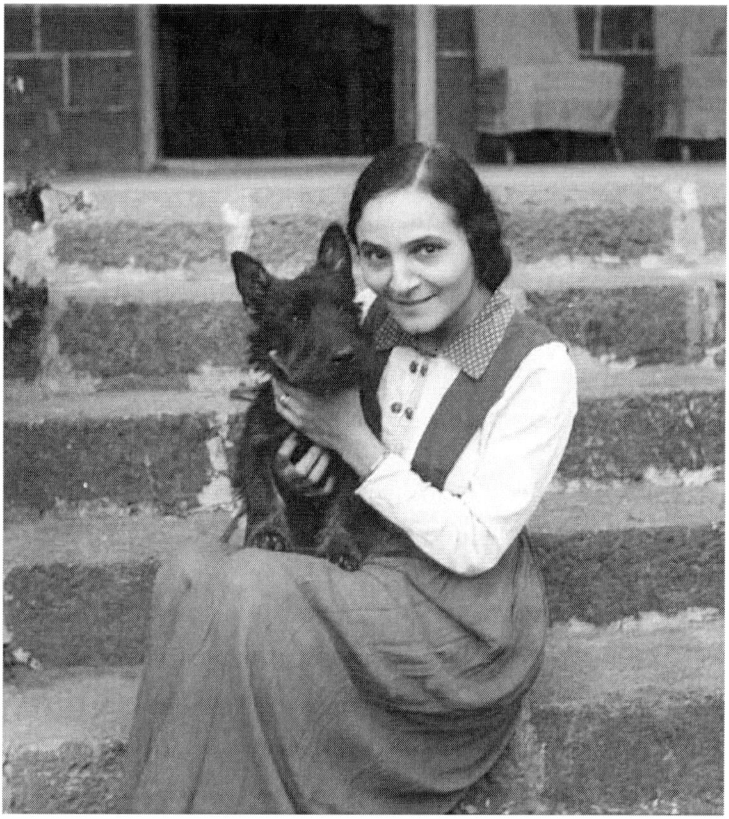

Mehera J. Irani, shown above with dog Cracker in Mahabaleshwar, was Meher Baba's chief woman disciple. Baba said she was the purest soul in the universe and loved him as he ought to be loved. The photo was taken on the occasion of meetings with Baba in Mahabaleshwar in late 1950.

Baba owed had to be repaid. Donkin was to try to raise this amount plus 10,000 rupees for the travelling expenses on his trip. William, as a Westerner, was the logical person to make the trip. His family connections in England would provide him with support during his stay there. William also received a small regular allowance from his family, which his mother had insisted be maintained when he went off to India in July 1939. A portion of these funds would have helped him make the journey.

On July 26 William left Satara for Bombay and flew from there to London on August 5, 1950. After a stay in England, he flew on to the US on August 26.

Bal Natu describes the effect of such sudden changes on those involved in the New Life in *Glimpses,* Volume II:

"This was ... the time when the companions physically endured much beyond their normal limits, and as such they had to face inner crises. Why did the companions choose to suffer and be with Baba? Because they had complete freedom to leave Him. A so-called free man shackled with rationality shall call this madness, but the liberated spirit of a lover shall regard this as a benediction. To learn the secrets of living a spiritual life, one has to know the art of dying to the past continually – an avenue leading toward the Eternal New Life."

While in Satara, Baba issued a general circular to all his Old Life disciples and devotees saying he would hold a special meeting in nearby Mahabaleshwar on October 16, 1950. This meeting marking the one-year anniversary of the start of the New Life would last from 7:00 to 11:00 a.m. and allowed the Spiritual Master to re-enter the Old Life for this short period. No one at this gathering was to talk to Baba about any of their Old Life affairs.

At the beginning of October, Baba left Satara and travelled the short distance to Mahabaleshwar, where he was to stay again at the Aga Khan's bungalow.

There were two main highlights of the October 16 meeting as described in *Glimpses,* Volume II:

First, "Baba asked forgiveness of God for not being able to live the New Life as He wanted to. He pardoned His companions for all their weaknesses and lapses committed in the New Life and in return He asked them to forgive him if He had done anything which had hurt their feelings."

The second event was Baba's Sermon, which William first read in English to the assembly on Baba's behalf. The sermon provides further insight into the teachings of Meher Baba:

> Being just now in the "Old Life" for these few hours, I will tell you what I feel to be the established Divine facts:

Essentially we are all one. The feeling of our being otherwise is due to ignorance. Soul desires consciousness to know itself, but in its progress toward this Goal which it cannot realize independently of creation, it must undergo the experience which it gathers as the individualized ego and which is all imagination. Thus it is faced at the outset with ignorance instead of Knowledge.

Dual forms and illusionary creations are the outcome of ignorance: birth and death, happiness and misery, virtue and sin, good and bad – all are equally the manifestation of this same ignorance. You were never born and will never die; you never suffered and will never suffer; you ever were and ever will be, as separateness exists only in imagination.

Soul undergoes experience through innumerable forms such as being king and beggar, rich and poor, tall and short, strong and weak, beautiful and ugly, of killing and being killed. All these experiences must transpire as long as the soul, though it is one in reality and undivided, imagines separateness in itself. When soul is bereft of the impressions of these illusionary experiences it becomes naked as in its origin, to become now fully conscious of its unity with the Over-soul which is One, Indivisible, Real and Infinite.

The soul becomes free of the binding of impressions through various paths. And Love is the most important of these paths leading to the realization of God. Through this love, the Soul becomes entirely absorbed in God, ultimately forgetting itself completely. It is then that all of a sudden Knowledge comes as swiftly as the lightning bolt which burns to ashes all that it falls upon.

This Knowledge uproots illusions, doubts and worries, and apparent sufferings are instantaneously replaced by everlasting peace and eternal bliss which

> is the Goal of all existence. Soul now free from its illusions, realizes its Original Unity of Being.
>
> Let us not hope, because this Knowledge is beyond hoping and wanting. Let us not reason, because this Knowledge cannot be comprehended or thought of. Let us not doubt, because this Knowledge is the certainty of certainties. Let us not live the life of the senses, because the lusty, greedy, false, impure mind cannot reach this Knowledge. Let us love God as the Soul of our Souls and in the height of this Love lies this Knowledge.
>
> The divinely Perfect Ones can bestow this knowledge on anyone they like and whenever they like. May we all gain this Knowledge soon."

At this meeting, William and 10 others agreed to continue with Baba as New Life servant companions. This group would not be part of the smaller group that Baba would soon choose to continue to accompany him physically on his New Life journey.

As 1950 came to a close, frantic activity appeared to be the norm for Meher Baba and his close followers. Shortly after the October 16 meeting, Baba set out on a one-month tour of other parts of India, despite his continuing poor health.

When Baba had returned to Mahabaleshwar, a small evergreen was dug up and decorated with handmade paper ornaments as well as a miniature cottage made out of cookies, icing, and sugar. Kitty Davy relates the Christmas 1950 celebration:

"There in the midst of the jungle in India, Baba had this wonderful surprise – a Christmas tree and wintry Christmas cottage! I can still see that sweet, gentle smile on Baba's face as He stood by it on Christmas morning. It was these small things, which brought forth Baba's not-so-frequent smile during this period when his suffering was acute."[134]

In the third week of January 1951, Baba and a few companions left Mahabaleshwar for Hyderabad. William did not accompany them on this mast/poor tour, for his doctoring skills were needed to help other followers who remained in

Mahabaleshwar. Baba at this time said that his servant-companions would remain with him only until June 10, 1951, indicating the strict rules of the New Life would be relaxed at that time. After this, Baba would continue his travels with only four close mandali members.

Activity within Meher Baba's global network continued at this time:

"A telegram arrived from Elizabeth Patterson in the United States in which she stated that there were some difficulties involved in Baba's proposed visit to the Myrtle Beach [spiritual] Center in 1951. Baba asked Donkin to cable back, 'Baba's plans are changed. Instead of leaving in July 1951, He will leave in February 1952. Do not worry and rest assured that Baba wants to come and stay for one year.'"[135]

Baba also announced later in February that he was entering a 100-day period of seclusion. Fifth-plane mast Ali Shah was also brought to Baba for a three-week period from February 15 to March 5. Baba began the seclusion period with a week-long fast, and after that he took only one meal a day.

During this time Baba had short gaps in his seclusion to see his mandali and close followers. Early in March, William encountered a personal dilemma that Baba dealt with directly. Bhau Kalchuri in the *Lord Meher* series describes the trial William faced:

"During this seclusion period Dr. Donkin received a telegram from London informing him that his mother was seriously ill. He did not tell anyone about it and appeared his congenial self. No one knew of it and, even if they had, no one would have told Baba. Donkin did not wish to inform Baba. On one occasion Baba sent for him and in the course of the conversation asked him, 'Is there any news from home?'

"Whenever Donkin got mail from the family in England, according to the conditions of the New Life, he would not open it. But on this occasion he read the telegram because he wasn't sure who it came from. He worried after that he had broken one of Baba's orders.

"After remaining quiet for a few moments in answer to Baba's question, Donkin said, 'Yes, news has come from home.'

"He could not tell a lie, so he acknowledged his mistake and told the news about his mother. Baba directed him to pack a suitcase and start for London immediately. On March 7, 1951, Donkin flew to London from Bombay."

This was William's second visit to London in eight months. These returns to the West must have been a true culture shock for him. They were perhaps also a time for him to step back and examine his life with and dedication to Meher Baba. William was free to walk away from Baba any time he wished. Baba would often say to his followers, "If you do not believe in me it is better that you leave me rather than hypocritically remain."

With his mother out of immediate danger, William returned a short time later to India and Mahabaleshwar.

The reasons for Baba's 100 days of seclusion were unfathomable to his followers, and the experience took a physical toll on him.

"This period was my first experience of seeing Baba so helpless and in such great physical pain," Kitty Davy would later write in *The Awakener* magazine.

Dr. Goher, a close women mandali, who served as one of Baba's doctors along with William and Dr. Nilu at the time, broke down in tears over his condition. Baba asked her why.

"She replied through her tears, 'Because we have done all we can and that has not helped.'

"Baba's reply to her was that it did not help him to see her so upset – that all was as it had been ordained, and our part was to keep cheerful and happy."

A later description of the seclusion process from Bal Natu sheds a little light on its purpose and the reason it was so taxing.

"At night Baba would spend a certain amount of time in complete darkness and another stretch of time in glaring light. [He may have indicated at the time that]... he was dealing with prevalent forces of darkness and the impending days of spiritual sunshine? Baba never explained the significance of this particular method of work which was adopted only once to accomplish the required spiritual results."[136]

Baba did indicate that a "revolutionary change" would be one outcome of the 100-day seclusion.

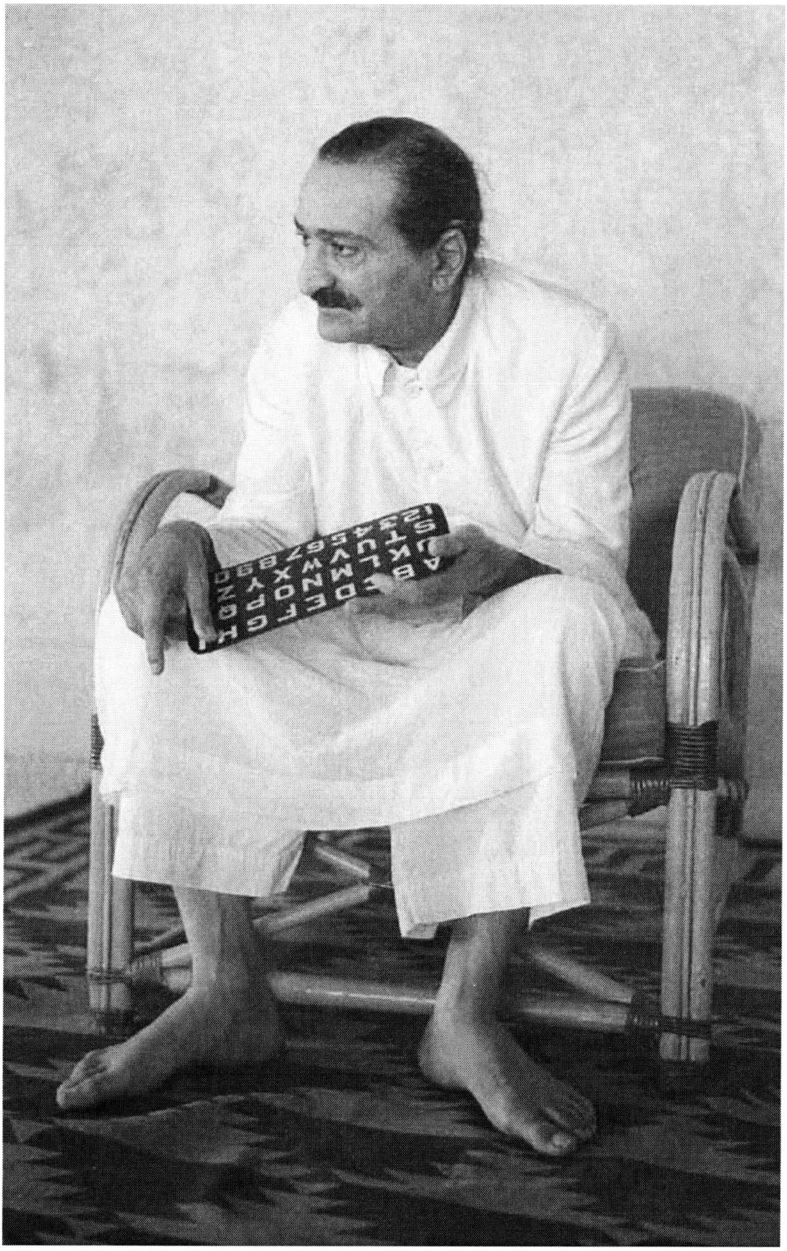

MSI Collection India

Meher Baba during an informal discourse session at Mahabaleshwar in the early 1950s. Baba and the mandali visited this rugged and lush area of India many times.

"God will, out of His infinite wisdom and grace, make me take a Step which will ring an extraordinary revolutionary change in my life and in the life of ... all those directly or indirectly connected with me."[137]

Baba's global followers encompassed a wide spectrum of the world's major religions. Baba held the essence of these religions in high regard, but was highly critical of the trappings and traditions which grew out of each as history unfolded.

Baba's followers belonged to 16 different world religions in the early fifties. On many occasions the Hindu, Muslim, and Christian followers were asked to recite the important prayers of their religions at Baba's public gatherings.

William almost always would be the one chosen to recite from the Christian tradition, including Baba's favourite writing, the Sermon on the Mount.

While Baba believed that a common thread of love, understanding, and brotherhood was at the heart of the major religions, he did not accept the external differences that had developed from the founding of the religions, as they led to conflict, strife, and even warfare. He saw the common thread in the words of Jesus, Mohammed, and Buddha, and considered these men human manifestations of God in different eras and different places.

Baba said his intention was to bring all of the world's religions together "like beads on one string."

In June 1951, Baba invited his followers to Hyderabad for a three-day gathering. On the final day,everyone gathered together with Baba to hear about the "God-determined Step."

The most important part of the "Step" was complete annihilation – mental and physical.

Dr. Ghani read out a number of points associated with the annihilation process. A time frame of October 16, 1951, to February 16, 1952, was to be adhered to. Baba invited any of his companions to join him in the process. He said he would have absolutely no responsibility and might have no concern whatsoever for anyone accompanying him.

Baba urged all followers who chose not to join him to hold fast to their love and faith in him. He said he would be pleased if only one or none of his followers chose to accompany him.

After the points of this new phase of Baba's life were outlined, William on behalf of Baba read out a declaration. In essence it stipulated Baba's commitment to the annihilation process.

Later the same day the group gathered for Baba's description of Manonash ([annihilation of the mind) – the most important aspect of this newest phase of his life.

Baba said initially he would be away for a four-month period and warned those who were considering going with him to seriously weigh the cost. No one who wished to join should expect any material or spiritual benefit from Baba; and those with him could face sleeplessness, sickness, and starvation.

In his explanation of Manonash, Baba said mind, which is chained to sanskaras (impressions), is the barrier to true realization. He said the human consciousness is really Infinite and Eternal, but for individuals to experience this original state, mind must go.

The discourses associated with Manonash are extensive and challenging. The personal interpretation that Western disciple, Kitty Davy, gives in *Love Alone Prevails* reflects a perspective she achieved years after the 1951 Hyderabad meeting:

"During this period, I did not give much thought to what Baba meant by His term 'Manonash' – the annihilation of the mind. It was not until many years later that my consciousness began focusing on the purpose and meaning of this important phase of Baba's work and I began recalling His various statements and explanations.

"On one occasion in the early years, Baba stated that He had come to bring about a revolution in man's thinking and that this change of direction in man's thinking was the slowest of all revolutions.

"At a later time, Baba gave a compelling discourse on the dual function of the mind. According to Baba, the first function of the mind is that of thinking, reasoning and intellect. What's known as the heart is actually the second function of the mind itself, with its emotions, feelings, creativity, and intuition.

"As I understand it, it would seem that the aspect of the mind that Baba meant by 'Manonash,' implies the breaking up of the mind's intellectual tendency, which has been gaining momentum for centuries and had reached its zenith – creating a separation at the expense of the mind's second function, its heart quality.

"The intellectual tendency of the mind now had to give way so that a oneness of experience could be created. To quote Baba, 'Do not listen to the voice of the mind. Listen to the voice of the heart. The mind wavers, the heart does not. The mind fears, the heart is undaunted. The mind is the home of doubts, reasonings, and theories. The heart when purified becomes the dwelling of the Beloved. Rid your heart of low desires, malice and selfishness, and God will manifest in you as your own Self.'"[138]

William's response to Baba on being asked to take part in the Manonash stage was short but decisive:

"Baba, my heart will go with you, but my body shall stay at Hyderabad."

The Manonash phase sounded as tough as or even more gruelling than the past New Life year of "helplessness and hopelessness" that Baba's companions had endured. It's a fair guess that many companions and followers, including William, were reluctant to endure more hardships. The direct companions on his past journeys especially had suffered. But Baba – living the same life along with them – certainly had suffered as well.

While Kitty Davy's explanation gave insight on the desired outcome of Manonash, the process was intricate and difficult to fathom for many. Baba explained the challenge in a discourse:

"The real goal of life is not the death of the ego but the death of the mind.

"When Mohammed or Jesus or Zoroaster talked of being born once and of dying once, it was of the mind [and not of the body]. When mind dies totally, the false ego becomes Real I [i.e., false individual ego is completely effaced and Real I manifests].

"In reality, ego is not born and as such it does not die. Ego [as witness consciousness] is always Real. It is only due to mind that ego acts and feels limited and false.

"Mind takes the body according to its good and bad impressions. Taking up and giving up of bodies [reincarnation] is not the mind of the ego taking birth or dying. Every time when body is discarded, mind survives, impressions remain. These impressions [sanskaras] press on mind to spend them by taking another body. So mind takes another body according to the impressions; ego witnesses. And another body, and another.

"While you are in sound sleep, ego, mind, and sanskaras are there. Sanskaras wake up mind. They say 'Go on, spend us.' Waking up from sound sleep is, in a way, an everyday birth for the body. When one body is left, another body comes up though there is a time lag between the giving up of one body, and taking up another.

"Mind exists even when a new body is not given to the ego; it is the mind-state of heaven or hell. But mind has to die while it is in a human body, retaining full consciousness. This is the goal."[139]

It seems that Baba's followers at the time, including Kitty Davy, were expected to digest the deliberations associated with the Manonash period and be open to a process. Manonash literally means passing out of the separate self (mind) to abide in God.

Bal Natu, trying to relay his own conviction of the Manonash phase stated in *Glimpses,* Volume II:

"Any Baba lover, as an ordinary man; may dare say that Baba out of his compassion for those who are ordained to the orbit of His Love, took on himself this additional binding [of Manonash] so that its consequent consummation could help His dear ones break the shackles of their minds to get closer to Him, in His own time.

"One has not to forsake one's rationality after coming to Baba. As long as one has a mind one is apt to have views whether to express them or not. However after sincere and honest efforts there comes a blessed moment when one cheerfully accepts one's inability to understand the hidden meanings behind the actions of the God-man and one totally gives in. Baba lovingly reveals a glimpse of Himself in the heart of such a person that quiets the mind. The more the heart is emptied of dogmatic interpretations, the more it is filled with the light of His renewing Love. Then the apparent contradictions and paradoxes do not bother such a lover. It is love alone that counts."[140]

Bal Natu also listened to Baba's explanations on various forms of meditation to achieve Manonash. After relaying Baba's discourse on meditation methods, at its conclusion he said in the same volume of *Glimpses*, "During this meeting Baba did not explain further regarding the path of meditation. But as this subject is of great interest to some seekers of God, I quote below some excerpts from a discourse which Meher Baba gave in later years:

"'The direct Path to God is the Path of Love. Love is not derived from meditation – it has nothing to do with it. Love is a grace of God. One in many has it, and it is all sufficient. Love does not depend on anything but itself. Love without meditation is enough – meditation without love is not.

"'That is why Sadgurus or Perfect Masters do not set meditation for their disciples as a necessary routine. Rather they stress the aspect of love and selfless service. The masters of the Path, on the other hand, not having reached the Goal themselves, advocate meditation to the aspirants following them.'"

William's commitment to his life with and love for Baba is reflected in an article he had published years earlier. Speaking of two paramount features of life with Baba, he wrote, "Of these, the first is the endless golden thread of His infinite Love woven into all His activities and orders, and the second is the vividness and freshness of His instruction.... There is no dusty bookish atmosphere about Baba's teachings; it is a living vibrant reality, which stirs every disciple to the very depths of his soul."[141]

Kitty Davy had the opportunity to ask Meher Baba directly on one occasion how one could successfully annihilate the mind. He replied, "It is only through the grace of the Master, through love. All you can do is to take My name and My love is always with you, helping you."[142]

Kitty said an important aspect which came out during Baba's Manonash and New Life periods was his ongoing reminder of man's need at all times for God. In her book Kitty related another comment from Baba on the meaning of love:

"Love has no limit, but the mind is in the way. This obstacle cannot be removed without My grace.... Only love for God works the miracle, because love is beyond mind and reason."

William's reluctance to physically accompany Baba on the Manonash phase doesn't appear to have sparked any guilt feelings with him. At least none have been recorded. He would have known at the time that many others shared this reluctance and the followers undoubtedly would have discussed Baba's proposition among themselves.

Baba himself was struggling with just who out of the final group of 15 he was going to accept into the Manonash phase. In the end Eruch, Pendu, Baidul, and Gustadji were chosen.

That life with Baba was a continuously changing experience is reflected in the fact that he would soon need William to work in another arena anyway. Plans were moving quickly for Baba's trip to the United States in February 1952, and William continued to be a key correspondent, keeping in touch with Elizabeth Patterson in Myrtle Beach, South Carolina.

Baba would have also indicated to William that he would travel to the US ahead of the main party to ensure everything was in perfect order for the group's arrival at the new Meher Spiritual Center.

As the fall months of 1951 approached, Baba was deep into his Manonash phase, which was to last until his planned departure for the US. The four chosen companions were given approval to accompany him on the Manonash journey.

Baba put great emphasis at this time on the symbols of the world's major religions, including a model of a church as a symbol of Christianity. Alabaster models of the symbols were actually made and kept in Baba's cabin along with pictures of the various human manifestations of God who led these religions. William became involved in reciting Christian prayers, while other mandali members did similar service for their own birth religions.

In November, Meher Baba ordered the women and men mandali, including William, to leave Hyderabad and return to Meherazad. Baba also indicated that he would conclude his Manonash period on Tembi Hill in Meherazad, which serves as a backdrop to his residential headquarters there.

Baba began his Manonash journey in mid-October and took five weeks to reach Tembi Hill (later called Seclusion Hill).

A sari dries on the grass in the foreground of Seclusion (Tembi) Hill, where Baba spent considerable time in seclusion late in 1951. William Donkin designed and cleared the first path up the hill overlooking the residential compound at Meherazad.

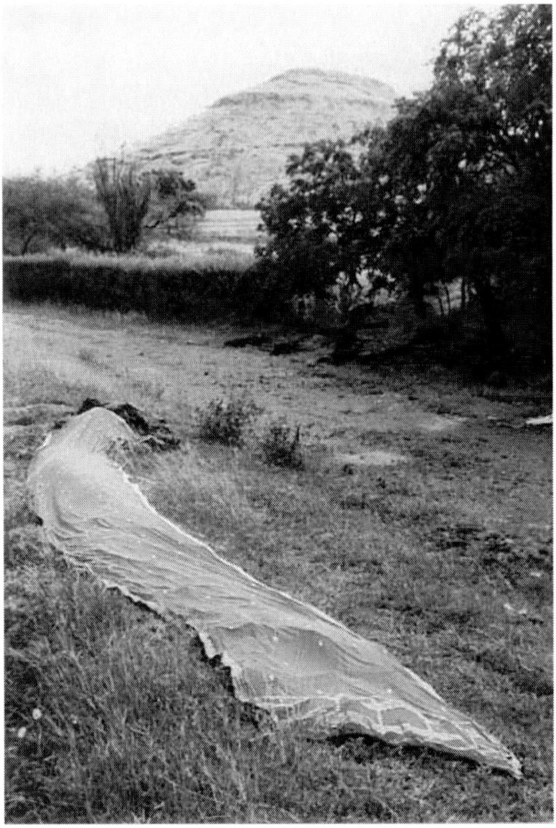

S of L

The departure from Hyderabad is recalled in Bhau Kalchuri's book *Meher Baba's New Life*:

"Adi Sr. and his assistant drove up to Hyderabad from Ahmednagar with two cars.

"As soon as Adi arrived in Hyderabad, the process of packing and loading the cars ensued, and when completed [a number of mandali, including] Donkin crowded into one car while the women occupied the other.

"Arrived the next night at Meherazad. Quite a surprise as when the companions set out in October 1949 they were told to give up all thought of seeing Meherazad again.

"As soon as Donkin was settled in, Padri enlisted him to clear a path for Baba and the companions up Tembi Hill, which was full of stones. Padri swept away the debris at the summit, where Baba planned to stay." Preparations were made to provide accommodation on Seclusion Hill for Baba. He had previously stayed on the hill for 13 days in December 1947. On November 13, he and his four companions completed the final 12 kilometres of the New Life journey and arrived at the base of the hill without passing through his residential compound adjacent to the hill.

Baba asked only to see Mehera and Mani briefly at the base of the hill before he ascended it. Baba stayed on the hill for three weeks. His four companions also stayed on the hill in tents, experiencing extreme heat during the day and taxing cold at night.

Baba asked that his followers try to contact a "pure being" to aid his work, and efforts were initiated to find a good mast, but none was located. After December 23 Baba relocated from the hill to a specially built cabin in the Meherazad compound. A mast was finally located and brought to Meherazad, where Baba spent a certain amount of time each day with him.

Baba continued to make use of the alabaster religious symbols. The five models were: a temple (Hinduism); mosque (Islam); church (Christianity); pagoda (Buddhism); and fire temple (Zoroastrianism). Prayers of the different religions were again recited, with William again delegated to read Christian prayers.

William undoubtedly was looking back on his New Life experience two years after it began. Close mandali Bhau Kalchuri provides insight into William's involvement in Plan 1-B:

"[He is] duty bound to serve the Beloved in caring for others. Dr. Donkin for example, at Baba's urging, joined this plan along with Gustadji and Kaka, both of whom were in poor health at the time.

"Baba appointed Dr. Donkin as head of the plan, and he became responsible for providing for them. To fulfil this role, he set up a medical clinic in Dehra Dun, and with the earnings, he maintained the three of them.

"The plan contains the model for an individual or a collective mode of life, which, as a way of serving the Beloved, provides care for the needy, the disabled, and the helpless. Its spirit is of selfless service to others.

"It becomes the duty of those in this plan to strive to serve the 'Beloved in others,' which is different from the service one finds in the world, where others are served as individuals. Although those in this plan are free to undertake other activities in their service to Baba, they are first duty-bound to care for others in some way, as in the case of Dr. Donkin, who took care of Kaka and Gustadji.

"This plan is quite flexible. It can be adapted, for example, to a household situation, in which several people may wish to join together collectively, whereas others may wish to carry out the plan individually.

"Both approaches can be accommodated simultaneously, each person concentrating on his or her own duties. For instance, although one person choosing the individual approach may work separately, he may decide to pool his earnings with those who are working together collectively in order to support a special project devoted to Baba."[143]

At this time, Baba also had a list of 124 "departed ones" read out to him – Eastern and Western devotees, 87 men and 37 women. The males started with Baba's father, and his name was followed by his childhood friend Dr. Ghani. The list of women included Baba's mother, followed by the Western women mandali Nonny Gayley, Nadine Tolstoy, and others.

At the end of January 1952, Baba lit the sacred dhuni (fire) to mark the end of the New Life. A circular (one of the New Life series) issued six months before the conclusion of the New Life had summed up this phase. In the circular Baba declared that the New Life would be kept alive by those

"Who live the life of complete renunciation of falsehood, lies, hatred, anger, greed, and lust; and who to accomplish all this, do no lustful action, do no harm to anyone, do no backbiting, do not seek material possessions or power;

"Who accept no homage, neither covet honour nor shun disgrace, and fear no one and nothing; by those who rely wholly and solely on God, and who love God purely for the sake of loving, who believe in the lovers of God and in the reality of Manifestation, and yet do not expect any spiritual or material reward;

"Who do not let go the hand of truth, and who, without being upset by calamities, bravely and wholeheartedly face all hardships with 100-percent cheerfulness, and give no importance to caste, creed, and religious ceremonies.

"This New Life will live by itself eternally, even if there is no one to live it."[144]

The above circular gave those who had been directly and indirectly involved in the New Life a barometer by which to judge their own standing in relation to the discipline involved. The statement also gave all those who followed Baba a blueprint for future behaviour.

11

Western Journey of 1952, Baba Sheds Blood

The dust was rarely allowed to settle around Meher Baba. William was extremely busy in January and early February 1952 planning Baba's journey to the United States.

William and Baba held daily discussions about the trip, even though Baba was in semi-seclusion up until he left for the West. William stayed at Meherazad rather than Meherabad to make the constant dialogue easier. Fellow Western disciples Kitty Davy and Rano Gayley were also staying there.

David Fenster relates in the book *Mehera-Meher,* Volume II, that "while helping with the details of the Western trip, Rano had to take some time off of this duty to undergo some minor surgery at the Salvation Army Booth Hospital in Ahmednagar.

"William at one point suggested that Rano travel ahead to America with him and have a post-operation check-up in the US, but Baba didn't go along with the idea.

"'What about me?' Baba asked. He apparently did not want to lose Rano's service in organizing the trip."

William's work included obtaining travel visas for the 15 devotees who would accompany Baba. On top of this duty he had to tend to the medical needs of the group and prepare himself to leave early for England and the US at the end of March, more than two weeks before the main party flew out of Bombay. The dates for the main party's departure were in constant flux.

It had been 15 years since Baba had been to the United States. The anticipation of Baba's visit is reflected in William's letter to "Elinor" [Elizabeth Patterson and Norina Matchabelli] before his own departure for America:

"Baba had so much work to do and interviews to give when he came out of seclusion on February 16 that I suggested it would be better to give Baba an extra 10 days before flying to America – in short, to change Baba's present provisional booking for March 31 to approximately April 10. Baba thought this might worry you and make you doubt that he meant to come. He therefore wants you to cable your approval of April 10th or your disapproval...."[145]

William immediately received this cable from Elizabeth:

"Baba asks whether the 10th of April suits us – anything! Everything suits us as long as he comes."

Baba issued a circular to his close followers in the West at about this time that outlined his intention to travel to the United States, England, and Switzerland. He stipulated that there should be no publicity associated with his trip to the West.

The departure date for the main party was shifted again to April 18 and complications were countless. Baba himself was ill, Norina had experienced a bad fall in Myrtle Beach, and Rano, whom Baba had asked to look after the main group during the journey, had fallen sick.

William stopped briefly in England en route to the US, but while there, received a cable from Baba reminding him to leave for the US by April 1.

The strains that Baba's demands sometimes put on his close disciples are reflected in William's family situation at the time. His mother Phoebe had died on March 25. William had been in England for her final days and the funeral, but was expected to leave quickly afterwards for the United States to help prepare the way for Baba's visit. He did manage to go on a short mountaineering adventure in the United Kingdom with his father, Sydney Bryan, before leaving. Baba's departure from India was not without some inner turmoil for mandali members who remained behind.

Eruch was one of Baba's main Eastern mandali, and Baba had asked him to make the journey to America. However, Eruch was exhausted from the New Life travels, as one who

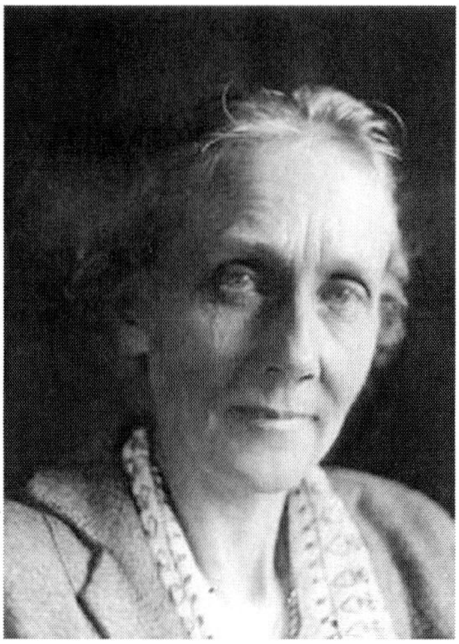
Donkin Family

Phoebe Donkin

stuck with Baba until the very end. He begged Baba to excuse him from the overseas journey on the grounds that he thought he would be useless because of his condition.

Baba was not pleased, but offered Eruch the alternative of travelling throughout India spreading Baba's message. Eruch was reluctant to do this, believing that he was not a good speaker. In the end, he agreed to the India alternative duty.

In a further complication to the predeparture turmoil in India, Baba insisted that the large travelling party go to Bombay a week before their flight was to leave. After shifting accommodation a couple of times to find somewhere suitable to stay, the group finally made it to Santa Cruz Airport in Bombay, where about 100 people saw them off as they began their two-day flight to the United States.

The flight would touch down in Cairo; Rome; Shannon, Ireland; and Gander, Newfoundland, before reaching Idlewild (now Kennedy) Airport in New York.

At the New York airport, following Baba's wishes, only a small group met them, which included Elizabeth Patterson, Margaret Craske, John Bass,* Delia DeLeon, and William.

Bass saw Baba for only five minutes after a lapse of 21 years, and related, "I felt such great Divinity in Baba's presence. I don't know how to describe it. It is something never felt before or afterwards. The feeling of Baba's terrific power and energy, at the same time a certain peace permeated....[146]

A train took them from Penn Station in New York to Florence, South Carolina. The trip to Meher Center from Florence

* John Bass was a Baba follower who lived in New York City. He was introduced to Baba in 1932 by Norina. He was an active member of the New York group until his death in 1970.

was made by car. When Baba arrived on April 20, his first stop was to visit the house that had been built for him overlooking a lake, the dunes, and the ocean beyond. Norina Matchabelli was waiting at the house to greet Baba, whom she had not seen for three years.

Other mandali members were put up in various cabins on Center grounds. Women mandali Mehera, Mani, Meheru, and Goher stayed in the Guest House cabin, which today is still reserved for women only. William was housed in the Caretaker's Cabin, and the remaining mandali stayed in other nearby cabins.

While Baba was planning to meet his close followers at the Center, he was already looking ahead to a cross-country road trip to California, as well as a stay in New York after his return from the West Coast.

William was, of course, drawn into Baba's various plans. He, along with Eastern disciples Adi Sr. and Sarosh*, were directed to Conway, South Carolina, to take the test to obtain their US driving licenses. William was also appointed to serve as the link for communicating with Baba's close US followers, who were all anxious to see their Spiritual Master. Ivy Duce describes her first contact with the India contingent after they arrived:

"The tremendous fluidity one has to have in connection with Baba showed up suddenly on the morning of May 6, when Dr. Donkin phoned that Baba wanted us to come down a day earlier. Charmian and I packed hurriedly and took with us Francis Brabazon from Australia and Enid Corfe**. We were greatly excited at the idea of seeing Baba again...."[147]

Baba's appearance was a shock to Ivy, who had not seen him since her visit to India four years before. Both Ivy and her daughter burst into tears, and Baba admitted, when they could not be convinced that he looked fine, that his frailty was linked to "the hardships of the New Life."

---

* Sarosh K. Irani was Adi K. Irani's (Adi Sr.'s) cousin. He met Baba in 1922. He was a businessman in Ahmednagar (Sarosh Motor Works and Sarosh Cinema) and for a while was Mayor of Ahmednagar.

** Enid Corfe was an Englishwoman who met Baba in the 1930s and stayed with Baba and the group at Portofino, Italy, in 1933 and in India in 1937. She was incarcerated in an Italian concentration camp during World War II, lived for a while in the US, and then moved back to England.

Other close Western disciples there to meet Baba at Meher Center included Darwin and Jeanne Shaw and their children, who had travelled down to South Carolina from Schenectady, New York. Darwin and Jeanne had met Baba in 1934. The couple was instrumental in the early development work at Meher Center, where Darwin served as caretaker for a period of time.

William continued his daily job of informing the various Western followers of their appointments with Baba.

William also became involved in an incident with Rano's relatives. Rano's "brother Clifford had been upset when Nonny [their mother] died in Bangalore, India, 13 years earlier, thinking that if Nonny had been in the West something could have been done to save her. Rano had asked [William] to write Clifford a letter explaining that they had done all they could medically."[148]

Rano had not seen her relatives in the US for many years and now was given the opportunity to reconnect with them. The circumstances for the reunion reflect the close and exacting relationship Baba forges with his disciples.

"Before the trip [to the US], Clifford had written demanding Nonny's ashes. Rano had been in tears that Nonny had to be dug up and taken back to America – but Baba had told her not to worry at all. She had brought the urn with her.... Now she asked Baba how long she could have to visit her family.

"'You decide,' Baba said. This was a quandary. If Rano stayed too long, Baba would have said, 'Oh, you want to be with them more than with me.'

"If she went only for a few days, the family would say, 'Why did you bother to come at all?'

"Rano had been in India for 15 years, so it was decided 15 days would be sufficient.

"Rano received another concession from Baba, asking that she be under no restrictions. Rano was afraid Baba might say no alcohol or impose some diet restrictions."[149]

Bal Natu in *Glimpses,* Volume III, provides brief descriptions of the encounters Baba had with various followers in the small Lagoon Cabin, which was built at Meher Center specifically for intimate contact with the Spiritual Master.

Communicating with Ivy Duce, Baba asked, "Ivy, do you love me? Will you stick to me to the end, at whatever cost?

"Yes, Baba," she replied.

Most of the interview with Ivy Duce dealt with Sufism Reoriented, as Ivy was the murshida* of the order. Baba gave her specific directions in regards to Sufism Reoriented:

"Listen very carefully, because for the first time I am taking a personal interest in Sufism. I am serious about the reoriented Sufism, and we must be so honest as to have its results appearing all over the world.

"There are three things that always hinder Truth. First is temptation – very, very few persons can overcome temptation; the temptation of money, fame, power, lust, leadership, are disastrous, very binding and very few escape it; second, vagueness about things; and third, dishonesty."

When Baba visited the US in 1952, he had indicated he would stay a year. Many followers who travelled to Myrtle Beach to meet him put their lives on hold for various amounts of time. Australian devotee and poet, Francis Brabazon, had travelled from his homeland. Although he may have expected to spend a long time with his Spiritual Master, Baba told him on their first meeting that he was to return to Australia before July 10.

William's role as a link to Baba's lovers was reflected in Baba's comments to Western women Filis Frederick** and Adele Wolkin, who were invited to come to Myrtle Beach for a week:

"I have heard so much about you both from Elizabeth, Norina, Donkin and Margaret [Craske], and I heard you from within. I feel so happy that at last I have seen you."[150]

Filis and Adele had stolen a peek at Baba when he and the group were boarding the train for Florence, in New York at Penn Station. Filis relates the story:

"We hid behind the big pillar high on the third balcony. Adele looked down:

---

* "Murshida" (or "Murshid" for a male) means spiritual guide or teacher, and is the title given to the head of the Sufi order.

** Filis Frederick first heard of Baba in 1943 from Norina Matchabelli. She first met Baba in Myrtle Beach in 1952. She was the editor of *The Awakener*, a magazine devoted to Meher Baba, and helped many young people who came to Baba from the 1960s on.

"'Oh there's Baba! And there's Mehera! And Donkin!'

"Though we were far away, Baba smiled, gestured upward and we were told later, spelled on the alphabet board what became our Baba signature – 'Filadele.' Of course He knew we were there. But I suddenly realized I was disobeying Him – none were to contact Him before Myrtle Beach. So I didn't look. I went home feeling very upset by my disobedience."[151]

Meher Baba was always an early riser, and his life at Myrtle Beach followed this pattern. He would leave his house at 5 a.m. and walk to the Guest House to breakfast with the women mandali. Then he would continue on to the main dining hall [Original Kitchen] to check that everyone was present. After a brief stop there he walked down to the beach with the women mandali only. On the beach, Baba walked some distance ahead followed by small groups of women who were busy gathering seashells – all trying to find the prettiest. On his return from the beach at about 9:30 a.m., Baba would then go to the Lagoon Cabin to commence his day of intimate meetings with individuals.

The days were not without periods of recreation and levity. Baba and others would often play croquet and groups would go rowing on the lake. Baba also encouraged the telling of jokes to lighten the more reflective moods associated with his meetings and spiritual discourses.

Bhau Kalchuri relays a light-hearted moment in his *Lord Meher* series involving William and English woman mandali Delia DeLeon, which occurred in April.

"Delia was terrified of snakes, and the Myrtle Beach Center was full of them and poisonous ones too. Being old acquaintances from London, one day Donkin played a naughty trick on her. He had killed a small snake; and coiling it up in a circle, placed it on Delia's plate covered with a white cloth. She was horror-stricken by the sight that met her eyes – but everyone else was roaring with laughter."

Baba would also often get involved directly in such antics. On the evolutionary track, Baba said snakes were stuck and would only advance if killed by a human, but insisted that the person take his name while doing so.

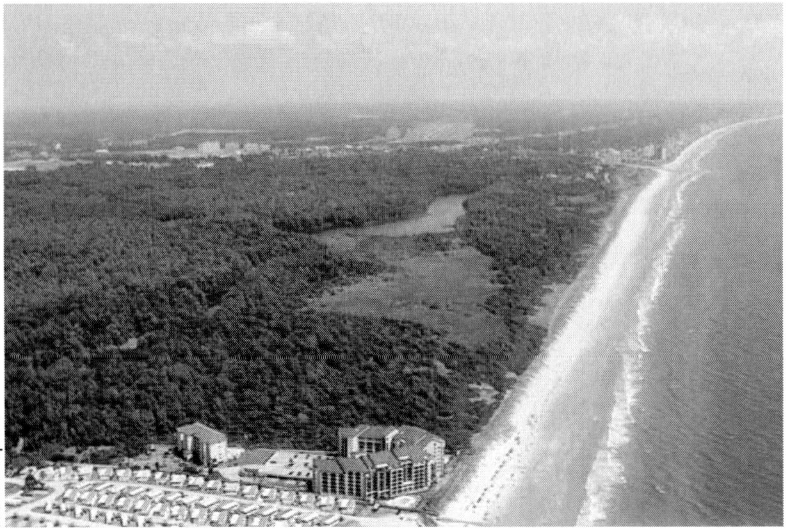

The 500-acre Meher Spiritual Center beyond the condominium complex was founded in Myrtle Beach, South Carolina, in 1944. Elizabeth Chapin Patterson and Princess Norina Matchabelli developed the property, which includes virgin forest, a number of lakes, and over a mile of undeveloped oceanfront. The property was designated a wildlife sanctuary in 1980.

A large group session was held at The Barn* when Baba visited Meher Center. The cypress-boarded structure was located between the central part of the Center property and the beach.

"On one day more than 1,500 people were invited to meet Baba briefly at The Barn. To speed up this process, visitors were handed a two-page mimeographed sheet titled, 'Baba explains:'

"Matters concerning His Silence, miracles, healing, and other topics were briefly touched upon. To quote one, 'God is not to be learned, or discussed, or studied, or argued about. God is to be contemplated, felt, loved and lived.'"[152]

"And another, 'The purpose of every kind of Yoga [search for Truth], Karma Yoga, Dynan Yoga, Raj Yoga, Bhakti Yoga, is

* The Barn was a mule barn that Elizabeth Patterson found in Conway, South Carolina, during the development of the Center during World War II. She had it moved to the Center and reconstructed board by board to be used for group gatherings during Baba's stays there.

to lose the limited self by forgetting that self through selfless service to others, through meditation, through love for God, and gain the unlimited self.'"

Baba wanted the large group of visitors to move quickly "to see Him, touch His hand, and pass on."

Elizabeth, sitting on Baba's right asked, "How can you help each when they pass so quickly?"

Baba answered, "If they linger longer, the mind begins to work and I want to touch the heart.

"There was a constant stream of men and women and children passing by. Some were deeply moved and left weeping, feeling Baba's divine love and compassion that shone forth from His penetrating eyes. Among the group were a number of black people, and it was remarked by those present that Baba always rose from his seat when a black person entered The Barn."[153]

Although only about 500 people actually met Baba in person through the invitation to the large gathering, many made major efforts to get there. Four dancers from the Metropolitan Opera in New York had learned about Baba from their instructor and long-time Baba mandali Margaret Craske. The group went so far as to charter a small plane and fly through a storm from Minneapolis (where they were on tour) to Myrtle Beach.

Although Baba had completed his meetings at Meher Center, the dancers – Loren Hightower ("Tex"), Zebra Nevins, Cathryn Damon ("Skipper"), and Sura Gesben – all were granted an audience with Baba because of the desperate measures they had gone through to meet him. Tex Hightower would later recall that the whole time Baba was expecting them, the dancers were flying through the storm. Hightower says Baba kept asking if they'd arrived yet, continuously returning his focus to them during the proceedings at The Barn.

The dance group flew back to Minneapolis in even worse weather. The plane had to land 60 miles from their destination and the remainder of the trip was made by car. The dancers not only missed rehearsal but a live performance as well, and their director immediately fired them. A higher manager at the theatre, however, later decided to keep them on.

The large darshan held at Meher Center on May 17 ended Baba's public appearances there and plans were soon set in motion for his road trip across the United States.

On May 19, 1952, William, along with four Eastern mandali, left in Elizabeth's Plymouth station wagon for the 3,000-mile trip to Meher Mount* in Ojai, California.

En route to California, William and his group received a humorous poem in a cable, which read in part:

"Avoid all temptation, and most of all lust,
Do not talk faltu [gossip] but of Baba, if talk you must
... I do not doubt you, but warn you in living faith and
trust."

A note was appended to the poem:

"Dear Don:

"Read this to the others. I want you all to feel assured that it is not doubt which makes me write this, but just that I was in the mood to send you a verse, and it is to avoid unnecessary complications unconsciously made.

"Baba"

The poem and note might have been timely in that suddenly William and the four other of Baba's close mandali found themselves on their own. They all knew, of course, that Baba would not allow sex outside of marriage, and they were also aware that Baba did not tolerate backbiting, which is often the end product of gossip.

On May 21, Meher Baba's main group packed two cars in Myrtle Beach in preparation for the trip west. Baba was to go in the Nash driven by Elizabeth Patterson. In the same car were Mehera, Mani, and Meheru. A second car, driven by Eastern man mandali, Sarosh, included Kitty, Dr. Goher, Rano, and Delia.

---

* Meher Mount is a property at the top of a mountain in Ojai, California, that was acquired by Jean Adriel and Alexander Markey and dedicated to Meher Baba. Agnes Baron lived there and was its custodian for many years.

The two-vehicle convoy stopped at Columbia, South Carolina, the first night; a small town near the Tennessee border the second night; and in the Ozarks on the third night.

Elizabeth, driving the lead car, recalls the May 24 morning:

"It had rained the night before and Route No. 64 was slippery, oil-slick.

"The shoulder of the road was not wide and there were ditches on either side. As we came up over the crest of a small hill a car came along driving on the left side of the road, going at a good clip.

"I started to slow up. The car continued without slowing up right at us on the left side of the road.

"At any instant I expected him to turn ... at the last instant he saw us and put on the brakes, whirling around and taking up the entire side of the road. The point of contact was my bumper which made him whirl all the more."[154] Delia DeLeon, travelling in the second car, describes the accident when she came upon it:

"Baba, Mehera, and Meheru had been thrown out of the car and injured.

"Baba and Mehera were the most seriously injured, Mehera with head injuries and Baba with a broken leg and arm.

"Elizabeth, pinned behind the steering wheel, was also badly hurt with broken arms, wrists and ribs. But Mani, who had been sleeping, seemed unhurt and so were the occupants of the other car.

"Horrified, we rushed to the spot and I recall so vividly the extraordinary expression on Baba's face – His eyes not seeing the immediate, but far away....

"He was bleeding freely on the ground. I had with me a little pillow and I gave it to Sarosh to put under Baba's head ... so it became stained with His blood*."[155]

Ironically the dentures William had coaxed Baba to get before leaving India caused one of his serious injuries. Baba wore the dentures only reluctantly and often only the upper or lower one alone. At the time of the accident the lower denture cut deeply into his upper gum, causing a deep wound

* The unlaundered, blood-stained pillow is on display in a Plexiglas case in Baba's House at the Meher Center in Myrtle Beach.

in the gum that afterward made eating and drinking difficult and painful.

Luckily the small town of Prague, Oklahoma, was just seven miles from the accident scene, and the injured were quickly taken by ambulance to the medical clinic there.

Those travelling in the second car immediately began contacting other Baba lovers across the United States, in India, and elsewhere in the world.

William and the men with him had already reached California. William was asked to fly to Oklahoma right away to help. The rest of the men mandali were to follow in the car.

"My God!" [William] declared. "They'll never get there. Adi doesn't know the route.... They'll end up in Alaska."[156]

Finding a seat for William on the airplane at the last minute was difficult, but Agnes Baron, who ran Meher Mount in California, told the airline that "a very important person" had been injured and was waiting for his personal physician.

Mandali member Sarosh also contacted Ivy Duce and her daughter Charmian, who came immediately, as did Margaret Craske, who came from New York.

Kitty and Rano stayed at the medical clinic to help Dr. Ned Burleson* treat the injured while other members of Baba's group took up residence in a nearby motel.

On her arrival, Ivy Duce helped Delia begin sending out cables to all those who would want to know about the condition of Baba and the others.

"Kitty Davy could not be pried away from the room where Elizabeth and Mehera were, except to take a quick bath in the adjoining bathroom. She stayed at her post night and day, stretching out on the floor between the beds in the middle of the night for a short while," said Ivy in her book *How a Master Works*.

The scene at the medical clinic and the demands on Dr. Burleson must have been stressful. His thoughts described later in *The Awakener* magazine are indicative of the situation:

---

* Dr. Ned Burleson ran a clinic about seven miles from the accident site. He treated Baba and the injured women mandali there. Fifty years after the accident, the Avatar Meher Baba Heartland Center was established, comprising two properties, the Burleson House and the Morrison House next door.

"When I finally got around to attending to Baba, I was surprised to see an individual who was injured as badly as he was, still smiling.

"I was also astounded to find he did not speak a word or make any sound denoting discomfort. I assumed that he could not speak, but was informed soon that he did not speak because of a wilful act."

The doctor said the most attractive quality about Baba was "the way he would look at me with those big brown eyes as if he were reading my mind."

Continuing with the magazine article:

"Later I determined that the most astounding quality was that something which made it possible for him to receive such profound devotion and loyalty from so many fine and educated people.

"The quality cannot be forced. Such devotion can only be possible because he deserved it or earned it."

Dr. Burleson referred to Mehera as the beautiful young lady with the "worst" skull fracture he had ever seen.

William and the other men mandali began an exhaustive routine of attending Baba each day and overnight at the hospital. Mehera's injuries were much more severe than Baba's, and there was genuine concern that she would not survive.

"Goher was all the time coming and telling Baba about Mehera," said Adi Sr. "Mehera's condition was hopeless. Every doctor was pessimistic.... Baba was so much concerned about Mehera. When Goher talked to Baba about her, we were not to be present. There was no talk about Mehera in front of us. No thought, no sight, no topic about her in our presence."[157]

Plans of course took a major turn because of the accident. Baba immediately asked Ivy Duce to go to California to explain his inability to meet with those waiting for him.

William's medical specialty in orthopaedics was suddenly drawn upon with Baba's broken bones. The condition of Baba, Mehera, and Elizabeth did eventually improve enough to move them back to South Carolina.

On May 29, Dr. Burleson sent a cable to India to quell concerns there:

"Irani family all doing well. None will die, none will be permanently disabled. We shall send them home to you ultimately as well as when they left except for their unhappy experience."

William and Rano flew from Oklahoma to the East Coast. There, Yaupon Dunes, Elizabeth's house in Myrtle Beach, was prepared for Baba and the others for their convalescence.

After 12 days in Prague, Oklahoma, the group left for South Carolina on June 4. Some travelled by car, but Baba, Mehera, Kitty, Goher, and Elizabeth travelled the 1,500 miles in two ambulances.

When Baba arrived at the Yaupon Dunes house, an incident provoked him that indicated that only the body was injured, but not his, at times, tenacious nature.

Adi Sr. had waited with William at the house for Baba and the others to arrive in the ambulances. But before Baba arrived, Adi had gone off somewhere leaving only William to greet Baba and the others. Baba was furious at Adi when he showed up later.

"Unable to control his temper, Adi retorted loudly, 'I will get on a plane and return to India this afternoon, if you want!'

"'You should have been here," Baba berated him. 'You should have waited.'

"Adi responded, 'but how am I to know the exact time of your arrival?'

"And so it continued…."[158]

The incident showed that Baba continued to use turmoil to bring deep-seated emotions to the surface, and also indicated that Baba sometimes got back as good as he gave. Although in the end Baba came out boss and all was forgiven.

Another incident, also revealed in the *Meher-Mehera* three-volume series, showed the toll the accident had taken on Baba and his close ones.

"While Mehera was gradually improving, Mani was having her own problems dealing with her anguish, so evident in the letter she wrote to those in India:

"'Without having much physical injury, except for a hurt knee,' she admitted, 'I suffered terribly within – seeing Baba's suffering, seeing Mehera's suffering, finding that I hadn't a share in it. I was feeling very down, depressed.'

"One day when Mani was in Baba's room, he noticed her downtrodden state. 'What's the matter with you? Your cheeks are gaunt. There are dark circles under your eyes. Don't you sleep?'

"Usually the women never see the men, but that day Baba told Rano to summon William. William came in, but did not look at Mani, and she did not look at him; William looked at Baba, and Mani looked at the floor.

"'Look at her,' Baba instructed him. 'She is black under her eyes; her face like this (Baba made a frown). Do something about the bags under the eyes. Give her a nice tonic and some pills to make her strong.'

"William made no reply."

"'Didn't you hear me?' Baba asked."

"'I heard you Baba,' he said, 'but no amount of pills or tonics will help her. What she needs is rest and a change.'

"Baba looked at the others and remarked, 'He's mad. I've always said so. I said to give her tonic and pills, and he talks of irrelevant things like rest and change. You're a barber not a doctor!'

"So William prescribed vitamins and a tonic. It did not help Mani at all. On the contrary, it meant more work for her. Baba told her to take the pills at 8:50 a.m., 10 minutes before breakfast, and the tonic 20 minutes after lunch at noon. This was in addition to the other small orders which Mani already was observing every day.

"'It was more meditation on Baba,' Mani explained. 'It's almost nine; I must remember to take my pills. Then Baba asked, "It's 12:20 have you taken your medicine?"'

"I would rush to take it. I had to be watching the time always, ... Baba would ask .... It resulted in more work."

Kitty was in charge of cooking and feeding the group at Yaupon Dunes. Eastern mandali Sarosh drove her to town each day to fetch groceries, and William continued to apply his medical skills to help in the recovery of the injured.

Baba was driven at one point to the hospital at Duke University in Durham, North Carolina, to check on his injuries. Baba and Mehera, who was also to be examined, travelled with Dr. Goher in an ambulance, while a car carrying William, Mani, Meheru, and three Eastern men mandali followed.

The pot always boils with Baba, and an Eastern disciple later relayed to Ivy Duce an incident at the Durham hospital:

"The doctor who was in charge wouldn't let anyone spend the night with Baba. Sarosh protested, 'But someone has to spend the night.'

"Even Dr. Donkin wasn't allowed, or Dr. Nilu, although they were both physicians. The doctor said, 'It is hospital policy that no one can spend the night with him. This is our policy and it is going to be strictly adhered to.'

"When this was related to Baba, he said, 'I'm going to leave. I am not going to stay here.' The mandali said, 'Baba, you can't! You're in serious condition and the doctors say that you must stay here for observation or until you get better.'

"So Sarosh went to the doctor and said, 'Look here – I know what your rules are, but you know that this is a Spiritual Master who always remains silent. And if you do not let one of us stay here, what happens if he gets ill and dies and no one can understand what the problem is? If he can't explain to them what it is that pains him or what he needs, then the hospital will get a bad name and it could be condemned severely by others for it.'

"The doctor thought it over and replied. 'You know, I am going to make an exception in this case. One of you may spend the night with Meher Baba – but only one at a time.'"[159]

Although the large cast on Baba's leg was replaced with a lighter one at the hospital, this one caused itching. It was removed at Baba's request, and the leg wrapped in a supporting bandage, before the group returned to Myrtle Beach.

While recovering in Myrtle Beach, Baba was also in touch with Ivy Duce and put the final touches on Sufism Reoriented. In one note that Baba wrote to Ivy, he said, "Sufism Reoriented is fundamentally based on enlarging the concept of Sufism and making it all-embracing for the nature of its knowledge and practice – yet maintaining the original value of Sufism...."

In another letter to Ivy, he wrote, "I want you to be certain that Sufism Reoriented will be bereft of the Mohammedan aspect to become universal instead....[160]

Elizabeth Patterson, who was still recovering, began to receive messages through Mani from Baba each day regarding upcoming plans, although for a month after the accident Kitty estimates Elizabeth saw Baba only twice.

It was at this point that Kitty received a hint from Baba that her life was to undergo a major shift in geography and service.

"I recall being in Baba's room when, out of the blue, He announced that someone was needed to stay in Myrtle Beach and help Elizabeth and Norina. [Elizabeth would be convalescing for months, and Norina, who was expected home from the hospital, was recovering from a severe heart attack and nervous exhaustion].

"The choice, according to Baba, was between Rano and myself. Baba turned to me and asked if I would be willing to remain and not return with Him to India. Without hesitation I said, 'Why, yes, of course, Baba.'"[161]

On urgings from his followers, Baba agreed to make a brief stopover in New York before taking the overseas flight to England. Prior to his departure on July 14 to New York, William had been working with Baba on gradual load-bearing exercises for his recovering leg so that he would be in better shape to meet his followers in New York and the UK.

Before Baba went north to New York, a number of his Western followers had already left for England, including William, who was to ensure arrangements for Baba's visit to England were in order. Another reason for William's early arrival in England was to consult with an orthopaedic surgeon he knew there about Baba's injured leg. Margaret and Delia also returned to England at this time.

An acquaintance of a Baba-lover in New York offered the group the use of her home at 14 Cohawney Road in Scarsdale for their two-week stay in the area. Ivy Duce maintained an apartment in New York, and it was here that Baba met many new people as well as his long-time followers.

July 18–20 were the heaviest days of darshan. Despite Baba's injuries, he was radiant as ever when welcoming people. Bal Natu describes the scene in *Glimpses,* Volume III.

"During the interviews a simple sentence from Baba, sometimes just a broad smile, a handshake, or non-verbal gesture, would convey to each visitor His love and personal concern."

July 19 was the first time that Don Stevens* met Baba personally. Don would go on to write a number of books about Baba, and was also instrumental in editing Baba's classic *God Speaks,* which would be published in 1955.

Before leaving Scarsdale, it was made clear to Kitty that she was going to serve Baba by helping Elizabeth and Norina at Meher Center in South Carolina. To help soften the impact this had on Kitty, she was allowed to accompany Baba and the women mandali to London, where she stayed for a short time with her parents before returning to the US.

Baba and his party flew from New York on July 31, 1952, and lived at the Hotel Reubens for their six days in London.

Ivy and Charmian Duce also made the trip from the US to England to spend some time with the group in London. Ivy relates a Keystone Kops** type of incident that occurred when the Eastern men mandali failed to turn up at the hotel.

"She [Rano] checked at the desk and was informed that they had not come in the night before.... By then we were all scurrying about trying to find out what had happened. Baba sent Rano and Donkin out in a car...to see where they were. A number of phone calls were made. Baba was being very funny about the whole thing, because he would alternatively turn around to Delia and say, 'It's all your fault!'

"Then it was Rano's fault, and Donkin's fault, and the girls' fault, and the mandali's fault. Then it became Baba's fault, and lastly it was God's will."[162]

The men mandali were finally located. They had ended up going to Delia's flat in Richmond and found out from her brother what hotel Baba and the others were staying in.

Nothing remains smooth for long with the Avatar, however, and true to form Baba continued to use various events to alter and/or crush the egos of his followers. Charmian Duce recalls another uproar:

* Don Stevens (1919–2011) was a retired oil company executive and member of Sufism Reoriented. He assisted in editing Meher Baba's books *God Speaks* and *Discourses;* narrated and edited *Listen, Humanity*; and is the author of *Meher Baba, the Awakener of the Age* as well as several small books related to Baba.

** Keystone Kops were the focus of a series of silent film slapstick comedies about an incompetent group of policemen.

"Even though the Reubens Hotel prided itself on the service they offered – the lunch fare was offered at certain times other than 'Avatar time.' William and Kitty were dispatched to find something for the group outside of the hotel.

"Alas, Baba wasn't pleased with what they found. The fish was too dry; the soup was too weak. So we ordered tea all around. But that led to a debate, refereed by Baba, as to whether we should have bread and butter with the tea. Meanwhile, we discovered the luggage was all mixed up. It was chaos the entire morning, but eventually everyone got fed ... and everything calmed down."[163]

On his London arrival, William had immediately contacted Dr. Reginald Watson-Jones, a well-known orthopaedic surgeon, to discuss Baba's injured leg. On August 2, William and Dr. Goher accompanied Baba to see Watson-Jones. The doctor advised that Baba should start regular load-bearing exercises on the leg in a week.

While in London, the group also attended a number of entertainment outings that Delia arranged. "Margaret [Craske] had given me some money to get tickets so that Baba and the girls could see a few shows while in London. So I booked several, including the musical *South Pacific* (at Drury Lane Theatre); *Ranch in the Rockies*, an ice-stage musical (at the Empress Hall); and *Sweet Madness*, a comedy starring Richard Attenborough (at the Vaudeville Theatre).

"Baba came to each one. William sat with him. When we went to *South Pacific*, we women sat upstairs in the circle; Baba sat downstairs. They really enjoyed it."

While in London, William managed to visit his family briefly. Little is known about these early visits William made to Winterfold, the family estate in Surrey.

While the family knew of his wartime service in the India Medical Service, they were told little about his life with Meher Baba. Conversations when he was at home usually focused on matters related to his extended family in England. By the early fifties, his twin sister Mary and brother John had both married, and William had a number of nephews and nieces whom he enjoyed. His oldest brother Bryan remained a bachelor

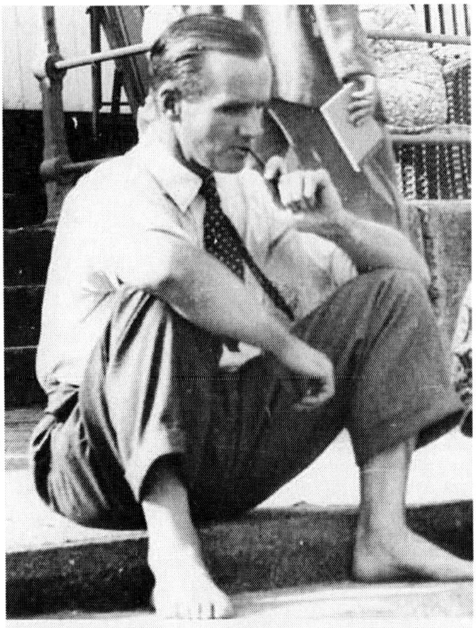

William managed to join other family members for a brief holiday at Frinton On Sea when he flew back from the United States to England in August 1952 en route to Switzerland. He is shown here alone in a reflective pose; enjoying a swim; and with his nieces and nephew and brother-in-law George Mathieson. The youngest Mathieson child is in the pram in the background being coddled by two aunts.

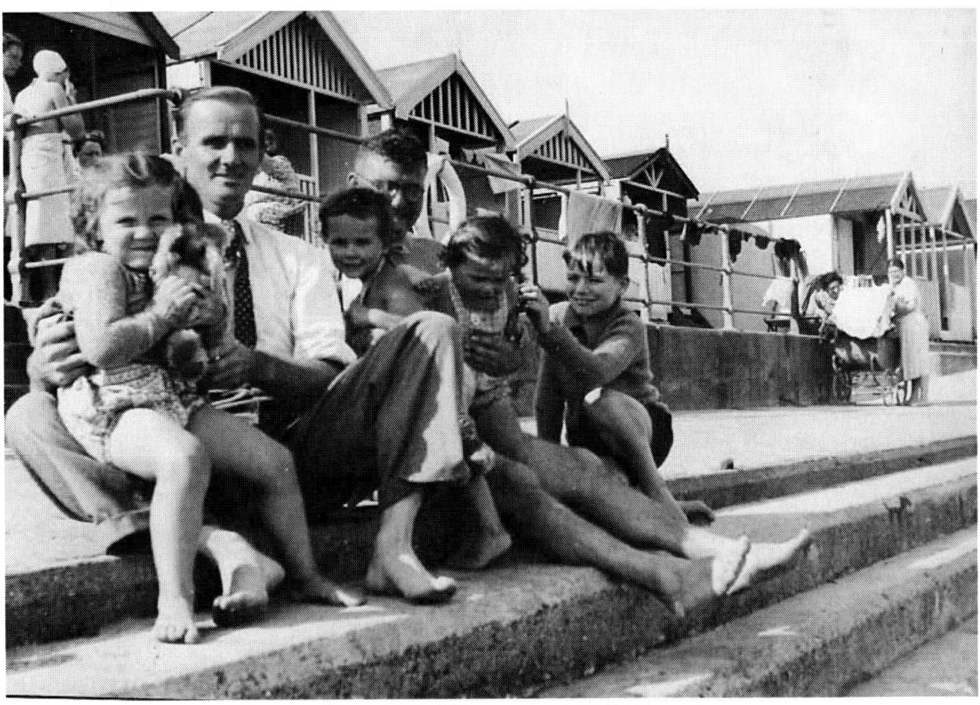

William's twin sister Mary probably took this seaside group photo.

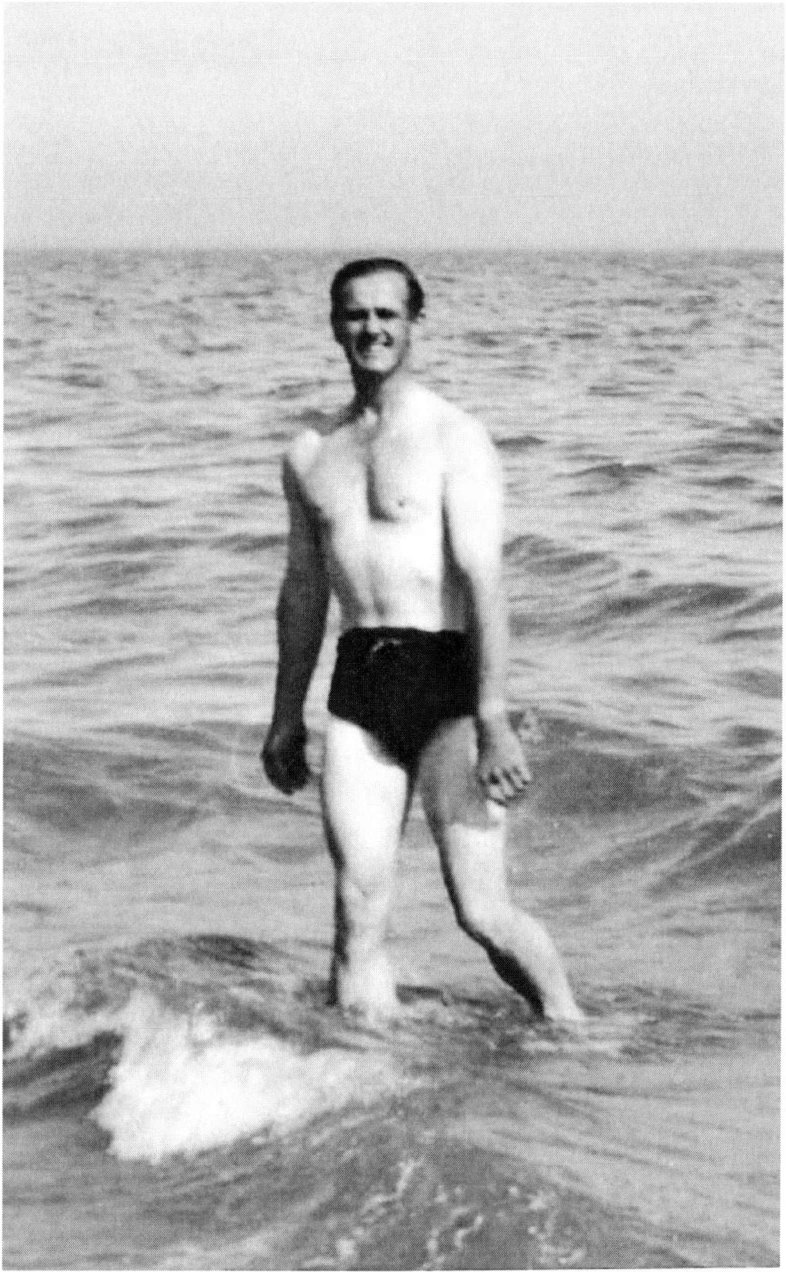

Donkin Family Photos

throughout his life. Any mention William made of India to the adults involved mainly stories of travel throughout his adopted country. For the most part the family thought William was simply working as a doctor in India.

Kitty Davy remained in London for five days to visit her brother Herbert, whom she had not seen for 16 years. Later on her way back to Myrtle Beach, Kitty stopped in Montreal, Canada, to visit her sister May, whom she had not seen for 25 years.

Another odd incident occurred when the party was to be transported to the London airport for the flight to Switzerland. Ivy drove the car containing Baba and Mehera. William drove his small sports car with Sarosh and Adi as passengers, and Rano, Delia, Goher, Meheru, and Mani followed in a taxi.

Ivy discovered she could not find the starter button for the car. Suddenly Rano, Mani, and Goher were rushing up the street to stop the men in William's sports car and ask them to come back and help. Before William arrived back at the car to help, Mehera's head had to be covered with a blanket as per Baba's order that she not see any men – an odd scene indeed. William finally was able to point out the starter to Ivy and the group proceeded to the airport.

Such oddball occurrences appeared to be a regular part of life with Meher Baba. Never a dull moment might actually be an understatement in describing these episodes, through which egos were being whittled down in various degrees. As Ivy Duce relates, "It is funny that when you are with Baba, even though you may protest violently upon occasion at an action, you will still realize the necessity of things going the way that they do.... As I have said before, Baba always picks the time when you are most exhausted and worn down to jump on you."[164]

Irene Billo met the group when they arrived in Switzerland on August 6, 1952. They drove in a number of vehicles to Locarno in the south of Switzerland, where Baba and the women mandali were put up at the home of Hedi Mertens,* another Swiss national and close Baba disciple.

---

* Hedi Mertens was a Swiss artist who was friends with Norina. Hedi and her husband Walter met Baba and became devoted to him when they hosted Baba on his visit to Switzerland in 1932.

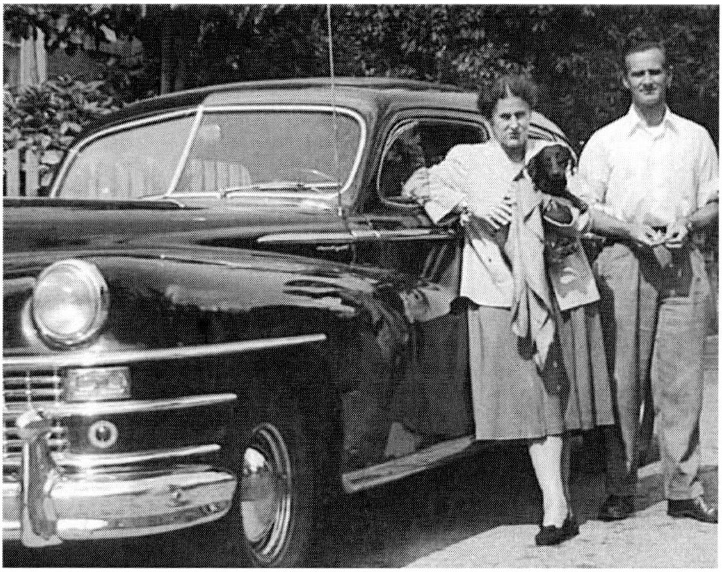

MSI Collection India

William Donkin and Irene Billo stand beside the car that Meher Baba used while travelling through Switzerland on his visit there en route back to India. The large car would have provided comfort to Baba and Mehera, who were recovering from injuries sustained in the Oklahoma accident.

"One of those permitted to visit the Eastern women at Locarno was Anita [de Caro] Vieillard,* someone whose company Baba always found amusing. Anita too had injured her arm and was wearing a cast, and she and Baba compared casts.

Anita came daily and took the women shopping and sightseeing around town. Before the Prague, Oklahoma, accident the original plan had been for Baba and the women to stay with Anita in France at her husband's family house in the country. The group had obtained French visas in Bombay before departing, and William had even stopped in France on his way to America to explain to Anita how to prepare for Baba's visit."[165]

* Anita (de Caro) Vieillard was an artist who met Baba in the 1930s. She married Roger Vieillard, a tennis champion from Paris. Roger also became devoted to Baba after meeting him when asking permission to marry Anita.

Another Swiss family, the Haefligers, were also close to Baba. Max Haefliger, although sceptical about Baba, read and was fascinated by Charles Purdom's book on Baba titled *The Perfect Master*. In July 1950, when William had been sent to London to raise funds to pay off the debt incurred in India, he had stopped in Switzerland en route, and Max Haefliger had contributed some money to the cause. William's visit had proved an ideal time for the Haefligers to learn more about Baba.

"This unexpected meeting deepened Max's link with Baba and he felt drawn closer to Baba, the Perfect Master. He was also much impressed by Donkin, whom he regarded as a perfect gentleman and a highly cultured Englishman."[166]

William's visit to the Haefligers had also fulfilled another mysterious purpose. He delivered a book called *Der Jungste Tag*,* written by Paul Otto Hesse. The translated title is "Doomsday" or "The Day of Judgment." Supposedly William had been acting on Baba's orders in delivering the book to the Haefligers, but the purpose was never explained.

On this visit to Switzerland, Baba thanked Max Haefliger three consecutive times for the donation he had made in 1950 during Donkin's visit. Although all appeared amiable in 1952, Haefliger would soon face a major upset in his life with Baba.

The Swiss stopover mainly provided Baba with an opportunity to rest. A local masseur came to the Mertens' house to massage Baba's arm and leg. William helped Baba with walking and weight-bearing exercises and efforts to get used to walking with crutches in the garden adjoining the house.

After a week in Switzerland, the Eastern men mandali who were accompanying Baba were sent back to India. William was the only male mandali member who remained to help Baba. Delia DeLeon, who had accompanied the group from England, also returned home to London.

An Air India strike a week later stymied the efforts of the remainder of the Baba party to fly to Bombay. They made the

---

* *Der Junste Tag (Judgment Day or The Last Day)* was a book published in 1949 by Paul Otto Hesse, which described the author's mystical revelation that after much destruction, there would be a significantly smaller world population that will be brought together in oneness, guided by "the Word" or inner voice.

trip from Locarno to Geneva hoping to fly out from there. This proved impossible and William was immediately called on to lay alternate plans.

In the process another uproar evolved. Shortly after William had been dispatched from the hotel to arrange visas for a new flight through Cairo and Karachi, word came through that the original Air India flight was back on.

But now William was inaccessible somewhere in the streets of Geneva. Rano and Charmian Duce were sent from separate locations to find him. The persistence of the search is reflected in the comments Rano heard when she visited one consulate:

"If anyone inquires again about this Dr. Donkin, throw them out!"

Charmian eventually located William at the British Consulate. He had not been successful in obtaining visas, and on his return to the hotel he learned that the Air India flight was on again.

In what would be a test to anyone's aggravation meter, Baba sent William and Rano out again on a fresh search to get six seats together on one flight. They were told wherever they went that this was impossible and couldn't be achieved for at least a week. William eventually gave up, but Rano persisted and eventually was able to get six tickets on an Air France flight, which would get them to India through connections in Paris and Karachi.

In the book *Mehera-Meher: A Divine Romance,* Rano says of the incident, "If you do your best, Baba always takes care of things." Rano never teased William about her coup in getting the tickets. Much later in her life she offered her opinion of William:

"You never crowed over Don. He was sensitive and had a dry humour. He was very nice; I enjoyed his company. But he had idiosyncrasies, like locking himself in his room once, when I had a message for him from Baba."

Charmian (Duce) Knowles relates another event that occurred when she was dispatched to pick up William in downtown Geneva. She was to use a Fiat Topolino – perhaps the smallest car in the world.

"I squeezed myself in and looked around; nothing was where I expected it to be. Nevertheless, I got it going and headed off downtown...." After a labyrinth experience on the streets of Geneva and dirty looks from a policeman direcing traffic, Charmian finally located the American Express office to pick up William.

"The Fiat was so low to the ground that when I looked out the window, I saw Dr. Donkin's feet and his legs up to his knees. Then I noticed there were three more pairs of legs! Not only was our six-foot Dr. Donkin there, but also Sarosh, who was even taller, plus two of the other men mandali.... Led by the intrepid Dr. Donkin, they crammed themselves in like luggage. We looked like one of those circus acts where numberless clowns stuff themselves into a miniature car."[167]

Charmian's mother Ivy was very astute when it came to assessing situations involving the different personalities of those associated with Meher Baba. Her opinion on William's fragile state during the airline ticket chase in Switzerland provides insights into the breaking points of close mandali members.

"I suspect that all this pressure and activity may have had a good effect on Dr. Donkin in keeping him grounded to earth.

"Having been with him daily during our first trip to India [January 1948], I found him greatly changed when he came to the Myrtle Beach Center in 1952. He seemed rather withdrawn and preoccupied. Even Mani remarked that maybe Donkin was becoming a mast.

"Although he was by nature a strong and very talented man, dedicated to Baba and the medical profession, I wonder if sometimes he was not indeed rather lonely, being the only [male] Westerner living among mandali from totally different backgrounds.

"There were a few times when it seemed that this strong mountain-climber was pushed to the brink of his capacity.

"Charmian witnessed a small scene in Switzerland upon entering Baba's room.... The doctor declared that he was through, that he could go on no longer, that he was leaving.

"He walked to the door and opened it. Just as he got through the door Baba indicated that he should be called back. One of the mandali simply called, 'Don!'"

"Donkin turned and Baba said, 'I want you to wheel me down the hall.'

"Don came back obediently and automatically guided Baba's wheelchair to where Baba wanted to go, and the incident was closed."[168]

William was not alone is facing trials living with Baba. An August 1952 letter from Rano Gayley to Kitty Davy, who at this point was living in the United States helping Elizabeth run the Meher Center in South Carolina, reflects her own anguish:

"I feel very much alone – Baba either finds everything I do wrong or ignores me completely. I don't understand what it is all about, but I hope I can bear up under it all ... I never seem to do anything right, just as in London. Well, be that as it may, I must grin and keep my chin up....

"All I can think is that Baba is trying to make it as difficult for me as possible, so that I need not feel too cocky at being with Him – or else my ego has too much of a capital "E" and needs more squashing."[169]

Baba's followers were not indisposed to share their feelings with each other. Charmian Duce, before her departure from Switzerland back to the US, posed intimate questions to both William and Rano about their relationship with Baba:

"I asked Donkin, Rano..., 'All of you are quite close to Baba and have been with him many, many years. How do you think it has changed you? Did you expect it to? Has anything happened? Have you gotten all sorts of evolution behind you?'

Charmian recorded the answers she received from these intimate followers, saying that William and Rano basically gave the same answer:

"Well as far as we are concerned, we've noticed a lot of changes. Our tempers aren't as bad as they used to be. We don't do a lot of the things we used to do, which were annoying. As far as our cognizance of our own evolution or anything like that is concerned, well, it just doesn't exist."

Charmian got right to the heart of the matter in asking "What are you here for?"

William and Rano replied, "Well we are just simply here as tools. A hammer doesn't have to know it's a hammer to strike a blow! People criticize us because we're not perfect, but we're not necessarily supposed to be perfect, because if Baba uses us for tools with which to set patterns for the world – or for his own purposes, whatever they may be – the world isn't perfect, and if we are supposed to represent it in any small way or on any scale, you can't expect us to be perfect.

"We have to represent what the world is like, or at least enough so for him to use us as different kinds of people from the world and as different expressions of things in the world.

"He can utilize the way we bring those things out, whether it's our anger or hurt [about] something, whether it's love, annoyance or anything else....

"Baba teaches us through living situations."

Charmian continues to offer her own take on these "living situations." In a passage in her book, *How a Master Works,* her mother Ivy writes, "He ... uses [situations] to teach lessons and bring out such better portions of us as we may have, and he also uses situations to disperse or bring into focus, so that they may be dealt with, such portions of our egos or being as might elude or hamper our involutions toward God.

"By ego I am referring to the 'false ego,' the ego which may cause one being to smite, hurt, hate, or injure – verbally, mentally, or physically – another human being...."

Charmian says further that, "Baba has always said that most of us are not evolved enough to complete our involution toward God-realization by the path of love, since it is the hardest way, considering human frailty, but that we could do it through the path of obedience, which one can swear to a Perfect Master."

Charmian stayed on in Switzerland for a few days before travelling to London and the United States. As Rano said to Kitty in a letter at the time, "Delia left on the 20th for London. Charmian was staying till the 26th then returning for a one-week stay in London. I think Delia is putting her up – she has gotten a glimpse of life with a Master not being a bed of roses."

12

Fiery Free Life, Darshans, Failing Health

Baba and the main group of followers finally arrived back in India on August 13. William, however, did not fly back with the group.

William apparently stayed on in Switzerland for a period of time, but was back in Meherabad on August 31. Baba asked that Adi Sr., Nilu, and William give an account of their trip to America and Europe to those who had remained in India during the four months they were abroad.

After the account, Baba said of the close ones who had accompanied him on the trip, "I found my mandali at their best ... and also at their worst!"

Although Mehera and Mani may not have known it at the time, they would never leave India again.

On Baba's return, he immediately wanted a report from his two Eastern mandali – Eruch and Pendu – about the tours through India the pair had taken on Baba's behalf for five months. Eruch outlined the various places the two men had visited, and after hearing the report, Baba said he wished "to visit many of the locations personally now, both to conduct mass darshans and to contact masts."

Many people whom Eruch and Pendu had contacted on their tour had read the book *Avatar*. American Jean Adriel* had

---

* Jean Adriel was one of the first Americans to learn of Meher Baba in 1931. She helped make the arrangements for Baba's stay at the Harmon Retreat outside of New York City on his first visit to America.

written this account of Meher Baba's life up until 1947, the year it was published.

Bal Natu in his book *Glimpses,* Volume III, says that on these tours the two mandali members were surprised at the response they received from people who had never even met Baba.

"For anyone's heart to awaken to Baba's love, a meeting with Him in person, in the gross world, is not essential. For that matter, all those who had Baba's physical darshan, although benefited spiritually, did not necessarily become Baba's lovers. The Avatar's outer physical contact, either with individuals or with the masses, is only in relation to His inner spiritual work, which is carried out on the different planes of consciousness, unknown and unnoticed.

"But coming to Him is an internal process. Baba as the God-Man resides in each heart. From within he draws us to Him so that we can finally see Him as He should be seen, instead of just seeing His physical form with our gross eyes. The outburst of love for Baba and the acceptance of Him as the Avatar of the Age by the people of Hamirpur and Andhra before having Baba's darshan testifies to this."[170]

Baba's Oklahoma injuries were still giving him pain and discomfort on his return to India. William tried his best to find solutions that would alleviate the suffering. He accompanied Baba to the hospital in nearby Ahmednagar for diathermy (heat treatment) and also was trying to get an appointment with a surgeon in Poona. The diathermy treatments intensified when William took Baba daily to a military hospital in Poona. He and Baba stayed for two weeks, returning to Meherazad on October 1.

Plans were underway to hold mass darshans in India during the final months of 1952, and 300 men were called from across the country to Meherabad to discuss the future gatherings.

At this time Baba, true to form, put a name on this phase of his mission– the Fiery Free Life. This phase had two aspects: one, impersonal, known only to Baba; and the other, personal, involving mast work, work with the poor, and mass darshans.

A special letter was presented to Baba's devoted followers giving them an opportunity to offer their money, property, service, or lives to Meher Baba.

The number of people who had become dependent on Baba had grown, and he remarked at one point, "How can we manage with so little money for so many people wanting to stay with me?"

After tallying the response to his letter, Baba observed with a wry smile, "It is easy to offer one's life to me, but it is extremely difficult for one to part with one's money."

Bal Natu relates in his book "that after receiving all the replies, Baba did not accept money or property even from those who wanted to give these to Him."

This was a tactic that Baba often employed. He would make a difficult request of his followers and then not require them to fulfil the request. The manoeuvre was used mainly to test his followers' love and obedience.

William continued to accompany Baba to the hospital for more x-rays of his leg. While Baba's other injuries from the accident in the US had healed, his left leg and arm were still giving him a lot of pain. A consulted doctor suggested that Baba practise walking on an uneven surface, so he began regular weight-bearing exercises under William's supervision at Meherazad.

By mid-October, Baba was able to walk independently with the aid of two canes.

Putting his health problems aside in November 1952, Baba, taking 25 followers with him, chose to embark on 35 days of mass darshans.

"Despite the pain and suffering which the accident had caused him, Baba sought out different people and visited many towns and remote villages.

"He traversed forests and hills, crossed rivers and streams, often going to places where no vehicle had ever been before. Wherever Baba went, crowds of people received him.

"They came on foot, horses, bullock-carts, and camels. In fact some said they had been waiting for several years to see him.

"Baba washed the feet of several poor people wherever he went and he bowed down to them and gave them money in gratitude, for he said that the poor were sharing the burden of the spiritual upliftment of humanity and were a great help in his work."[171]

All the while that Baba was in India, he kept in close contact with his followers in North America and Europe through letters and a series of Life Circulars.

Rano Gayley had taken over from William in writing letters on Baba's behalf to Kitty Davy and Elizabeth Patterson in Myrtle Beach. Those letters, as well as the Life Circulars, would be shared with other North American Baba followers. Kitty Davy describes the importance of the Life Circulars in her book *Love Alone Prevails*:

"His life depicted in Life Circulars is what pertains to His lovers in an act of settling them into the life of selfless service, love of God and an indomitable faith and courage to fight the battle of life. It does not provide material means of satisfying desires but gives inner strength to overcome desires with an affluence of conviction and generousness of heart."

The Life Circulars contained various other instructions. Followers were often asked to fast and maintain silence for short periods of time and to repeat the name of God most familiar to them audibly on specific occasions for one hour a day.

The orders were always to be carried out through one's ordinary everyday existence. Baba always insisted that his followers adhere to their responsibilities and not seek escape from the wheel of life. True liberation and God-realization, he said, should be found within the total fabric of life and not through escape to some perceived ideal situation or environment. He did, however, recognize and recommend retreating for periods of time to places where renewal and reconnection to the spiritual life could be achieved. The Meher Center retreat in Myrtle Beach, South Carolina, was established mainly for this purpose.

Just prior to the departure on the mast darshan tours, Baba brought a large group of male followers together in Meherabad for several days.

A large pandal (awning) was erected at Meherabad to provide shade and protection for the gathering from November 1 to 9. Trains carrying male followers from the north and south of India arrived at Ahmednagar and buses came from Poona.

At one point during the first day Baba asked all assembled to repeat one of the names of God from the world's major religions "quietly, in a very low voice, and think that God is within you and is listening to you."

Sacred scriptures were read from four different religions, including Christianity.

Baba's daily interactions with his followers were often carried out using three languages – English, Hindi, and Marathi.

William was usually called on to recite the English version of prayers, and it was during this period that William first read the Prayer of Repentance – one of two main Baba-related prayers* still recited to this day.

The prayer indicates what Baba expected of his followers :

The Prayer of Repentance

We repent, O God most Merciful; for all our sins; for every thought that was false or unjust or unclean; for every word spoken that ought not to have been spoken; for every deed done that ought not to have been done.

We repent for every deed and word and thought inspired by selfishness, and for every deed and word and thought inspired by hatred.

We repent most specially for every lustful thought and every lustful action; for every lie; for all hypocrisy; for every promise given but not fulfilled; and for all slander and backbiting.

Most specially also, we repent for every action that has brought ruin to others; for every word and deed that has given others pain; and for every wish that pain should befall others.

In your unbounded mercy, we ask you to forgive us, O God! for all these sins committed by us, and to forgive us for our constant failures to think and speak and act according to Your will.

---

* The main Baba-related prayers are the Master's Prayer (sometimes called the Universal or Parvardigar Prayer), which Meher Baba dictated in Dehra Dun on Thursday, August 13, 1953, and the Prayer of Repentance, dictated by Baba in Kuldabad in November 1951.

William recited this prayer in English on many occasions late in 1952. At one gathering, Baba bowed down to four of his mandali members, including William, while he read the prayer.

Baba depended on William each time he wanted the prayer or any new message related to a particular phase of his life read in English.

William recited two more explanations on the heels of the *Prayer of Repentance* that reminded followers that suffering was a part of the journey to God-realization, and that Baba's status had shifted to that of a devotee himself, to the point that he insisted on visiting the tombs of three Perfect Masters with whom he had a connection. These Masters were Sai Baba, Upasni Maharaj, and Babajan.

Consultation with the London orthopaedic surgeon, Dr. Reginald Watson-Jones, continued through the fall of 1952, as new x-rays of Baba's left leg were sent to him in England. Baba, whom William once described as a "terrible patient," kept constantly on the move during this time period, apparently oblivious to the extra strain the travels placed on his injured limb.

On one occasion in early November, Baba insisted that the mast Ali Shah be brought to him when he visited Meherabad. Baba had just given up the use of his crutches and wanted to bow down to the mast, despite concerns from his mandali. Dr. Nilu carefully supervised the occasion, and Baba was successful in touching Ali Shah's feet with his forehead.

Bal Natu, who visited Baba during November 1952, relates a discourse on anger that Baba delivered at this time to his followers:

"'These days I try not to get angry or excited. Whenever I am about to, I remember the words of Christ and say in silence, 'Get thee behind me, Satan.'

"'So, whenever you find that thoughts of lust, greed, jealousy, anger, money matters, or family matters possess your heart, say silently [as did Jesus], 'Get thee behind me, Satan,' and be at peace.'"[172]

While most of Baba's 35-day tour was restricted to smaller towns and villages, he reluctantly agreed to visit Delhi to meet with 3,000 students at a Sikh college. He delivered the following message to the students:

"India has gained its national freedom. Let us now try to gain our Spiritual Freedom beside which every other kind of freedom is a binding....

"The purpose of life is to realize God within ourselves. This can be done even whilst attending to our worldly duties. In the everyday walks of life amidst intense activities, we should feel detached and dedicate our doings to our Beloved God. Enough has been done to make people food-minded. They must now be made God-minded."

William's time with Baba during late 1952 appears to have been sporadic. He went on some of the tours, but Baba did not include his name among the large group of male mandali in his party. William was also very busy trying to find a way to alleviate the pain Baba still experienced in his left leg. This quest undoubtedly taxed his belief in himself (i.e., ego) as an orthopaedic doctor, particularly when he often saw how the leg pained Baba.

The orthopaedic surgeon in London who had viewed the latest x-rays on Baba's leg said that the bones had not set as well as they should have. In *Glimpses,* Volume III, Bal Natu conveys Baba's response on hearing the discouraging news:

"What the surgeon writes is true. In addition, it seems that the local doctors are unable to say why I have a fever. They think that it might turn into anything! But in spite of whatever the doctors and the surgeon state, I will carry out the programs the way they have been chalked out."

The tours took place during late 1952 and early 1953.

In the villages Baba visited, community members often raised the topic of politics because of India's recently achieved independence. Baba traditionally stipulated that his followers should not be involved in politics. While he accepted that the ideals of political parties were noble, he said they were not as important as man's search for his true Self. In late 1952 he reminded his followers that they should also maintain a critical perspective on religion.

"So, I love and adore all religions, but I am of no religion. Nor do I seek to establish another religion or add to the numberless illusions that divide man against man. No religion was ever intended to be anything more than the Gateway to God as Truth; but every religion has, in the course of time, got converted into a veil, obstructing the undimmed perception of that One Truth. As soon as the Truth of direct inner realization is intellectualized and formulated, it gets enmeshed in creeds and dogmas. They have a tendency to bind the soul in the very attempt to emancipate it. They cover the Truth in the very act of seeking to express it."[173]

Little mention in published sources is made of William's activities in late 1952 and early 1953. His father Sydney Bryan had passed away in England on November 12, 1952, eight months after his mother had died and just two days before William's forty-first birthday. His oldest brother, Bryan, inherited both the Donkin engineering business and Winterfold.

William received some unsolicited attention on one of the trips when the group stopped in the Indian state of Andhra Pradesh* in January 1953. Because he was the author of *The Wayfarers,* he was considered an important person. This was a source of amusement to William, and he got into the habit of pre-empting any obeisance that was offered to him by saluting the person he was meeting before they could bow down to him.[174]

Baba decided to send William back to Meherazad when the group was visiting Andhra, perhaps to shield him from the attention and any possible ego build-up that *The Wayfarers'* publication might be fostering.

William's departure on January 24 coincided with the arrival of Bal Natu, who joined the party for a week. Meher Baba was constantly aware of the cost and logistics of providing for his followers who accompanied him on tour, and having William leave when Bal arrived may have in part been to keep the expense sheet balanced.

The pattern of the tours involved scores of devotees meeting the core group at various stopovers. Sometimes this

---

* Andhra Pradesh is a Telegu-speaking state bordering on Maharashtra and on the southeast coast of India. Andhra Pradesh's capital and largest city is Hyderabad.

happened without invitation and became overwhelming. Bal Natu describes one scene at Eluru* in Andhra Pradesh:

"Over a thousand people had assembled on the railway platform with the expectation of having a glimpse of Baba's radiant face. This delayed the train for one hour."

Many of these devotees were from Hamirpur,** where Baba exerted a major influence. The large group pleaded with Baba to allow them to accompany him to nearby Andhra Pradesh where a large public darshan was planned.

William's moment of fame in Andhra is ironic – Baba's Indian followers seemed drawn to the published words of Western followers who had written books about Baba's work.

The chief host for the Andhra mass darshan had turned to Baba after reading Englishman Charles B. Purdom's 1937 book *The Perfect Master* in the early 1940s. American Jean Adriel's *Avatar,* published in 1947, a year before William's book, *The Wayfarers,* also caused a stir in India. Both Purdom's and Adriel's books were biographies of Meher Baba, written and published in the middle of his public life and work.

The Andhra darshan turned out to be a major public event. It is estimated that 15,000 people passed before Baba at the gathering. In addition to the mass public gathering, Baba also made personal visits to the homes of his close ones.

"On entering a home, Baba would be welcomed by the members of the family and by all their neighbours who had gathered there.... Baba made no distinction as to caste or creed, high or low. He went to the high officials of the town and to the humble homes and hovels of cobblers and sweepers as lovingly and spontaneously as if He were one of them."[175]

Baba's pace on this tour was frantic. At one point he joked that "the 19 house visits he was to make had turned into 90."

---

* Eluru is a city in Andhra Pradesh bordering on the freshwater Kolleru Lake approximately 40 miles from the Bay of Bengal. It is known for producing tobacco, palm-oil, and cocoa crops and the manufacture of carpets by expatriate Persians.

** Hamirpur town and district is considered the most literate, best educated area in Himachal Pradesh in the lower Himalayas of northern India. The town lies to the east of the mountains where the land undulates, but the north/northeast sections of the district feature bare, rugged hills with deep ravines.

Baba also continued to issue various instructions and discourses to his devotees during the time away from Meherazad.

On January 26, 1953, at a meeting with his close ones, he asked all of them "to abstain completely from any lustful action until the end of April 1953."

Sensing reluctance among the followers, he added, "Try, I will help you."

Also during this tour Baba also stated, "I am God in human form; I alone am Real; all else is Illusion. Love me from the depths of your hearts."

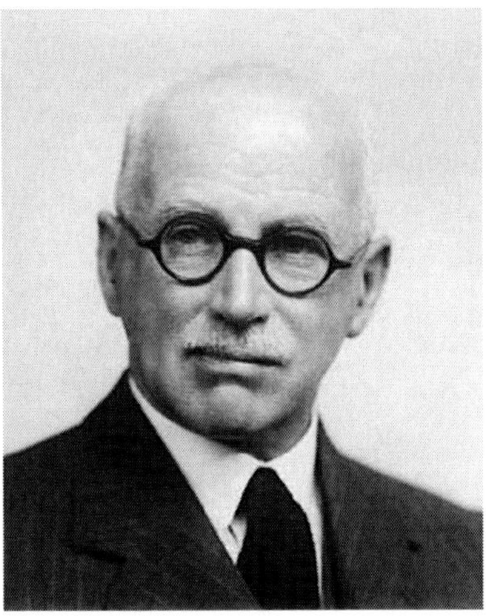

Donkin Family

Sydney Bryan Donkin

For his lovers who came for the tour from Hamirpur in northern India and had to return before Baba left C.R. Reddy College,* the site of the mass darshan in Eluru, Baba comforted them saying, "If you have love for me, distance or being away from my physical presence doesn't matter. I am in you and the Universal Mind can give anything, to anyone, at any time. Just follow these instructions: Love me; don't deceive; don't commit misdeeds, I will be with you."

On January 30, Baba and company were back at Meherazad and Meherabad, after 35 days of touring in the north and south of India. William immediately became involved again with his "difficult patient," and on February 4, he, along with three Eastern women and three Eastern men mandali, accompanied Baba to Poona for an x-ray of the left leg, which was still bothering him.

* C.R. Reddy College is a popular engineering college established in 1945 in Eluru in the state of Andhra.

The group returned to Meherazad the same day. Preparations were already underway for a trip and extended stay in northern India at Dehra Dun, the town where William earlier had attempted to set up a medical practice. Before leaving for the north, Baba summoned Western devotee Irene Conybeare,* who was staying in nearby Poona. Irene was another Westerner who was writing a book – *Civilization or Chaos.*

Irene would write later in *The Awakener* magazine about a question-and-answer session with Baba at this time:

"At Pimpalgaon [Meherazad], there was an opportunity to ask questions. So now was my chance.

"'Baba!' I said boldly, 'Where do the flying saucers come from?'

"Baba's face relaxed in a broad smile.

"'I would not answer that question for anybody, but you only! They do not come from any other planet....'"

After two weeks at Meherazad, Baba and a group of six female and twelve male disciples, including William, left for Dehra Dun on February 15, 1953.

They would spend nine months in Dehra Dun, where Baba wanted to remain in seclusion. Two houses were rented. The men stayed at 107-A Rajpur Road and Baba and the women mandali at 103-A Rajpur Road.

Although William was given his own room in the men's house, very little has been divulged about what he did during his stay in Dehra Dun, even though Baba appeared to be engaged in important work there.

World turmoil was ongoing in the early fifties. While much of Europe was attempting to recover from World War II, the Korean War of 1950 to 1953 saw various superpowers supporting either North or South Korea.

Many of Meher Baba's followers worldwide were also experiencing difficulties, but Baba was cutting off correspondence with everyone – particularly those who wanted answers or his

* Irene Conybeare was from an intellectual and rationalistic British family. She heard of Baba from Will Backett in 1940 after having some mystical experiences. She met Baba briefly in 1941 and wrote several books, including *In Quest of Truth* and *Civilization or Chaos.*

opinion on their problems. He insisted that they all face their difficulties with "grace and fortitude."

Oddly enough, Baba did take time to offer advice to Irene Conybeare on her book. Irene had been working with Ramjoo,* one of Baba's men mandali, on the content of the book and disagreements had arisen between the two. On February 27, Baba dictated a letter of clarification to Irene regarding content of the book. It reads in part:

"There is no difference in consciousness of the Avatar and a Sadguru or in their perfection....

"Both are one with God. Both experience infinite power, knowledge and bliss, and both use these aspects of Sat-Chit-Anand** for the universe.

"The difference is in the scope of their working. Sadguru works for the selected few in a chosen way and for the universe in a general way. Avatar works for the selected few in a special way and for the universe in a chosen way."[176]

It was during the Dehra Dun stay that Bhau Kalchuri joined Baba permanently. Bhau later served as Chairman of the Avatar Meher Baba Trust*** for many years, and was author of many Meher Baba books, including the multi-volume *Lord Meher* series.

Bhau had met Baba a number of months earlier at Saoner and Nagpur. At the time Bhau was involved in completing three master's degrees – in public administration, chemistry and physics, and law. Baba asked Bhau bluntly at their meeting, "Will you obey me 100 per cent?"

Bhau immediately replied, "Yes."

On successfully completing his examinations for his master's degrees, Bhau came to Dehra Dun to join Baba forever in

---

* Ramjoo K. Abdulla, one of Baba's mandali, had been raised an orthodox Muslim and joined Baba at the age of 23 in 1922. Baba asked Ramjoo to keep a diary from January 1922 to January 1925 that recorded Baba's interactions with and training of the earliest mandali.

** Sat-Chit-Anand is most often translated as Truth-Knowledge-Bliss or alternatively Existence-Knowledge-Bliss.

*** Avatar Meher Baba Trust was established by Baba in 1959 to provide for his disciples who were dependent on him and to care for his Tomb and the property at Meherabad.

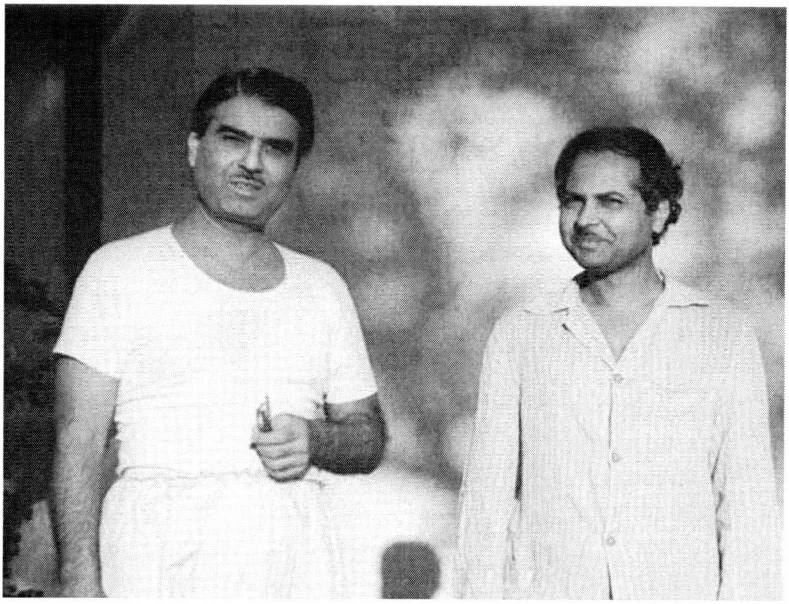

MSI Collection India

Bhau Kalchuri, right, joined Baba in 1953 as a mandali and wrote many books relating to Baba, including the 6000-page biography Lord Meher. *Later in the fifties Bhau's wife Rama and children Sheela and Mehernath became part of Baba's family. Mandali Eruch Jessawala, left, was with Baba constantly and was the main interpreter of his hand gestures.*

March 1953. After that, Bhau's wife Rama and children Sheela and Mehernath lived under Baba's watchful eye.*

During Baba's stay at Dehra Dun, he took time to strengthen his relationships with his close followers there. A public darshan was also held for all of his lovers in Dehra Dun and for seven hours they filed past him

Baba at all times stressed honesty. On one occasion in Dehra Dun an atheist came before Baba. His response: "Everyone is an atheist till he finds God by actual experience. It is better to be an atheist and be honest in words and deeds than to pose as a lover of God and lead a dishonest life. God is independent. He needs no worship; He only needs that we be honest."[177]

* Rama, Sheela, and Mehernath lived in Khushru quarters (the Trust Compound) and Baba said of the children that he was their real father.

Baba also continued his contact with masts and the poor while staying in Dehra Dun. He did not hesitate from seeking even more seclusion while staying in northern India and on April 10 left Dehra Dun and travelled 22 miles further north to stay for seven weeks at Mussoorie,* "the queen of hill stations in India."

Baba had hoped to deal with correspondence while staying at Mussoorie, but soon abandoned this and asked Adi Sr. to issue another circular informing his followers not to write to him for any reason from May 15 until the end of September 1953.

There is no mention that William was included in the Mussoorie trip.

Although the decision that William would have his own room away from the rest of the mandali appears to have been an arrangement that Baba agreed to, the doctor's frustration was evident in a supposedly small episode which erupted after the group's return on June 30. The dialogue is taken from the pages of Bhau Kalchuri's *Lord Meher*:

"[Dr.] Nilu complained to Baba, 'Donkin is discontinuing his subscription to his medical journal from abroad, which I need, as you have told me to keep up with the latest developments. Tell him not to do so.'

"Baba's reply: 'Let us consult Hafiz and see if Nilu's wish is to come true.'

Baba asked another mandali member to bring a volume of Hafiz's work and open it at random. Some sentences were read in Persian and translated.

"It seems Nilu's desire will be fulfilled," concluded Baba.

William was not convinced. "Hafiz says nothing about medicine or a journal."

Baba responded, "Anyway, until the end of 1953, don't stop the journal."

William then complained to Baba, "You had in the beginning made grandiose plans [about opening medical facilities], which until now have not been put into effect."

---

* Mussoorie is a hill station about 20 miles from Dehra Dun in the foothills of the Himalayas. It grew from a hunting lodge built by a British officer in 1826. It has green hills, breathtaking vistas, and beautiful waterfalls.

Sidestepping a direct answer, Baba had Hafiz consulted again, commenting, "Ask Hafiz again when these two doctors will leave me alone."

After the second Hafiz quote was read, William again noted, "But no reference is made about medicine or a hospital."

"The time is coming soon," Baba replied.

Although the session ended on a lighter note a short time after with more Hafiz quotes and an agreement to continue William's subscription to the medical journal, the fray indicated that William was certainly internally frustrated at times.

Baba had indeed indicated, before William graduated from Barts 14 years earlier, that he would need a surgeon and that a hospital was included in the long-term plans for Meherabad.

William's delicate state is understandable. Both of his parents had died in England the year before. He was continually plagued in not finding a solution to the pain in Baba's left leg. And in the move to Dehra Dun, Baba was no longer giving William jobs to do, while freely allocating various responsibilities to other mandali members.

Baba's emphasis on eliminating the ego of followers is worth another glance. William struggled through medical school thinking that his skills would be put to good use in India. Early on, however, William realized that predictability was not a part of life with Meher Baba. Soon after arriving in India both William and Dr. Nilu were referred to as "barbers" rather than doctors on more than one occasion. It is possible that William also witnessed or heard about the deflating ego session Baba had with Dr. Goher, who joined the ashram after graduation from medical school in Delhi. He basically told her not to assume any lofty attitude because of achieving her medical degree.

In *Lord Meher*, Bhau Kalchuri gives his own opinion on William's situation at this time:

"Donkin was a gifted, diligent doctor, but after the New Life period Baba had not given him any specific duty and it was therefore difficult for him to pass the time. Baba's inner work for him was of course for the best; but outwardly Donkin remained ill at ease. For him to be without work was a penance."

Although the mood appeared serious in Dehra Dun, William was still capable of carrying out his signature pranks.

Life with Meher Baba was always filled with many pets – dogs, cats, goats, deer, parrots monkeys, and even horses. While in Dehra Dun, Baba had presented his chief woman disciple Mehera with a pet horse, Sheba. When Baba decided to move with the group from Northern India, one of their stopping places for a period of time on their way back to Meherazad was Satara.

Mehera tells a Satara story about William and Sheba in her book about the ashram pets, *Baba Loved Us Too: Stories of Meher Baba and His Pets:*

"One day Dr. Donkin was waiting at the gate for Baba's call. Feeling bored, he lit his cigar.... The aroma of the tobacco wafted

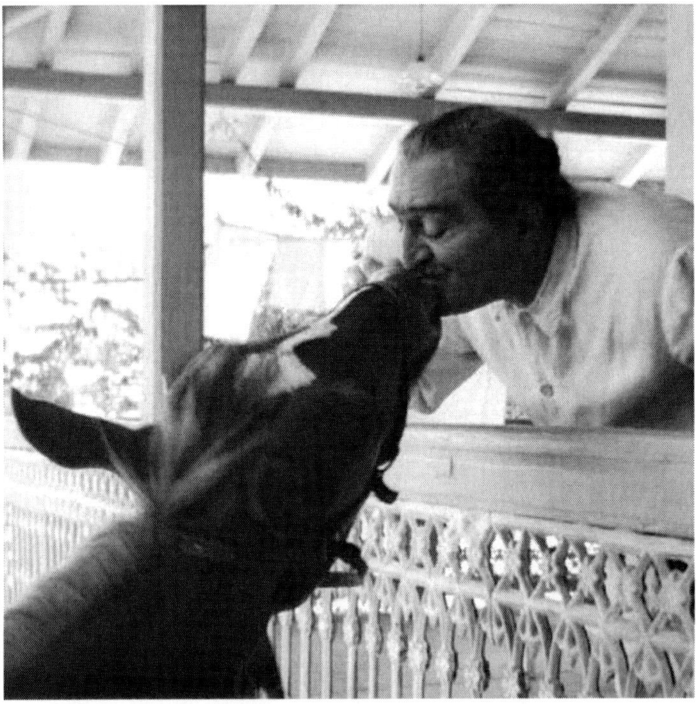

MSI Collection India

Sheba, who enjoyed tobacco treats from William Donkin, gets a kiss from Baba. Sheba was a gift from Baba to Mehera. A wide range of pets was always included in the ashram life.

its way through the air to Sheba in her stable.... She started rubbing her lips against the screen window.

"The strange sound attracted Donkin's attention. Curious, he walked over to Sheba. As Donkin watched Sheba rub her lips against the screen he got an idea: perhaps Sheba would like some tobacco.

"Dr. Donkin slipped a few shreds of tobacco through the holes in the screen and, would you believe it, that lady of many tastes gobbled it up!... Sheba began rubbing her lips once more against the screen, letting Donkin know she was ready for an encore.

"After that, Sheba and Donkin were fast friends ... and Sheba would [get] ... the stumps of his cigars or a pinch of his pipe tobacco."

From mid-August until September 2, 1953, Baba was involved in a specific work and he did not wish to be disturbed. Part of the daily routine during this time was to have the Master's Prayer, which Baba had dictated August 13, recited daily, and William was asked to read the prayer in English.

The Master's Prayer and the Prayer of Repentance are the two main prayers issued by Meher Baba in his lifetime. While the Prayer of Repentance dwells on its title subject, repentance, the Master's Prayer's direction toward divine beings or divinity is more lofty, almost unworldly and beyond understanding.

The English version reads as follows:

The Master's Prayer

O Parvardigar, the Preserver and Protector of all,
You are without Beginning, and without End;
Non-dual, beyond comparison, and none can
    measure You.

You are without colour, without expression, without form, and without attributes.
You are unlimited and unfathomable, beyond
    imagination and conception, eternal and
    imperishable.

You are indivisible; and none can see You, but with
Eyes Divine.
You always were, You always are, and You always
will be;
You are everywhere, You are everything; and You
are also beyond everywhere and beyond
everything.

You are in the firmament and in the depths;
You are manifest and unmanifest, on all planes
and beyond all planes.
You are in the three worlds, and also beyond the
three worlds;
You are imperceptible and independent.

You are the Creator, the Lord of lords, the knower
of all minds and hearts; You are omnipotent
and omnipresent. You are Knowledge Infin-
ite, Power Infinite, and Bliss Infinite.
You are the Ocean of Knowledge, all-knowing,
infinitely knowing, the Knower of the past,
the present, and the future, and You are
Knowledge Itself.

You are all-merciful and eternally benevolent;
You are the Soul of souls, the One with infinite
attributes.
You are the Trinity of Truth, knowledge, and Bliss,
You are the Source of Truth, the Ocean of Love;
You are the Ancient One, the Highest of the High;
You are Prabhu and Parameshwar, You are the
Beyond-God, and the Beyond-Beyond God,
You are Parabrahma, Allah, Elahi, Yezdan, Ahura-
mazda, and God the Beloved.
You are named Ezad – the only One worthy of
worship.

Little is known about William's activities between the final months of 1953 and mid-1954.

During the fall of 1953 in Dehra Dun, Meher Baba began to refer to himself more as the Avatar of the Age, especially to his close followers. This proclamation often included discourses or directions. An example excerpted from one discourse:

"Mere intellectuals can never understand me through their intellect. If I am the Highest of the High, it becomes impossible for the mind to gauge me, nor is it possible for my ways to be fathomed by the human mind.

"I am not to be attained by those who, loving me, stand reverently by in rapt admiration. I am not for those who ridicule me and point at me with contempt. To have a crowd of tens of millions flocking around me is not what I am for. I am for the few who, scattered amongst the crowd, silently and unostentatiously surrender their all – body, mind, and possessions – to me. I am still more for those who, after surrendering their all, never give another thought to their surrender.

"Those who have indomitable courage to face willingly and cheerfully the worst calamities, who have unshakable faith in me, eager to fulfil my slightest wish at the cost of their happiness and comfort, they indeed truly love me."[178]

Baba appears to be heightening the demand on his close followers. In taking on the mantle of Avatar, he essentially was saying he was a human manifestation of God comparable to Zoroaster, Rama, Krishna, Jesus, Buddha, and Mohammed. The excerpt above is only a part of what Baba said at the time.

Charles Purdom, close English follower and author, says of Baba's lengthy declaration, "This was the most explicit direct and the fullest public statement made by Baba about himself. It is the equivalent of what is said in the Upanishads*:

"'Brahman is all, and Atman is Brahman. Atman the Self.... I am Atman, the Spirit himself...'

"To make such a declaration required the highest degree of courage."[179]

---

* The Upanishads are Hindu scriptures that constitute the core teachings of Vedanta. They were not written over a period spanning from the middle of the first millennium BCE through the medieval and early modern periods.

13

Three Incredible Weeks, A Tough Lesson

During the early months of 1954, Baba toured Andhra State giving darshan to more than 200,000 lovers.

On one occasion he relays how specific he was in *The God-Man* about the attitude followers should display in working for him:

"When you spread my eternal message of love to others, show them first that you really love me. Do not merely make them read my books and messages; do more.

"Live such a life of love, sacrifice, forgiveness and tolerance that others will love me. If instead of doing the real work of love, you start organized propaganda for me, it is absurd. I need no propaganda and publicity, but I do want love and honesty. If you cannot live the life of love and honesty, you should stop working for me. I am quite capable of doing my Universal Work alone."

At the time Meher Baba said, "There are about 220 men and women from the East and West who have so completely and utterly surrendered to me that they would do anything I say."

William was undoubtedly included in this group. Early in 1954, plans were afoot to invite a group of 20 of Meher Baba's close Western male followers to take part in what would eventually be called the Three Incredible Weeks.

William was at last given a specific job – to be completely responsible for the health of the visiting male devotees.

Before this visit occurred, early to mid-1954 was devoted to Baba's visiting Baba's followers in India. He used Mahabaleshwar and Meherazad as alternating home bases. On these trips the mandali who travelled with him were strictly Easterners. Just as Baba had depended on William as a Westerner for his travels to England and the United States, he now turned to his Indian mandali and lovers to organize and assist him on travels in their home country.

On February 7, 1954, Baba and nine men mandali left Mahabaleshwar for Hamirpur. William stayed behind at the Aga Khan bungalow with the women mandali and three other Eastern men mandali. Returning on March 6 from Poona to Mahabaleshwar, Baba related the news of his one-month tour to William and the women mandali.

The group of Western men arrived September 10 at Ahmednagar to begin their Three Incredible Weeks. They included citizens of England, France, Switzerland, the United States, and Australia – all countries where Meher Baba had travelled and had followers.

Charles Purdom, who arrived with a small British group ahead of the other larger group of Western men, writes to his Swiss friend Max Haefliger about the Bombay arrival:

"Donkin came to meet us and has been very helpful, but is very busy helping to get the previous (Western) women's quarters at Meherabad ready for the visitors from abroad."

If William had felt distant, useless, and alienated from Meher Baba before the group arrived, his spirits would have been buoyed by the trust Baba placed in him to look after the visitors' health care.

Baba told the assembled men shortly after their arrival, "Don [William] is in charge of your health, if you have any difficulty tell him."

A day later, Baba led the Western men on a walk up Seclusion Hill. On the way he showed them William's small medical facility. "This is Don's dispensary, and I have nothing to worry about regarding health, because here is the doctor and he is most dear to me. The faith and love with which this dear son of mine has stuck to Baba is unique. As I told you yesterday, it anything bothers you, if the slightest thing is wrong with you, tell Don."

These words to the 20 Western male visitors certainly would have had a resurrecting effect on William. For the most part he had been at loose ends since the end of the New Life period. His emptiness was tempered somewhat when he was called on to help organize Baba's trip to the West in 1952, but the responsibility of the Western male visitors in September 1954 probably came at a time when his morale was teetering.

Meherwan Jessawala, who was a young man at the time, recalls William's dedication in taking care of the Western 55visitors:

"Every morning he would clean the latrines. Before anyone got up, he would clean them with his own hands. He never spared himself. He worked behind the scenes. [He] never liked attention and wasn't the least bit ostentatious."[180]

Charles Purdom describes in his book, *The God-Man,* the arrivals and accommodation setup for the Western men:

"The original intention was that all should stay as guests of various devotees in Ahmednagar, but Baba had decided it would be more convenient and more in accord with his purpose, for us to be under one roof at Meherabad. Up on the hill is the large two-storey stone house that had served for years as a retreat for his secluded women disciples, in which Baba had been the only man to set foot with the exception of the doctors. The upper storey had been converted for the occasion into a dormitory; two other rooms were on the ground floor, where there was a large lounge.

"At the rear was erected a refectory under a corrugated iron roof, a little beyond the kitchens with a cook and assistants, also five Indian-type bathrooms and washstands, with running cold water and mirrors for shaving, and five toilets. Early in the morning buckets of hot water were brought to the bathrooms as required. The meals were varied and tasty; clothes laundered, pressed or cleaned as necessary; outgoing mail was posted and incoming mail delivered. Medicines were supplied for those who needed them."

Later in his account Purdom said, "Baba proved that a Perfect Master was also a perfect host."

Baba immediately took the group for a tour of local places associated with his work. The Western men also witnessed a mass darshan attended by 10,000 Indian devotees.

While Baba told the men "I am your Master, but I am also your friend," the group's visit was not without heartbreak. Shortly after gathering them together Baba asked them their thoughts.

One group member, Max Haefliger from Switzerland, found himself quickly embroiled in turmoil when Baba asked him to say something. "I don't understand anything about you, but I like your people," said Max.

"That means you don't like me?" asked Baba.

Max said something about liking Baba sometimes.

"So you like my people all the time," said Baba, "and you like me sometimes."

The dustup did not stop with this brief exchange. Later Baba turned to Max and said, "Max, you don't like me; anyway, I like you all the same, all the time."

Baba was undoubtedly trying to teach Haefliger something in the exchange.

Charles Purdom, who considered Haefliger a close friend, describes the drastic conclusion of this chain of events when members of the group were granted private meetings with Baba.

"After I had seen Baba, and in view of what had passed earlier between him and Max, I thought I should have a talk with the latter before his interview, but somehow, I failed to do so, although Max was the last to see Baba.

"When we met immediately after, he said to me, 'Baba is sending me home.'

"'When?' I asked.

"'At once,' was his reply. 'I am packing now. Baba and I have agreed that neither of us will say why this has happened.'"

Purdom was devastated about the expulsion of his friend.

"Max went away, leaving me with a heavy heart, for he was the man I knew the best, with whom I had most in common of all those present; I had been looking forward to our being together during the fortnight. A certain amount of gloom settled upon the entire company as we gathered in the lounge after our evening meal, but no one referred to what had happened."

Purdom must have enjoyed a good rapport with Baba; because two days later Baba gave an explanation to the group about Max's leaving:

"First I want to tell you in a few words about Max. I have had a note from Charles asking me if I would say something to explain his departure, for it has distressed him.

"In the interview he told me something we both promised not to disclose, and gave a description of his state of mind since he met me two years ago. He then told me that he really did not want to come, but something had made him do so.

"'And now, Baba,' he said. 'I leave it to you, whether to go immediately or to stay until the meeting.'

"I told him to go. He felt very sad, but I told him to go immediately. He will accordingly leave Bombay on the 22 September. He is a very fine man, and I love him very much. Today he sent me a telegram saying, 'Dear Baba, I humbly apologize for having disappointed you and ask your forgiveness.'

"I cabled in reply, 'Don't worry, My love and blessings.'

"This I tell you because dear Purdom wanted to know why Max left."[181]

While the explanation still was far from complete, it must have provided some solace to group members.

Ivy Duce in her book *How a Master Works*, published in 1975, continues the thread of Max's life after his sudden departure from the Three Incredible Weeks in September 1954. Writing about his years after 1954, she says, "Actually Baba in his inimitable manner had in this way given to Max an experience that proved a catalyst through which Max realized his true love for Baba. He has maintained a firm connection with Baba ever since, making great sacrifices to come to Baba's sahavas in Myrtle Beach later....

"Lud [Ludwig Dimpfl, who had attended the Three Incredible Weeks] later filled me in on the story of Max, who lived in Berne, Switzerland, and whose behaviour at the 1954 sahavas was always inexplicable to me, since whenever I had seen him either in Switzerland or at Myrtle Beach, he was a very strong Baba devotee.

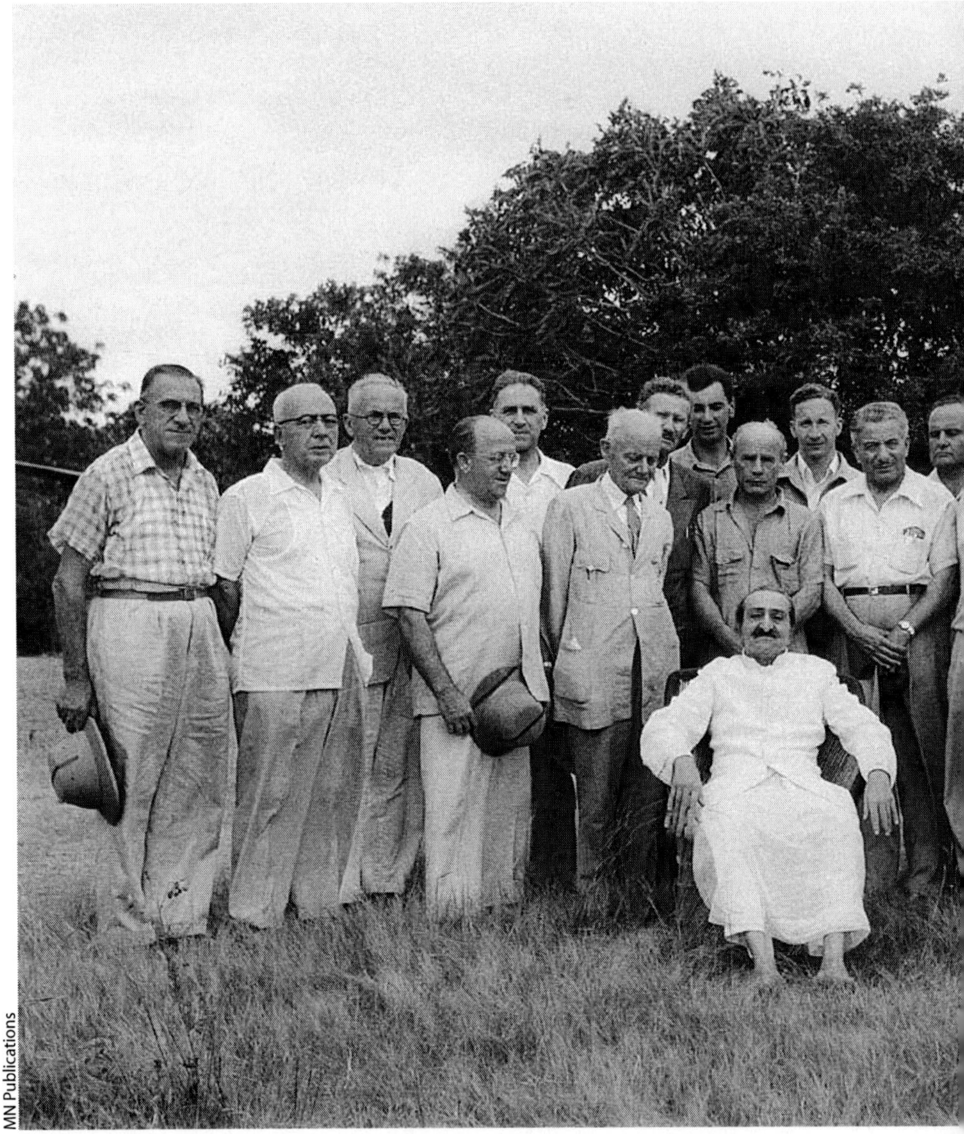

MN Publications

Meher Baba is shown at the Samadhi with the Western men who spent Three Incredible Weeks in India with Baba in September 1954. Dr. William Donkin, who was responsible for the health of group members during their India visit, is at the far right in the photo.

The Western visitors included, back row from left: John Bass, USA; Ben Hayman, USA; Charles Purdom, UK; Malcolm Schloss, USA; Frank

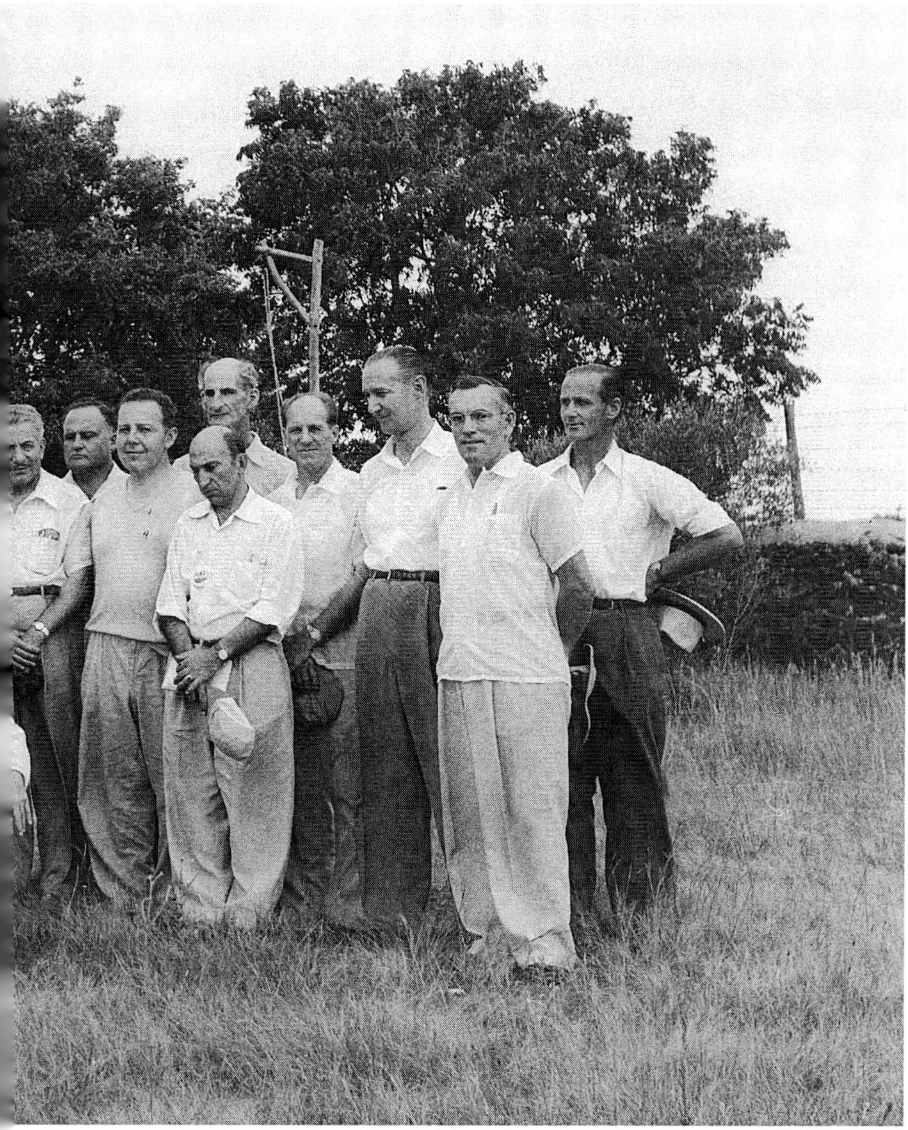

Hendrick, USA; Bill LePage, Australia; John Ballantyne, Australia; Fred Frey, USA; Fred Marks, UK; Darwin Shaw, USA; Phillipe Dupuis, France; and Frank Eaton, USA. Middle row, from left: Fred Winterfeldt, USA; Will Backett, UK; Francis Brabazon, Australia; Joseph Harb, USA; Lud Dimpfl, USA; and Dana Field, USA. Another participant, Alexander Markey, USA, is not shown in the photo.

"Lud related that when Max first heard of Baba he was a stockbroker in Switzerland and his first thought upon hearing that Baba knew everything was that this would be a gold mine of information for a stockbroker. Hence, when Max finally met Baba he took advantage of the situation and asked the Master what would be good stocks to buy. Baba mentioned several stocks and Max bought them, and all of the stocks proceeded to grow in value. The next time Max came to Baba he again asked him what stocks to buy and Baba said to him, "'Sell your stocks.'

"Whereupon Max went back to his job and sold all of his stocks, plus all of the stocks of his clients. The market kept going up and the clients were furious because of his bad judgment. He then went back to Baba and complained about what had befallen him.

"Baba replied,'I told you to sell your stock. I didn't tell you to sell your clients.'"

Max himself confirmed this story when he visited the Sufi Center in the fall of 1972.[182]

The Haefliger story reflects the tough road Baba lovers had to adhere to in following their Spiritual Master. The successful stockbroker was suddenly left with egg on his face when he prematurely sold off his own and his clients' stocks. Throughout his life Baba said he was out to destroy egos, because these egos interfered with the growth of Divine Love in his lovers. Haefliger's prowess as a stockbroker was shattered.

This compares in some ways to William and his desire to be a worthwhile doctor. Baba did not always grant the wishes of his lovers. The experience was painful for many, but he warned them many times that following him was not a journey for the faint-hearted.

Despite reverses, for a few of the Western male followers the Three Incredible Weeks were just that. Baba emphasized to group members that they should be completely natural, and although it was difficult for many, any feeling of distance and stiff correctness in behaviour began to dissolve during the first week.

At one point during the men's stay Baba distributed a circular to them titled "Meher Baba's Call," which read, "Live not in ignorance. Do not waste your precious life span in differentiating between and judging your fellowmen; but learn to long for the love of God. Even in the midst of your worldly activities, live only to find and realize your true identity with your beloved God."

While William was in charge of the overall health of the men, he was also given other responsibilities. On one occasion William read to the group a Christian prayer that he himself had compiled from several sources just for the occasion. William followed the reading of his unique prayer with the reading of Baba's *Prayer of Repentance.* Zoroastrian and Moslem prayers were also read on this occasion.

William also spoke on one occasion, using a microphone to convey what Baba said was an important message:

"Baba wants to use a simile about the atom bomb. Just as an atom bomb, which in itself is so small, when exploded, causes tremendous havoc, so, when He breaks His silence, the universal spiritual upheaval that will take place will be something that no one can describe. It will happen in a second, at a time when nobody expects it. Just as when an earthquake takes place suddenly, when no one is ready and no one can do anything, but everyone in the affected area feels it, so the breaking of My Silence will create a spiritual upheaval and everyone will feel it in his heart."

Throughout his spiritual mission Baba made numerous promises to break his silence, but vocally never did. He lost followers along the way who tied their hopes and spiritual inclinations to the promised nirvana which was expected to accompany the breaking of his silence.

Even today debate continues about the breaking of Baba's silence with some followers believing individually that Baba has broken His silence in their own hearts.

The Three Incredible Weeks spanned September 11 to 30, 1954. A part of the experience for the Western men was a mass darshan on September 12 involving thousands of Indian Baba lovers. A number of the Western men later reflected on this event and their stay with Baba.

From Lud Dimpfl of the United States:

"On September 14 we gathered around him and introduced ourselves. After this Baba spelled out on the board, 'I want you to be completely natural with each other; not strained.'

"Never have I desired more to do something and felt so unable. How does one act naturally? The feeling of distance and need for correctness did start to dissolve. It was a dissolving rather than anything forced. Baba does not move a person by repelling him from avenues which he should not follow. Baba is simply attractive."

From Dana Field of the United States:

"I assure you we have been welded into a unit by Baba, and there is only love and peace.

"Dr. Donkin is close to Baba, although very different. He is our medic. Very handsome and healthy, but also apparently gentle."

Dana Field also offered insight on his own shortcomings:

"Baba forgives and we understand each other. The least smell of intellectualism, which for him is synonymous with hypocrisy 'bothers' Him. He told me to balance mind and heart, with heart having precedence. It is a wonderful lesson, especially having Baba's own example of awakening rather than teaching."

From Philippe Dupuis of France:

"The main teaching I got from India ... was ... that spiritual life is no fun, no adventure, not part-time, not excitement! It is like modern wars. It is total! It is not to be thought only but lived. The best way to do it is to give up everything – forget everything; be ready and glad to die at the feet of one's Master, if you have the grace to have one....

"The poor mind of ours is the main obstacle. It seems only the Master can put it aside for us and unlock our heart – which is the secret of all secrets."

From Joseph Hamad Harb of the United States:

"I cannot and I shall not ever forget the first time He ever embraced me within His loving arms. It was a most unforgettable feeling – so comforting, so peaceful, so delightful that my gratitude for this supreme privilege was of such indescribable feeling that the tears welled up and overflowed with joy and happiness. I loved Him and didn't want to take my arms away from Him. I wanted more and more of His embracing.

"Baba will go to any extreme of physical exertions to find and awaken those souls with sincere or utmost yearning for God-Realization."

From Will Backett of England:

"He walked round the table to place both hands on our shoulders, and the gentle firmness of his touch gave deep significance to that simple gesture.

"There was much laughter when he circumnavigated the long table to find where he could best tickle each one, joining in the fun Himself, for he likes us to be bright and happy always. At the Ping-Pong table provided for our relaxation, He was a doughty opponent with unique grace and speed. He also showed us a different game of marbles, awarding a prize to the winner and applauding his skill or luck, as part of the deeper game of Divine Love, which is the Master's real sport."

The Three Incredible Weeks had an extraordinary effect on the Western men who attended. Baba tried hard from the start to put all the men at ease. On one occasion he said that while he was a Perfect Master, he was also their friend and one of them.

A few days later he reminded the group, "I am what I am even if the whole world bows down to me or turns against me. It does not matter; it is no one's fault. To know Baba is not a matter of eating ladoos [Indian sweets]; one has to die to oneself to know me. It is not just a joke: [this] Love."[183]

William was a constant attendee in the activities of the Three Incredible Weeks. Baba would continually ask the Western men about their health and advise them to take even minor concerns to William. Specifically Baba asked Darwin Shaw to gargle after every meal and when awakening in the morning and when he went to bed at night. Darwin was told to see William if his discomfort did not clear up.

The Western men left India after September 30, 1954, for their various countries in the West. A letter written later to close Eastern Baba follower Savak Kotwal by Western participant Alexander Markey reflects his feelings about leaving India:

"You, the dear Saroshes [Sarosh and Villoo] and Don [William] had transformed the ashram into the most glorious abode in the whole of India. I shall forever remember it with thanksgiving."[184]

Another member of the Western group, Lud Dimpfl, carried the manuscript of Baba's book *God Speaks* with him to the United States. Baba had asked Ivy Duce and Don Stevens* to edit the book. The two were caught off guard by the request, but decided to set aside two weeks at Ivy's house for the editing. They were also asked to do the preface and introduction for the book, and while both thought this job would be left better to someone with more authority, they agreed to take on the task.

"We had expected to ask some famous person or writer like Dr. Donkin to do this work, so it was quite a surprise," Ivy said in her book *How a Master Works.*

The returning Western men and others in the Baba community were shocked to hear of the sudden death of group member Malcolm Schloss shortly after he returned from India. He was found dead October 7 on the bathroom floor of the New York apartment he was staying in. Malcolm had spent a few days in France on his return trip working on the final draft of the book *Three Incredible Weeks*** with Charles Purdom of England, another participant in the trip.

A note from Baba on Malcolm's passing reads, "Inform all concerned that most fortunate Malcolm passed away from you on most important day of seventh in unique circumstances after embracing Baba and completing Baba's work [the printed account of the sahavas]."

Charles Purdom wrote of Malcolm's death and their work together assembling the book on the India experience. In a let-

---

* Don Stevens met Baba in the 1950s and helped edit Meher Baba's books *God Speaks* and *Discourses;* narrated and edited *Listen, Humanity*; and wrote *Meher Baba, the Awakener of the Age* as well as several small books related to Baba.

** The book *Three Incredible Weeks with Meher Baba* was published in 1979. It is a compilation of the diaries of Charles Purdom and Malcolm Schloss (kept at Baba's request and originally published in The Awakener) and accounts of other participants published in The Awakener as an article called "Facets of the Diamond."

ter he sent to Fred Winterfeldt* of New York, who also attended, he said, "What an experience we had!

"I thought something was going to happen to Malcolm. It is very dangerous to be near Baba. I am sure we shall all suffer from it in one way or another – suffering and profit from it will be the proof of what we really got from Baba.

"It was a marvellous experience. Our report of it [Malcolm's and mine – largely his except toward the end] does nothing like justice to what we went through. I wish it had been possible to rewrite it. It was really like an addition to the Gospels, and needs to be written as well as they are.

"To interpret our experience and what we heard is no easy matter. Baba, though a man and living in the human world, lives also and speaks in the divine world and is to be understood in the divine, not the worldly sense.

"That is very hard. And that is why he says, 'Love Me!' Only if we love him can we understand at all. And he says love *me* – because that is easier for us than if he said 'Love God,' which all the preachers say every Sunday and nobody takes any notice. It was a wonderful experience to be with so many men of different experiences and thoughts and temperament and to be so much at harmony. And I shall never forget you."

---

* Fred Winterfeldt learned of Baba in New York from Ivy Duce in 1948. With his wife Ella (together called Fredella by Baba), he hosted the Monday Night Meetings in New York City for many years. When they retired, they moved to the Meher Center where they greeted guests at the Gateway.

14

Heightened Activity, More Blood Shed, West Again

While Baba was creating his own turmoil with the men from the West, natural global elements were churning on an equally large scale. Hurricane Hazel, one of the worst eastern North America storms of the 20th Century, hit the East Coast of the United States with a vengeance in October 1954.

In *Love Alone Prevails,* Kitty describes the effect of the hurricane on the Meher Spiritual Center's 500-acre beachfront property in Myrtle Beach, South Carolina:

"The hurricane was due to hit the coast around 9 a.m. [October 15] and Elizabeth saw waves said to be 60 feet high. Elizabeth had decided that the basement of Yaupon Dunes would be the safest place, so I prepared hot coffee and tea and Elizabeth, Norina, and I took a picture of Baba and the radio with us. Elizabeth's father had selected the highest land on which to build the house and we were quite safe there...."

Elizabeth later wrote to Mani of the hurricane experience, "Hazel came at the time of the full moon and it was also high tide when it struck, but at the same time a wonderful thing happened.

"The wind and rain that preceded the actual hurricane shifted from the ocean side and struck from the land side, so at the height of the hurricane the wind blew against the waves of the ocean which kept them from piling up on the land.... If it can be explained 'scientifically,' it was that some places were struck as it were, 'in the face' and Myrtle Beach was struck 'in the back.' Other beach areas further up [north] were all but demolished.

"The Center must have had at least 200 trees blown down throughout the woods and across the roads, but [there was] no damage done to the buildings...."

Elizabeth explained in her letter to India that there were eight separate breakthroughs along the Center beach and salt water poured into Long Lake affecting fresh water fish there.

"The lake will freshen up again as there is no inlet from the ocean that we have not filled in. I had bulldozers on the Center beach filling in wherever necessary and I personally supervised the work to make sure it was done well.

"At high noon on the day of the hurricane, the storm subsided almost more quickly that it came. All of a sudden, it had passed by and the sun came out and has been out almost every day since."

Hurricane damage to the south and north of the Meher Spiritual Center was major. More than 1,200 homes were destroyed in the adjacent beach areas.

At the beginning of December 1954, Baba began semi-fasting, taking only one meal a day. He and his followers spent much of the month in partial fasting. Baba himself observed a strict seclusion during the month, coming out only to celebrate Mehera's and Christ's birthday on December 25.

When not in seclusion, Baba was very much involved in the planned publication of *God Speaks.* Ivy Duce and Don Stevens were busy editing the manuscript which Lud Dimpfl had delivered to them in September on his return from India. Both editors had other obligations – Don to his oil business work and Ivy to running Sufism Reoriented. Ivy points out that their editing skills also ran somewhat at cross purposes to each other.

"I was trained in earlier methods of classical English, while Don had become accustomed to the modern practice of omitting as much punctuation as possible."[185]

To further complicate the final work on the book, William was working with Baba's sister Mani on Dr. Ghani's rough notes, which had been dictated to him by Baba. Some of this material was also destined for the pages of *God Speaks.*

Baba had hoped that *God Speaks* would be published in May 1955. The final manuscript was turned over to Dodd, Mead and Company on March 14, 1955, but the publisher insisted that a fall publication date would be better than May.

Throughout the first half of 1955, Baba underwent several periods of seclusion, travelled, fed and bathed the poor and lepers, and again worked with masts. He issued orders in April stipulating that he would be "in retirement" for three months – May 1 to July 31. He insisted that no one was to visit him or communicate with him directly or indirectly for the three months.

"All those closely connected with me, all those who love me, and all those who care to follow my instructions must be scrupulously honest; must strictly abstain from sexual actions; and must try to spread my message of Love and Truth as far and wide as possible during the period of crisis for three months from May 1 to July 31."[186]

As Baba often did throughout his lifetime, he again gave his followers the opportunity to leave him and live life on their own terms. Specifically, if they stuck by him, he dictated four crucial points to achieve "Mastery in Servitude," his lifelong motto:

> The things of lasting value for the Path are
>
> Divine Love,
> Obedience to a Perfect Master,
> Absolute sincere and wholehearted service to others,
> True renunciation of all worldly things, leaving no room for thoughts other than of God, the only Reality.

There is little information on William's activities during 1955. He was still involved in various medical responsibilities for Baba's health and the other mandali and also working with Mani on the additional material for *God Speaks*.

In October 1955, Don Stevens made his first trip to India where a sahavas program was planned. Another Westerner, poet Francis Brabazon, arrived from Australia on November 1.

It was on this occasion that Baba delivered another glowing reference to William when introducing the mandali to the new Western visitors:

"Donkin, for 16 years he has been with me. He is a doctor holding his degree from an English medical school. When the war broke out he served in the army as a major. Out of his salary, he used to send money to me every month. After the war he re-joined me. He has stuck to me throughout. For an Englishman to stay here and adjust himself to our conditions is difficult, but he has done it."[187]

In late 1955, from November 3 until December 3, Baba held a series of sahavas programs at Meherabad and during the four-week period gave various discourses. On one occasion he stated, "I have already told you that love for God and obedience to a Master are beyond the reach of man on his own and that complete surrender is almost impossible. The best thing is for man to purify his heart."[188]

In a cable dated December 20, 1955, Baba informed his followers in the West that he would again visit England and the United States in the summer of 1956, accompanied by Adi Sr., Dr. Nilkanth Godse [Dr. Nilu]; Eruch; and Meherjee Karkaria. William would not accompany Baba on this trip.

In mid-January 1956, Baba's darshan in Satara, India, attracted 30,000 people. Baba handed out prasad for 10 continuous hours. (Prasad is small, usually edible, gifts from a Spiritual Master.) In a letter that his sister Mani wrote of the occasion, "The program lasted from 8 in the morning till 6:30 in the evening [except for a little water once, Baba partook of nothing during this time]. Baba did look very tired when He returned, but the next morning worked as usual."

In early July 1956, Baba and the same four men mandali departed on their western tour. They stopped for a number of days in England, and then travelled to New York City, where they spent seven days. A reception that included 135 people was held at Manhattan House.

While Baba was away William's impish nature found expression back in India. While in Satara, he and Bhau Kalchuri decided to play a trick on Savak Kotwal, who thought himself quite the ladies' man. William purchased a beautiful sari and Bhau dressed up in it, complete with makeup. Savak, noticing this "strange lady" under some duress in the ashram, offered to help her. As Baba frowned upon such interaction between the sexes, when another mandali member discovered the pair together Savak came under some sharp criticism.

When Bhau took off the disguise and revealed himself later, it was Savak's turn to criticize the culprits who had tricked him.

In the US, Baba and the group travelled to Meher Center in South Carolina from New York, staying there for six days. They then went on to California and later Australia, finally arriving back at Satara, India, in mid-August.

Later in the year in November, Baba made an unusual request, asking every Baba-lover in the world immediately to write a short letter directed to Baba, adding that none should expect a reply.

As November closed, disaster loomed around the corner for Baba and four of his men mandali. On December 2, 1956, while driving back from Poona with the mandali, Baba's party was involved in an automobile accident. Eruch was driving. The car suddenly went out of control, struck a low stone culvert, turned over, and landed in a gully. Everyone in the car was thrown out and seriously injured.

Baba and Vishnu were taken by a passing motorist back to Satara and a truck later brought Eruch, Pendu, and Nilu to the hospital in Satara. Nilu never regained consciousness and died before arriving at hospital. Eruch suffered broken ribs and Pendu's leg was badly damaged.

The injuries to Baba were serious. His head and face were badly hurt, his tongue torn, the right hip damaged, the upper rim of the acetabulum* was fractured.

Doctors William and Goher as well as another orthopaedic surgeon were immediately summoned. X-ray photos were taken. The possibility of an operation was discussed, but Baba refused the suggestion. He was quickly moved to Poona where better medical facilities existed.

While the healing of the fracture seemed to progress, Baba continued to be in great pain.

---

* The acetabulum is the concave surface of the pelvis where the head of the femur (thigh bone) meets with the pelvis.

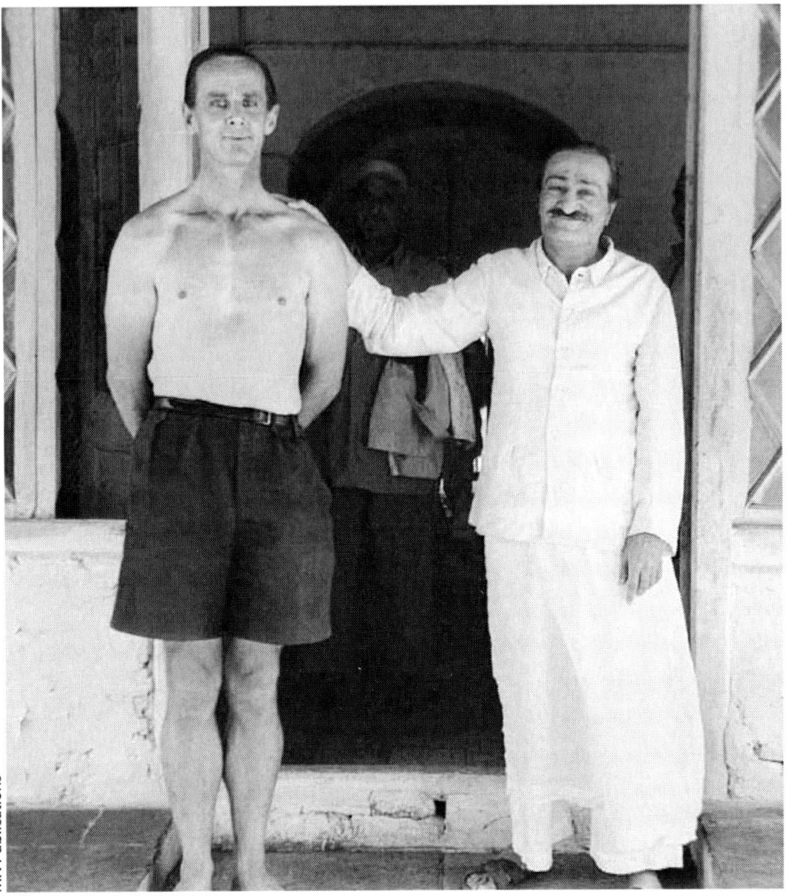

Meher Baba and Dr. William Donkin are shown in Satara in February 1955. While Baba would often take the mandali to the limits of their patience, there were also times when praise was showered on them for their fortitude and service.

As an orthopaedic surgeon, William was brought very much into the forefront of Baba's recovery process. He had been responsible for summoning the osteopath from Poona to Satara.

Although it was advised that Baba's pelvis and entire right leg be put into a cast, this became unmanageable when a week after the accident the pain became very severe as muscle spasms set in.

When Baba was moved to Poona, he stayed at a bungalow named Silver Oaks at 3 Salisbury Park Road. The women mandali and William stayed at the same residence.

An incident had occurred in Satara before the accident that bears relating.

"Baba had sent Don [William] and Goher to visit a few Indian Christian missionaries who were doing social work in the area. The missionaries liked the two doctors, but could not understand why they were staying with Meher Baba. They told William they 'were praying for him.'

"Mani once confronted a missionary, casually remarking, 'you know, we love Jesus Christ more than you.'

"'The missionaries in Satara were doing wonderful work,' Mani remarked, 'but they couldn't understand about Baba. They could somehow feel something reflected in the people around Baba, like Donkin and Dr. Goher, who were mostly involved with them, but they couldn't stand the idea of Baba as Christ. We tried to help them understand, but then Baba had the accident....'

"'The man who calls himself God,' the missionaries said in scorn, 'He couldn't even save himself.'

"'Yet,' [continues Mani], 'as we were leaving for Poona, there they were, standing on the road with such reverence when they knew Baba's ambulance would leave. The ones who were more strongly opposed to the idea of Baba as Christ were standing lined up, with so much reverence on their faces. I actually wept.'"[189]

In mid-December, William consulted Dr. Samarendra Chandra Chatterjee, an orthopaedic surgeon from a military hospital.

The latest x-rays of Baba's pelvis taken on January 19, 1957, indicated the bone was healing properly.

During this time Baba apparently decided to drive home a lesson with Dr. Goher. Bhau Kalchuri describes the incident:

"One day, Goher told Donkin that Baba was in so much pain he could not move his leg. Donkin went to the military hospital and brought Dr. Chatterjee, [but Baba then appeared OK]. Chatterjee asked Goher why she sent for him. Donkin even chastised her for bothering Chatterjee. [It was Baba's way to contact Chatterjee and make Goher go through a humiliating experience.] Again, he was at work eroding egos."[190]

Shortly after the accident, William worked to obtain and prepare a special bed for Baba designed to help alleviate the pain from his injuries. Meherwan Jessawala, a young man at the time, recalls the extent of the search for the bed:

"Baba was very uncomfortable and Donkin was beside himself looking for an ideal hospital bed. He went to a flea market, and in what looked like a pile of scrap metal, he could see a hospital bed. He bought the whole thing.

"I thought, what is this, is it a real bed? I was amazed as there were no planks, just ironwork."

"He went to the timber market and got teak boards the right size for the bed. Then he designed a mattress, which was in four parts.

"My aunt stitched the mattress out of Egyptian cotton. He was very keen about getting it done. I was about Baba's size so he would get me to lie down and take measurements.

"'What fits me would fit the Lord,' he said.

"The old paint from the bed was scratched off, red oxide applied and a final coat of silver paint."

Meherwan says that when Baba finally tried out the new bed, "for the first time he felt extremely comfortable."[191] Despite his suffering, Baba insisted that events planned for 1957 would go on. In a special circular sent to his lovers worldwide in mid-December, he stated, "In this apparent helplessness I declare anew that everything except God is illusion and that the only way to be united with this Self of all selves is love, sacrifice, and unreserved and honest resignation to the Beloved's Will. I am the Self in all. I am the Ultimate Goal. So love me with all your honesty and being. After my seclusion is over [on February 15] I will be free from this helplessness. I will give my sahavas, darshan, and blessings to all."

In December 1956, Baba's sister Mani had begun a series of Family Letters[*], which would be sent to the Western family

* The Family Letters (also *Eighty-Two Family Letters to Western Followers of Meher Baba*) were written by Mani from December 1956 to August 1969 to inform the close westerners of Baba's and the mandali's news and activities.

of lovers and followers of Meher Baba. These letters continued until August 1969.

In addition to responding to the news of Baba's injuries and the pain they had caused, Kitty Davy writing from Yaupon Dunes and Meher Center in South Carolina in March 1957 voiced her disappointment at the slow progress in attracting new followers to Baba in America.

"In spite of the lovely weather, I feel depressed when I think of Baba coming here twice and the time Elizabeth and Norina have been here, and I now for five years. There should be more love and faith here for Baba, large numbers know of Baba and the number grows, I know; but where to look for that love and faith that means so much to Baba.... Results may not come with this generation down here."[192]

William continued to be instrumental in co-ordinating Baba's recovery. On January 20, Mani reported progress in her letter to the West. Baba was able to be transferred from his bed to a wheelchair – a gift from William. The new folding wheelchair replaced a cumbersome old wooden one. The osteopath who was still treating Baba issued orders that no weight-bearing exercises or attempts at walking with the aid of crutches should be attempted until early March, a full three months after the accident.

At the end of January, the former ashram base at Satara was shut down. Baba also was to be moved from Poona back to his compound at Meherazad in mid-February.

While Dr. Chatterjee said Baba's injuries were healing, the pain he was experiencing was extreme at times and indicated that the doctor's prognosis was less than accurate.

William's time was divided. He would make weekly visits to see Baba at Poona and then at Meherazad after Baba returned home. He was also put in charge of the recovery of Pendu, who was staying at Meherabad and still not walking three months after the automobile accident.

Mani's series of Family Letters – dispatched to Elizabeth, Norina, and Kitty at Myrtle Beach and then forwarded to other Western Baba followers – continued to reflect upbeat progress regarding his recovery. A storm was brewing regarding Baba's condition, however, and William would soon feel its force.

Programs involving large groups of followers continued to be planned and held. In mid-February, Baba received 800 poor people, giving them prasad and touching the feet of each one. He also was making plans for large darshan programs, which would attract thousands, in Sakori and Poona later in the spring.

Baba seemed to be continuously working on various levels. On one trip to Poona in April with the women mandali and four of the men, including William, Baba was engaged in a game of checkers with one of the men.

"An important government official came to meet Him. Baba, however, continued the game. The official looked confused as he could see nothing around him indicating any kind of 'spiritual behaviour,' and naturally did not understand Baba's actions… [which conveyed], 'Though to you I seem absorbed in the game, you do not know what work I am doing in the universe. My universal work continues every moment – while I eat, drink, sleep, play – constantly.'

"The official received Baba's answer without question and continued to watch the game.

"Occasionally Baba reached out and patted him. Later the official revealed to the men present that with every pat Baba gave him, he received an answer to a question that had just arisen in his mind. 'This has been the most memorable experience of my life.'"[193]

During this time, Baba was being coaxed to practise walking. William assisted him in using the crutches. But the pain associated with these efforts prompted caution. Baba's sister Mani writes in a Family Letter to the West on April 11, 1957, "It is obvious Baba has to remain outwardly inactive for longer, as the pain continues and has not diminished. Because of this the doctors have found it advisable to reduce the walking and weight-bearing considerably till further x-rays have been taken and further investigations prove that all is satisfactory."

Part of the investigations involved consulting again with Dr. Reginald Watson-Jones in London. Watson-Jones had examined Baba in London in 1952 after his Oklahoma accident. The doctor informed India that Baba's hip appeared dislocated and unless it was operated upon, it would never heal properly.

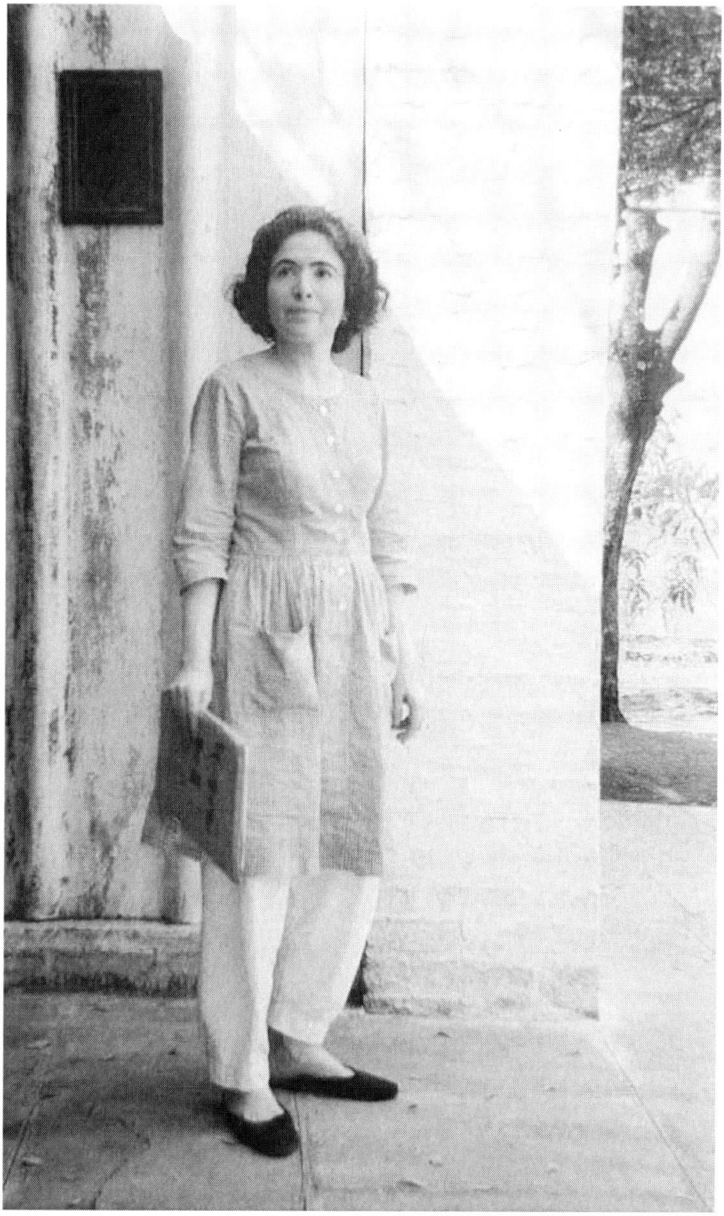

MSI Collection India

Mani S. Irani was a tireless worker for her brother Meher Baba. She served as chair of the Avatar Meher Baba Trust for many years and was responsible for writing the 1956–1969 Family Letters, which served as a link to lovers and followers in other parts of the world.

William suddenly found himself in the line of fire. Bhau Kalchuri describes the scene in *Lord Meher*:

"This was discussed on July 24, but Baba did not agree to the operation. He was, however, perturbed with Donkin for not sending all his medical reports at the beginning, as he had hinted he should. As a result, the dislocation in his hip had gone undetected for eight months. On July 25 Baba dictated to Eruch these cutting remarks in a letter to Donkin, 'If you had done so [sent Dr. Watson-Jones the medical records], I would not have suffered the unnecessary unbearable pain. You, doctors Chatterjee and Ketkar have made a mess of my case.'"[194]

William had to have been devastated by this admonishment from Baba – although now in his eighteenth year in India, he may well have welcomed any attention from Baba, favourable or unfavourable.

There are also accounts in *Lord Meher* that Eruch was feeling depressed because he had been driving when the accident occurred.

"Eruch felt guilty about the accident and Baba's pain. Baba told him not to fuss. Eruch said, 'Baba you used to walk fast. Now look, it's all gone.'

"'Who says that?'

"'The greatest surgeon in the world, Donkin, and all the other doctors say it.'"[195]

There are however many examples in various writings about Meher Baba that indicate that his close mandali, when not squabbling, supported each other whenever necessary. Bhau Kalchuri points out that when Eruch was feeling down about the accident, William discovered a passage in the book *King Jesus** that claimed Jesus had a limp. When Eruch read this he was somewhat reconciled that even Jesus had to suffer in a similar manner.

Throughout the latter part of 1957 and early 1958 Baba was busy planning another trip to the West, including visits to the United States and Australia.

---

* *King Jesus* is a 1946 novel by Robert Graves based on research on Jesus as a man. It claimed that Jesus was secretly the son of one of King Herod's sons, and that his mother Mary was also of royal lineage, making him literally a king.

While various levels of fanfare had accompanied Baba's two other trips to the West in the fifties, he insisted that there would be no publicity or even people meeting him at the airport when he arrived in mid-May in the United States.

William along with Eruch, Adi Sr., and Nariman Dadachanji* would accompany Baba on this Western tour.

Baba's disregard for his pain is evident in his decision to proceed with other large sahavas programs in India early in 1958.

At the end of the year, Dr. Harry Kenmore,** a blind American chiropractor, was in India attending to Baba. His treatment appears to have brought some relief. In a Family Letter of December 1, 1957, Mani relays Baba's own take on the situation:

"I tell Harry that as long as he is here and attending to Me, I will do what he says, and in his absence will try to carry out his instructions. But I cannot promise to carry them out fully because I have work to do.

"He has satisfactorily attended to his business and I have attended to mine. I have taken on this body for humanity's sake, and during the year I have to use My body for the work I have to do in My love for humanity. Therefore I must not take care of it to the extent of letting it interfere in My work. On the other hand I must take enough care so that it stands up to the strain of work that lies ahead of Me."[196]

In addition to sending the Family Letters to the West from 1956 until 1969, Baba's sister Mani and Mehera were also writing letters to "EliKit" (Elizabeth Patterson and Kitty Davy) at the Meher Spiritual Center. The content of the letters to the Center dealt with the operation of the South Carolina retreat and the planned Western visit in 1958, as well as fond commentary about the earlier years Elizabeth and Kitty had spent in India.

William again got involved in an embarrassing situation with Baba during the group's airplane trip from Bombay to the

---

* Nariman Dadachanji met Baba in 1929 and became a lifelong close disciple. He married his cousin Arnavaz (with Baba's blessing). Baba frequently visited, stayed in, and gave darshan in their home in Bombay, called Ashiana.

** After their 1956 meeting, Baba would call Dr. Kenmore to India to give him chiropractic treatments. Baba said he was a mandali and liked his recitation of the Master's prayer. Baba ordered him to hold annual public programs in New York for Baba's birthday (February 25) and Silence Day (July 10).

United States. The plane touched down briefly in Cairo and then went on to Rome where there was a four-hour layover. William tried his best to make sure that Baba was comfortable during this layover but his efforts backfired. Bhau Kalchuri describes the incident in the *Lord Meher* series:

"Donkin requested that the pilot radio ahead for a room in the Rome airport in which his patient [Baba] could rest during the layover. Speaking in Italian, Donkin impressed them that he was a British doctor in charge of a very important person. Two attendants met them at the airport with a wheelchair and insisted on escorting Baba. They did not speak English and only Donkin spoke Italian. They wheeled Baba onto a platform and while Donkin went to check about the room [an ambulance came and mistakenly took Baba and Eruch off to a hospital]. Donkin, Nariman, and Adi [Sr.] arrived [at the facility some time later] and after a couple of hours returned to the airport."[197]

While there is little mention of the exchange that occurred between Baba and William after this inadvertent side trip, it's a fair guess that any inflated ego William might have acquired trying to organize the good turn was squashed.

Although Baba rapped William on the knuckles often, there were occasions where Baba put the doctor's gentle nature to work. A brief side story which occurred before the group left for the West reflects this.

While Bhau Kalchuri was completely dedicated to Baba and stayed with him full time, he did have a wife Rama and two small children – Sheela and Mehernath. For a few years the family lived away from Meherabad, but they were finally allowed to move there in 1957. Sheela Kalchuri Fenster recounts one of her first memories of William:

"Once in the Meherabad hall when I was six or seven, Baba asked us, 'What do you like to do most?'

"I said, 'Baba I wish you were here when there is a full moon. I could hold your hand, and you and I would walk in the moonlight.'

"Baba instructed William, 'One night, take her for a walk in the moonlight.'

"Although Sheela protested saying she wanted only to walk with Baba, she eventually agreed to the walk when Baba said: 'I will be there. It won't be Don [William] who is walking with you.'

"A short time after, William did take Sheela for a walk under a full moon at midnight.

"'William took my hand, and hand in hand we walked.... It felt as if Baba were walking with me.'"[198]

The moonlight walk with Sheela would bode well in the relationship between William and her in the future. Sheela soon came to consider him her best friend.

William undoubtedly felt the relationship with Sheela was special. He had a large flock of nieces and nephews back in England close to Sheela's age. While very fond of them, he would see them only on rare visits to his homeland.

Amusing incidents often highlighted the growing friendship between the English doctor and young East Indian girl.

"William not only treated people, he was like a vet for my dog [and my later pets, also]. For example, William would come to our house and vaccinate Tipoo. Although William gave Tipoo an injection only once a year, whenever [he] came to the Family Quarters, Tipoo would see him, start howling, and act peculiarly as if he were about to receive a shot.

"I told Baba about it, and Baba came out of the hall to see. He had William approach Tipoo, who immediately lay down on his back and whimpered loudly. Baba laughed so much he had tears in his eyes and asked for a handkerchief."[199]

Since Baba's 1958 visit to the West was not to be a media event, no one met the group when they landed on May 17 at the airport in New York. They continued directly to Meher Center in Myrtle Beach.

Baba met followers for the first time on the morning of May 19 at the Lagoon Cabin – the small, intimate structure built specifically for brief meetings with devotees.

About 200 people were invited to the Myrtle Beach event, and later in the day a bigger group met Baba at The Barn, the large building that could accommodate all those attending the sahavas.

In an aside to one of those attending, Meher Baba said that this would be his final trip to the West and he would not be returning again.

Baba was experiencing immense pain in his damaged hip during the visit. At one point he discussed with William and the other mandali the possibility of cancelling the sahavas. In the end, however, he decided to stay fourteen days in the US and five days in Australia.

The process for daily communication once the party arrived at Myrtle Beach was for Eastern disciple Nariman Dadachanji to tell William the day's schedule. William would then convey the time Baba would be at the Lagoon Cabin and Barn to Elizabeth and Kitty, who would make sure the larger group knew.

William's role during the 1958 trip to the United States and Australia appears to have been as an organizer, doctor, and "fixer." He travelled to Myrtle Beach ahead of the group to see that everything was in order, and while there he was in constant communication with Elizabeth Patterson and Kitty Davy regarding the format of the sahavas.

On one occasion Darwin Shaw, one of Baba's close Western disciples, describes a co-operative job that he and William were dispatched to accomplish at Baba's House on the Center.

"One morning Baba told me to help Dr. Donkin ... to tighten the webbing on Baba's bed instead of attending a meeting in The Barn.

"This turned out to be quite a chore. Instead of springs, Baba's bed had, and still has, interwoven webbing as is used on Indian beds under the mattress. I felt that for some reason Baba wanted me to have closer contact with Dr. Donkin."[200]

Other Westerners also had unique Baba-related duties to perform. At this time long-term Western mandali member, Margaret Craske, was teaching ballet in New York City. A number of her dance students came with her to the sahavas and were chosen to carry Baba in a special chair during his stay at the spiritual retreat. The topics Baba raised in the discourses given at The Barn were serious, and he was not shy about asking for a major commitment from his followers:

"What I want is your love and obedience 100 per cent. I want one who does his best. In the time of Jesus, I said the same thing: leave all and follow Me! And the same in the time of Krishna and Zoroaster. I do not mean you have to leave all your responsibilities, but that My Will becomes yours. My will should be your pleasure. God is infinite honesty. To love God you must be honest."[201]

In addition to the serious spiritual discourses and explanations, there were also light, fun-filled occasions.

One event was a children's birthday party for about 40 girls and boys. Baba served lemonade to each child, embraced each one, and cut the cake. The children were later taken out for a boat ride in the gondola* on the lake. Baba also met a group of women and a group of men at separate times. With the women, Baba distributed gifts sent from Mehera in India, and at Baba's House he tossed the men candies as prasad.

Eastern and western music were played, including Baba's favourite, "Begin the Beguine," which he said had eternal meaning. The dancers from New York City also performed for Baba. An even lighter event occurred when a number of the men loosely called the "Alligator Club" entertained Baba with skits and jokes. The next day Baba said, "Yesterday's performance made me so happy – not just because it made me laugh, but because you all love me."[202]

Humour seemed to be high on the agenda during Baba's 1958 visit to Meher Center. Baba arranged that a rubber snake be placed outside of where Kitty was staying. Kitty promptly got a broom and began beating the "snake" all the while saying "Baba, Baba, Baba." Suddenly Baba and a few other mandali appeared from the side of the house in a full uproar.

In her book, Kitty gives an account of May 29, Baba's last day at the Center:

"He was driven to the Center beach and carried to the water's edge where He removed his sandals and dipped his feet in the water. The women took a turn carrying Him back to the

---

* The gondola at the Meher Center was an authentic one from the 1939 World's Fair in New York City. Elizabeth saw it advertised and bought it for the Center. Baba rode in it and it is still used on the Meher Center lake.

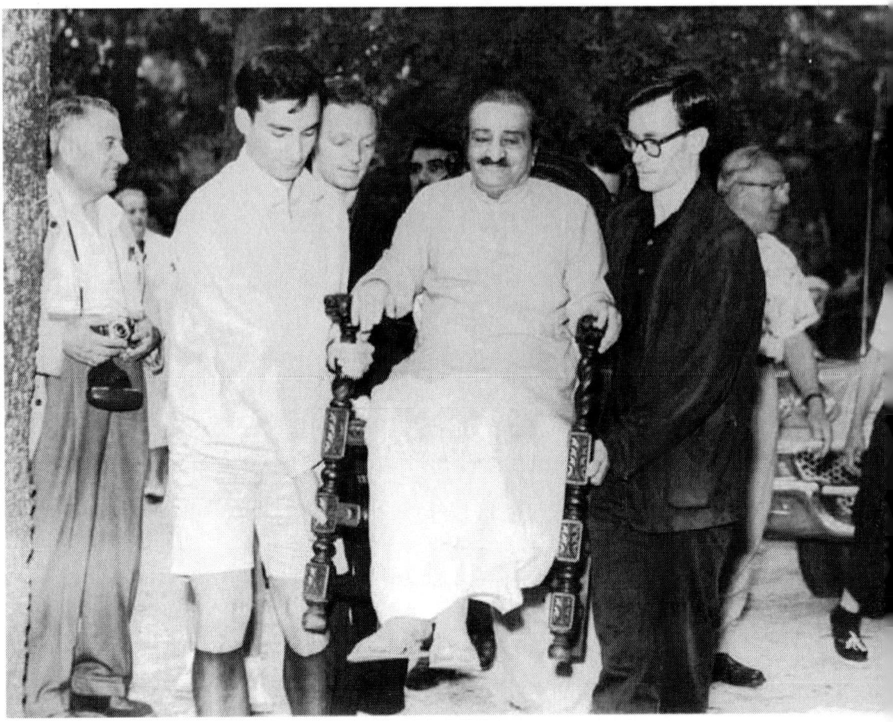

Carrie Ben Shammai Archive

car and Barn. Then He went to the Lagoon Cabin for the last few private interviews with various ones of the group."

When the group left Myrtle Beach for Washington to fly on to California, American Baba-lover Lud Dimpfl* accompanied them. Baba, William, and the other mandali stopped briefly at Dimpfl's home in Kentfield, California, an hour from San Francisco before flying onward to Australia.

The group stayed at Avatar's Abode,** the retreat on Kiel Mountain near Brisbane, Australia, for eight days. Again, Baba

---

* Lud Dimpfl was a scientist with Chevron and learned of Meher Baba from his co-worker Don Stevens. Lud met Baba for the first time in 1952, and later his wife and children also met and became followers of Baba. He was a member of Sufism Reoriented until his death in 1988.

** Avatar's Abode is a 99-acre property of great natural beauty on the summit of Kiel Mountain near Woombye on Queensland's Sunshine Coast. It has a panoramic view of the ocean to the east and over valleys, farmlands, and rolling blue hills to the west.

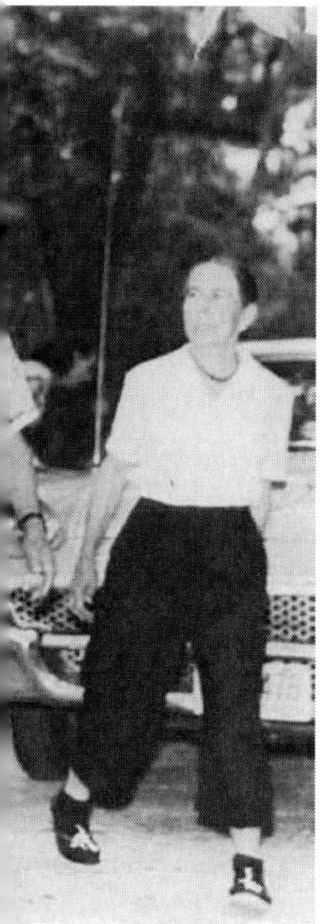

A group of men that included several dance students of Margaret Craske carries Meher Baba in a special chair during his visit to Meher Spiritual Center in May 1958. Mandali member Kitty Davy is shown at far right.

emphasized the importance of obedience in the discourses to his followers.

The program during the five days was a miniature version of what had occurred at Meher Center in South Carolina. Baba asked about the Australian centre and was told that it was his property. He instructed this to be changed so the Australian retreat would be held by Francis Brabazon. Baba refused to hold any property in his own name.

At one point during the Australian visit, Baba asked William to read the Prayer of Repentance to the gathering.

William also read out what Baba had said about the importance of sahavas, a Master's gathering for devotees:

"I want you all to remain happy in My sahavas. I am the ocean of Love. Draw as much of this love as possible. Make the most of this opportunity. It rests with you to draw as much love as you can out of the ocean."[203]

Baba went on to say through William that it was not up to the Master to explain to his lovers how to love, pointing out that a husband or wife does not explain to one another how to love each other.

"The easy way to receive it is to forget your home, family, and all worldly affairs when you are here, and be receptive to My Love."[204]

Baba (again through William) went on to say getting a good night's sleep was also important.

"I am God; if you remain drowsy in My presence, you will miss me, and your drowsiness will oblige you to remain absent from My presence in spite of daily attendance."[205]

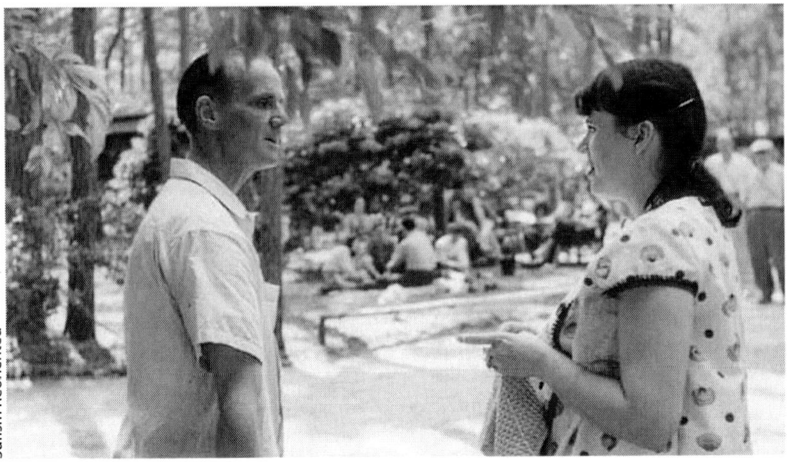
Sufism Reoriented

William talks to Charmian Duce Knowles during Meher Baba's 1958 visit to Meher Spiritual Center in Myrtle Beach, South Carolina. They would have had a lot to catch up on after not seeing each other for a number of years.

The next day, Wednesday, June 4, 1958, William delivered another discourse on behalf of Baba called "Love is the Remedy."

The discourse is given in its entirety here because it serves as the foundation of Meher Baba's way:

> Do not give undue importance to explanations and discourses. Words fail to give any meaning to Reality; because when one supposes that one has understood; one has not understood; one is far from understanding anything as far as Reality is concerned. Reality is beyond human understanding. The moment you try to understand God you "misunderstand" Him; you miss Him when you try to understand Him. Reason must go before knowledge dawns. All this is a show, fun, a play. Mind must go because the play lies in the mind. And the play is that mind must annihilate itself. Only manonash [annihilation of mind] takes one to Reality. There is a way to annihilate the mind. The way

> is love. Just consider ordinary human love: when a man or woman is deeply in love with his or her partner, nothing comes between them. They get totally lost in love for one another.
>
> There is neither admiration nor fault-finding. There is total absence even of exchange of thought: love prevails without thoughts. Mind becomes defunct for the time being: for in such intense human love mind does not come into play. The mind apparently gets annihilated for the fraction of a second when love and loving are at their zenith. This brings about a state similar to trance. If ordinary human love can go so far, what should be said of the height of Divine Love?
>
> I am the Ancient One, the One residing in every heart. Therefore love others, make others happy, serve others, even at discomfort to yourself; this is to love Me. I suffer for the whole universe. I must suffer infinitely; unless I suffer how could I ask My lovers to suffer for others? I am One with all on every level: I am One with all on every plane of consciousness: and I am beyond all planes of consciousness.[206]

Baba, William, and the other mandali left Australia on the night of June 7, 1958, to fly back to India. They arrived in Bombay on the evening of June 8.

15

Seclusion Deepens, East Meets West in 1962

Shortly after Baba returned to India, he began a period of seclusion which would last until November 1958. Usually during such a time he would issue various orders to individual mandali throughout the world. William was told to stay in Meherabad and often tended to the medical needs of other mandali. Eruch was also directed to remain in Meherabad, and both he and William were told not to expect to be able to visit Baba in Meherazad, which was only a short car ride away.

On Silence Day – July 10 – Baba did make an appearance at Meherabad, and at the time his Universal Message was delivered. The message is still prominent today in Baba's teachings. Before the message was read out, William recited the Parvardigar (Master's) Prayer in English, after which the prayer was recited in several other languages, including Telegu, Hindi, and Marathi.

Oddly enough Baba gave no directives to his followers in the West regarding maintaining silence and/or fasting on July 10, perhaps indicating that his followers should remember his talks on obedience. His sister Mani wrote, "Baba desires to give no instructions for the observance of this 10th of July – the 34th anniversary of His Silence; and leaves it entirely to the inclination of each concerned – i.e., it may be observed if and as we like, or not observed at all. No queries should be sent here in regard to this…."[207]

In August 1959, Mani observed that Baba was at times walking unaided and unaccompanied.

"We are not quite used to all this and can still find ourselves joyously startled when He suddenly gets up and walks over by Himself to another room. This is not only contrary to our most optimistic expectations, but contrary to the emphatic opinions and advice of eminent doctors and specialists who had been concerned in the matter and know the extent of the injury."

While life carried on in India in the fall of 1959, Myrtle Beach was walloped with another hurricane. Elizabeth Patterson and Kitty Davy moved from Elizabeth's Yaupon Dunes home to Pine Lodge on the Center property, hoping they would be safer since it is further distance from the oceanfront. The move to apparent safety took a bad turn, however, as Kitty outlines:

"During the evening of the storm, Elizabeth took a fall on the steps of Pine Lodge. There we were with no help available in the middle of a hurricane.... Elizabeth was immediately rushed to hospital and a cable was sent to India."[208]

Kitty followed up the cable with a letter:

"Dear Mani:

"I know you, Don [William], and [Dr.] Goher will be waiting patiently to hear the extent of damage to Elizabeth's leg.... It is a nasty break – a compound fracture.... Elizabeth will return home this weekend – the same wheelchair Baba used will be ready for her use – and she will have two crutches. She is looking well, is cheery, and accepts what is to be."[209]

While Baba was in seclusion for much of 1959 and 1960, a few Western visitors did gain brief audiences with him, some on invitation and others just by showing up. The blind chiropractor, Harry Kenmore, was one person whose company and healing advice Baba appreciated enough to welcome him more than once during these two years. A Navy man, Harry Dedolchow*, who was a member of Ivy Duce's Sufi group in the US, also dropped in on September 7, 1959. Dedolchow showed up

* Harry Dedolchow was a merchant seaman who learned of Baba in 1955 from reading *Avatar* by Jean Adriel and then meeting Ivy Duce. His ship sometimes docked in Calcutta, which gave him opportunities to meet briefly with Baba.

without advance notice and while Baba only agreed to see him for five minutes, the visit was extended to two hours.

Later in November, New York Baba-lover Joanna Smith, who was travelling in India, also came to see Baba. Mani writes in her diary of the visit, "She was overcome with happiness and love at the meeting and to see Baba walking so briskly as he personally took her round the garden. She asked Baba when He would come again to the West, adding, 'They must see you walk like this, Baba.'

"Baba's reply was a smile that was noncommittal."[210]

Later, at Christmas time, Don Stevens visited for a week along with his cousin Alain Youell.*

As Baba's usual pattern was to link Western visitors with his English doctor disciple, William would have had contact with these guests.

Life was not all happy reunions with other Westerners for William, however. In February 1960, Bhau Kalchuri was hospitalized for anal fistula surgery at Booth Hospital in Ahmednagar.

So strict were Baba's orders that William was reluctant to allow Bhau's own children to see him in hospital. Bhau's daughter, Sheela Kalchuri Fenster, describes their brief visit when permission was finally granted:

"William accompanied us. Baba had permitted us to visit Bhau for only five minutes. William was so obedient, he stood in the corner timing our visit; and after five minutes he said we had to leave."[211]

Sheela admits to sneaking in to see her father without permission on several other occasions.

"I used to skip school. My father was happy to have company. William came once when I was there. I hid at the back, as I knew William would be upset if he found me there."[212]

Bhau was later brought back to Meherabad and kept in Baba's Interview Cabin under William's care. Baba had given Bhau's children and wife Rama permission to visit Bhau, but William usually restricted the visits to only a few minutes.

---

* Alain Youell is a well-known psychologist and human development expert who has worked in the US, UK, Eire, Canada, India, Japan, China, Australia, New Zealand, and Thailand.

Sheela observed William's care of Bhau while he was convalescing and wrote of it:

"I was fascinated to watch how well William nursed my father. For example, William would carefully sterilize Bhau's clothing – boiling them – as well as his bed sheets, pillow cases, and towels, to prevent Bhau from being exposed to germs. The entire room was scrubbed with disinfectant daily. William spent hours changing Bhau's bandages. He did everything so meticulously, always."[213]

Baba's annual trip to Guruprasad came round again in March 1960. He indicated that he would take a number of the young boys who were working in Meherabad with him to Poona.

One of the youngsters, Motiram Kamble, recalls his disappointment at not being chosen and William's intervention at the time:

"Baba told me to stay at Meherabad. I started crying – disappointed that I was not also going to Guruprasad."

Motiram, who was 12 at the time, said William pacified him and said he would look after him. He would become William's lifelong servant, although he readily admits that William rarely treated him like a servant. Baba agreed to entrust Motiram to William's care and gave William instruction that he was never to beat the boy.

Motiram recalls the moment:

"William had a fiery temper and would at times throw all of his furniture out of his cabin and then later retrieve it. Baba entrusted me to him and ensured that William would not harm me."

The British doctor and Motiram would be together for nearly a decade.

"He [William] bought clothes for me. We went on trips to Poona and Bombay together. He would speak Hindi to me and always made sure I was able to stay in the same hotel."[214]

Later, in mid-1960, California Baba-lover Lud Dimpfl visited Meherabad for four days. He managed the side trip to India in the middle of being transferred to Iran by his company.

Mani describes Dimpfl's visit:

"He was immediately merged in Baba's sahavas – seeing Baba at work and in relaxation, Baba with the multitude and with the intimate few, sharing the different endearing facets reflected by Baba's mood of the moment. In short, being just one of the mandali, except that he carried around an 'I must surely be dreaming' look on his happy face. Baba seemed just as happy to have Lud with Him."[215]

Younger people who had never met Meher Baba also travelled to India from different parts of the world.

Irwin Luck, an American youth of 23, was one of those who came on his own after receiving special permission. He did not wish to return home, but in obedience to Baba's wish, did so after a few days with him. The cable Irwin sent home to his father after meeting Baba said, "Baba is all and more than what I said He was. Love to you and Mom."

Irwin recalls an amusing scene in 1960 involving William:

"I had diarrhoea. Baba was in his chair, I was on the floor, and Donkin was behind me. They were talking about me between one another and Baba kept blowing kisses to Donkin."[216]

Irwin again visited Baba in 1961 and 1962, on these occasions accompanied by his brother Edward. They became lifelong followers of Meher Baba and both live close to the Meher Center in South Carolina.

By the end of 1960 it appeared that Baba's periods of seclusion had become his way of life. Ivy Duce gives an indication of the mood this created among his Western followers:

"By December it was evident that Baba had simply undergone the first lap, or six months, of his seclusion and that it would continue indefinitely. He stated he would see absolutely nobody in 1961. Baba sent out word that from the 26th of December 1960 through the 15th of January 1961, he wished all his lovers in the East and in the West to repeat any one name of God 500 times daily for those 21 days; that during this period they should go on a fast; the men were given the option of fasting for any number of days but Baba said that the women should not fast for more than five days out of this period of 21 days. Yet Baba expected all of his lovers to accomplish at least one fast of 24 hours if they could not do more."[217]

Baba's increasing seclusion coincided with his failing health in the early sixties. William was often called on, along with Dr. Goher, to consult on Baba's various ailments. In late 1960 Baba was diagnosed with herpes zoster. His doctors suspected that he caught this bowing down to lepers and the poor in September. The ailment affected the right side of the tongue, palate, face, and the right ear. At the end of the year Baba suffered numbness in his face, which William and Dr. Goher diagnosed as Ramsay Hunt neuralgia, with two nerves in his face affected. It was decided to inject alcohol in the nerve. This worked, and Baba was able to eat comfortably again.

Concerns for Baba's health would become constant throughout the early sixties, and Baba sometimes hinted that the end of his life was approaching. While William was continuously alert to Baba's health, he was also expected to administer to the medical needs of his fellow mandali.

As Baba's birthday approached in February 1961, Baba had ended a period of seclusion and fasting. Both William and Dr. Goher were concerned at this time about Baba's diet and whether he was getting the right amount of calories and sugar.

Although seclusion was the watchword at the start of the sixties, Baba still allowed some of his close Western mandali to visit.

On February 10, Don Stevens arrived at Bombay, and William was sent to meet him. They drove directly to Poona. Baba also decided that William should accompany Stevens and Joseph and Kari Harb on a trip to Satara and Mahabaleshwar. The Harbs, from California, had learned about Baba through the Sufi movement in 1947, and Baba had given them permission to live for a time in India.

During the trip, William and Stevens went on an extra excursion. William thought his new American companion might be interested in seeing a band of wild monkeys, but the adventure quickly turned into a misadventure, and placed William in more turmoil with Baba.

"Wandering down a forest canyon, the two got separated. William warned Stevens about poisonous vines and then hiked on ahead. Shortly after, Stevens got ensnarled in such a vine and not being able to summon William, who was out of earshot, had to handle the plant to get free of it. The men later reconnected and William said he would make sure to clean Stevens' hands with antiseptic when they returned to Meherabad.

"The next morning in Mandali Hall, Baba noticed Stevens scratching his hand and said, 'Don, what is that?'

"Trying to evade the issue and protect Donkin, Stevens replied, 'I don't know Baba, just a little bit of a rash.'

"Baba then wormed the full story out of Stevens.'Where was Donkin?... Go fetch Donkin,' said Baba angrily.

"Furious, Baba asked Donkin for all the details. He was extremely upset, and lashed out at Donkin [entrusted with Stevens' welfare], for his carelessness.

"Both men came away from the experience somewhat scathed.

"'I wanted to crawl right underneath my cushion and disappear,' said Stevens. 'I liked Donkin very much and hated to see him raked over the coals for my own carelessness. I felt sick.'"[218]

Luckily for Stevens, Baba gave him one of his prized handkerchiefs shortly after the incident. Stevens was overjoyed and the itching on his hands and arms soon went away.

On January, 23, 1962, Baba's right-hand man and interpreter, Eruch, fell ill and was admitted to Booth Hospital for a tonsillectomy the next day. William attended the operation.

The tempo at the ashram was upbeat in the early months of 1962 over the planned November sahavas. This would mark the first time that Easterners and Westerners met Baba together in a large gathering.

There were strict rules laid out in advance of the occasion, which was to be held at Guruprasad* in Poona. A Life Circular issued on March 21, 1962, states in part, "Baba wants all concerned to bear in mind that His permission to visit Him at that time in November will be only for his lovers who are close to Him in His Love, and is not meant for the general public."

* Guruprasad was the palace of the Maharani of Baroda, Shantadevi, in Poona. She became devoted to Baba and gave him the use of Guruprasad whenever he wished – usually the summer months when it was very hot in Meherabad and Meherazad.

Contact with Baba at the gathering was only from 4 p.m. to 6 p.m. daily, but Baba did make extra time for his lovers travelling from outside of India.

"Lovers from overseas only will be allowed to visit Baba at Guruprasad Bungalow, Poona, each morning from 9:30 a.m. to 11 a.m. in addition to the afternoon session. Easterners must not visit Baba in the mornings."

The circular stated that Baba was breaking seclusion only for the darshan. No individual interviews would be allowed. Nor were personal problems to be brought to Baba. Westerners were responsible for their travel all the way to Poona.

"To the women, I would say wear comfortable skirts and footwear for the darshan hours, as the formal apparel of tight skirts and high heels will prove an inconvenience and a definite handicap for those wanting to take his darshan or preferring to sit Indian fashion on the ground."[219]

There was no let-up in William's medical duties in the early months of 1962. Mandali member Pendu had a prostate operation in April and was admitted to a local nursing home for many weeks of recovery.

During this period, Vishnu, a mandali member with Baba for over 40 years, died suddenly from heart failure.

Baba conducted a number of meetings prior to the massive East-West gathering of November. About 2,000 Baba-lovers where expected. Those attending would be aged six to ninety-two, and only 171 would come from the West. Thousands of others who lived close to Poona or had relatives nearby would be able to make day visits to Guruprasad for the darshan days.

The months of 1962 before the November sahavas saw more surprise visits from Westerners. Harry Kenmore, the blind American chiropractor, dropped in while vacationing in Poona.

In addition to the Family Letters sent out every eight weeks, Mani also kept up personal, ongoing correspondence with "Elikitruth" (Elizabeth Patterson, Kitty Davy, and Ruth White*) at Meher Center in Myrtle Beach.

---

* Ruth White had heard of Baba from Malcolm Schloss in 1945, met Baba in 1956 in Myrtle Beach, and travelled to the East-West Gathering in 1962 at the age of 92..

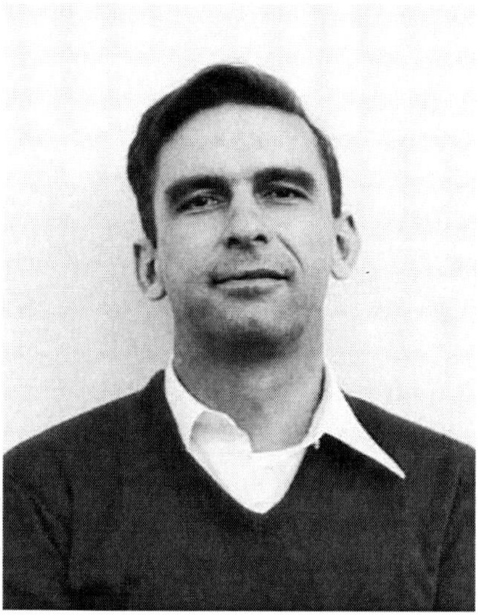

MN Publications

Don Stevens met Meher Baba in the early fifties and would become a staunch worker for his Spiritual Master. He has written many books about Baba including *Listen, Humanity* and also shared the job of editing *God Speaks* with Ivy Duce.

While Baba was strict about his seclusion, he was also sensitive to the needs of his lovers. Mani recalled that on one occasion, he agreed to see a few children of the Poona lovers.

"But instead of a trickle, 300 rushed through the open door. This was followed by two weeks in which he permitted his lovers to come to Guruprasad for one hour between 4:30 and 5:30 p.m., under the conditions that they should not bring offerings nor garlands; they should not bow down to him nor seek interviews nor advice on personal problems, nor expect spiritual discourses."[220]

To complicate the planning of the large gathering to be held in November, the Poona area was hit with heavy monsoon rains in July, which caused the collapse of two dams resulting in major floods.

"Nearly half of Poona was under six feet or more of water and the entire city was without water and electricity. The flood waters reached to within a few yards of Guruprasad where Baba was staying."[221]

Baba told William a unique story of survival that came out of the Poona flood – one that attracted worldwide attention through a widely circulated photograph. To escape the danger during the deluge, five men, two snakes, a mouse, and a cat sought a safe perch in a tree-top, where they remained for hours without harming each other. After the flood subsided they all went their separate ways.

While William oversaw Pendu's prostate recovery, he was called on frequently to deal with Baba's precarious health. In October, William was called to Meherazad to help diagnose Baba's symptoms, which included spasms and fevers. Despite their poring over updated medical books all day long, he and Goher could not figure out the cause of the strange afflictions, which failed to subside after several different medicines.

Despite Baba's ailment, "the show" (the East-West Gathering) was destined to go on. In the planning, three different doctors were directed to look after the medical needs of the "darshanites." William was designated to tend to any concerns expressed by the Western male visitors.

The difficulty of finding suitable accommodations for the 171 Westerners coming to Poona was expressed in a Family Letter of September 20, 1962:

"Suitable hotel accommodation for His growing number of Western Novemberites is beginning to cause some slight anxiety."

In a lighter vein, Mani recalled a halting English speech that mandali member Kaka* had made to Western followers, including William, who came to see Baba at Cannes in 1937.

"Now I want to talk about our Master's order. When Master passes order it must be obeyed. Never mind if you like it or not. There should be no discussion. When you follow the Master, every desire must be left. Somebody wants good food, somebody wants good bed, somebody wants go swimming, somebody wants to shopping – then what use coming to Master? Go holidays!"

Baba was not without displaying his own sense of humour or perhaps a legitimate concern during the preparation period for the East-West darshan. On one occasion, while talking to

---

* Kaka Baria first met Baba in 1928. He had been a mechanical engineer, automobile mechanic, and taxi cab owner before joining Baba permanently as a mandali.

William and another of the doctors about a bus trip the Westerners were to take from Poona to Ahmednagar, Meherazad, and Meherabad after the darshan, he said, "Please see that no one dies en route."

William and fellow mandali member Padri were both responsible for leading the Westerners on this tour after the conclusion of the East-West Gathering.

Baba was also very specific in telling the Western visitors to rely wholly on William for their medical needs. He was assisted by a female and male Indian doctor who treated all female and Eastern male patients respectively.

"It is Baba's wish that you must therefore promptly inform Dr. Donkin whenever you feel indisposed, night or day. In the daytime Dr. Donkin will make the rounds of your different hotels at least once, and will be at Guruprasad during the morning and afternoon gatherings there. At night he will be on call at Napier Hotel, and anybody needing any medical aid should without fail phone him at Napier Hotel.[222]

Ivy Duce, the Murshida of the Sufi Order in North America, recalls getting sick during the sahavas.

"I had the flu, despite all the flu shots I had taken in the USA before I left.... When Dr. Donkin came in he examined me and although I felt terrible to miss a minute with Baba, he assured me there was nothing as acute as the Poona flu and I should stay in bed for the day. I sank back on my bed of pain, feeling released from guilt. He went back to Guruprasad and told Charmian [Ivy's daughter], 'I have told your mother to stay in bed today, but I doubt if Baba lets her.'"[223]

In a letter Charles Purdom writes to his friend Max Haefliger about the gathering, he says:

"I have had stomach upset and a cough, but everyone seems to be ill a bit ... Donkin has been excellent but how thin and old he looks."

Despite Baba's insistence that there would be no discourses, he opened the darshan with a pointed statement:

"Suffering is a sign of having realized God: suffering is God's gift to men.... You are to become the dust at the feet of the Perfect Master, which means that you do not know your own self. You are nothing but dust. You are no longer your own.

"There is another point. God is indivisibly one and invisibly in each one.

"God is each one. What are the divisions, why are you separate? This is nothing but ignorance: there are no divisions, no separations. Think of God as the ocean, and as every drop in the ocean as the ocean itself. Every bubble is an appearance of separateness. The bubble of the mind does not know that it is the ocean until the bubble bursts....

"Long for union with God until you go beyond longing for union and long only for the will of Beloved God. Complete forgetfulness of self is to forget even that you have forgotten."

While it is difficult to convey the feelings of the 7,000 who attended or even the 171 Westerners' feelings, the experience of Kitty Davy, who had lived with Baba for 16 years before taking up her duties in 1952 at Meher Center in South Carolina, perhaps reflects the suffering, longing, and the will of God that Baba alluded to:

"In the afternoon, after we were again assembled in the hall, Eruch read Baba's Welcoming Message. This was followed by the *Master's Prayer* in English and a short message from Baba, including the statement 'May My Love make you feel one day that God is in everyone.'"

Here was a new challenge, thought Kitty. "I felt Baba was outwardly pushing us away from Him." Later that day Kitty had the opportunity to approach Baba directly. She recalls, "I remember that when it was my turn to come to Baba's chair, I asked Baba if I would be returning to India to stay with Him. Eruch translated Baba's gestures and said I was to remain in Myrtle Beach and help Elizabeth. I knew then, and I think that others too felt, that we were not going to see Baba again. In fact, Baba did say to one that we would not see him again.

"I think I would admit that this was the saddest day of my life; the sadness of realizing that I was definitely to return and wholeheartedly make my home in the West. Until 1962 there had still remained the glimmer of hope that one day Baba would call and I would return to India to live once again in close proximity to His physical presence." [224]

16

Courage Stressed, Purdom Dies, Darshan Cancelled

As 1963 unfolded, Meher Baba's followers worldwide began to see strong signs that he was restricting their access to him.

He first issued an order that the Meher Baba centres in India and elsewhere should not have any sort of celebration for his sixty-ninth birthday in February.

At the same time he asked his lovers to spread far and wide His messages "My Dear Children" and "My Dear Workers," which he had given during the East-West Gathering.

Mani's Family Letters to the West were to continue four to six times a year. Her next letter, February 15, 1963, was longer than the usual letters. Mani was perhaps trying to make up for the new rules of separation by painting as full a picture as possible of Baba at Meherazad.

She described the simple daily teatime the women mandali enjoyed with Baba:

"Mingling with snatches of conversation and the tinkle of teaspoons in cups is the music from our transistor radio – occasionally accompanied by heavy snores from our old Cocker-spaniel fast asleep in his corner by Baba's chair."[225]

Mani mentioned that at least one Western Baba lover had slipped in under the radar. Baba permitted Adele Wolkin from New York, a nurse, to be in India for three months working with the poor and needy at a Bombay hospital. When Baba called Adele to Meherazad to tell her she would best serve his purpose by returning to the USA and working there, Adele pleased her Master by saying, "Beloved Baba, I live to obey You."

While followers of Meher Baba were going through a topsy-turvy year with new rules, William was also facing major upheavals. Earlier Baba had issued what appeared to be almost an edict when he relayed to William, Padri, and others living in Meherabad, "Be prepared for whatever changes may occur in 1963."

Baba was warning even those in his backyard that in the future they were going to have less of his physical presence. The separation felt by those from afar was felt tenfold by those living in Meherabad. Despite its close proximity (15 miles) to Baba's residence at Meherazad, Baba would not visit Meherabad again after 1962. When he wished to send messages to those at Meherabad he would summon either William or Padri to Meherazad and convey his wishes to them to pass on.

What may have appeared to be a co-operative relationship between William and Padri in this dual duty was far from reality. The two male mandali were continuously at loggerheads, scrapping and arguing over issues such as water supply and cooking at Meherabad.

Despite the personal feuding, William was expected to faithfully carry on with his medical duties. Bhau Kalchuri's family (wife Rama and children Sheela and Mehernath) moved from Meherabad to Khushru Quarters in Ahmednagar (the city located between Meherabad and Meherazad) in June 1963. Strangely, Baba also ordered the family never to visit Meherabad again.

Sheela Kalchuri's childhood bond with William was strong and she immediately missed his company on leaving Meherabad. The Kalchuri family suffered a number of health problems in 1963, and William was constantly responding to their needs.

At one point during the year Sheela's mother Rama was hospitalized, and on another occasion both Sheela and her brother Mehernath were in the hospital. Sheela suffered from an ear problem, and William was involved in treating her and her mother.

Although 1963 was one of much seclusion for Baba, he did on occasion step out of this seclusion – one occasion being May 26 in Poona. Baba had been an expert cricketer in his youth, serving as wicket-keeper batsman, so he agreed when asked to host an awards afternoon for the Poona District Cricket Association. He did this at Guruprasad, his summer residence in the city.

"It was a field day for the cricketers. They received their trophies of shields, cups, and merit certificates from Baba's hands, along with His blessing of Love; they received His darshan and participated in the arti sung at the end of the function," his sister Mani wrote in the Family Letter of June 12, 1963. "As one who knows and loves cricket, Baba advised them to play bright cricket and not to make it boring for the spectators just for the sake of remaining unbeaten."

Newspapers covering the event made hay with various headlines:

"Go in for bright cricket says Meher Baba," the banner headlines on the sports page of *The Times of India* read.

A reporter at another newspaper wrote, "Avatar Meher Baba has devotees by the thousands, not only in India but in other parts of the world."

Baba's statement included, "I am happy to present these trophies today. When I was a boy in school and college I played cricket. Now I play my Divine Universal Game....

"It is good to excel in whatever one takes up, as long as with excellence there is a feeling of humility; for this leads to love of God, and to love God as He should be loved is the best excellence."[226]

William was called on to perform a unique duty during 1963. Merwan, the son of one of Baba's mandali, Sarosh Irani, was to marry Anita, a woman from Switzerland that he had met in England. His bride, Anita, wanted a small portion of the Indian marriage to include the Christian ceremony, and William was asked to give her away.

The couple and William kept in touch afterwards and on one occasion when William visited them in England he presented them with a small refrigerator as a present.

In another 1963 Family Letter, Mani made note of the religions, professions, and occupations of those attending one of Baba's gatherings at Guruprasad:

"The weekend mass of humanity gathered around Baba was always made up of men and women of diverse religions –

Hindus, Muslims, Zoroastrians, Sikhs ... Christians, and others; of different castes and creeds and from varied walks of life.... I once tried to make a list of the men sitting there, by their professions and occupations.... Among that group were a lawyer, a yogi, businessman, cricketer, medical doctor, clerk, bakery owner, army colonel, poet, wing-commander of the air-force, musician, university professor, former member of parliament, principal of college, typist, chiropractor, editor, shop-keeper, school teacher, bank accountant, cook, motor mechanic, geologist, priest, college student, pathologist, singer, and salesman."[227]

A new plan was initiated in the US to bring Baba's message to the many who would attend the World's Fair that would open in April 1964 and run for two years in New York. Jane Barry Haynes,* a young protégé of Elizabeth Patterson's, was busy organizing the Baba booth for the World's Fair. Baba lovers from around the world contributed the $7,000 cost of leasing 100 square feet of space. A quarter million copies of a short biographical pamphlet featuring his Universal Message were printed and made available free during the international event.

Books by and about Meher Baba were published in 1963. *The Everything and Nothing,* a collection of Baba's discourses, was one; the other, *The God-Man,* was written by British Baba-lover Charles Purdom. This was another biography of Meher Baba that updated Purdom's earlier biography, *The Perfect Master,* published in 1936.

As the year 1963 concluded, arrangements were being made for a gathering of 250 women at Meherazad on December 23 (Mehera's birthday). Mani aptly commented on the occasion, "If the women Baba-lovers have had cause to feel disheartened over the fact that the men are always given more opportunities to visit Baba then they now have cause to rejoice; for Baba has fixed an 'All Women' day."[232]

Though in seclusion, Baba issued statements when a major world event occurred. On the assassination of John F. Kennedy in

* Jane Barry Haynes was an actress who ran a theatre in Myrtle Beach. She learned of Baba from Elizabeth Patterson and first met him with her three children in 1958. She eventually was involved in running the Meher Center for many years.

November 1963, Baba wrote to his world family, "He was a great man, good and sincere. Dying as he did has not only made him immortal in mankind's memory and history, but it has also given him a great push forward spiritually. However, although he was assassinated because it was ordained to be, it is not a good thing and it portends more suffering ahead for the world."[228]

As 1963 gave way to 1964, Baba continued to be involved in universal work known only to him. His hip pain continued and it provided some relief to him to host occasional music programs at Meherazad and to even take part in rousing card games.

One card game, called Larisque,* would involve 26 players – each with two cards. On one occasion up to 40 followers played using two decks. The game was hilarious and there was always an uproar over who had or had not cheated.

"I don't see how anyone's argument can be heard for they all talked at once – until Baba, pink in the face from silent laughter, gives a loud clap that brings the clamour to a sudden halt. However, the best part is reserved for the last when the game is over, and the losers bend over together and rub their noses on the ground before Baba; and that I fancy is the part many of them look forward to most!"[229]

Baba explained that the reason for playing the game of cards was threefold:

"The burden of my universal work gets lightened;

"The minds of the players are focused on me in a most natural manner;

"Those who lose have to rub their noses on the carpet before me, the Highest of the High. This is a privilege filled with significance and thus the losers become winners."

Baba's seventieth birthday was celebrated February 25, 1964. While the occasion was subdued at his Meherazad residence, tensions and a surprise radio broadcast occurred at other birthday events in India and beyond.

The president of India, Sarvepalli Radhakrishnan, read a birthday message from India's capital Delhi. For the first time

---

* Larisque is a card game where the players sit in a circle of two alternating teams of 13 players each. The losing team (always the one Baba was not on, as he was known to cheat) would have to rub their noses on the carpet before Baba.

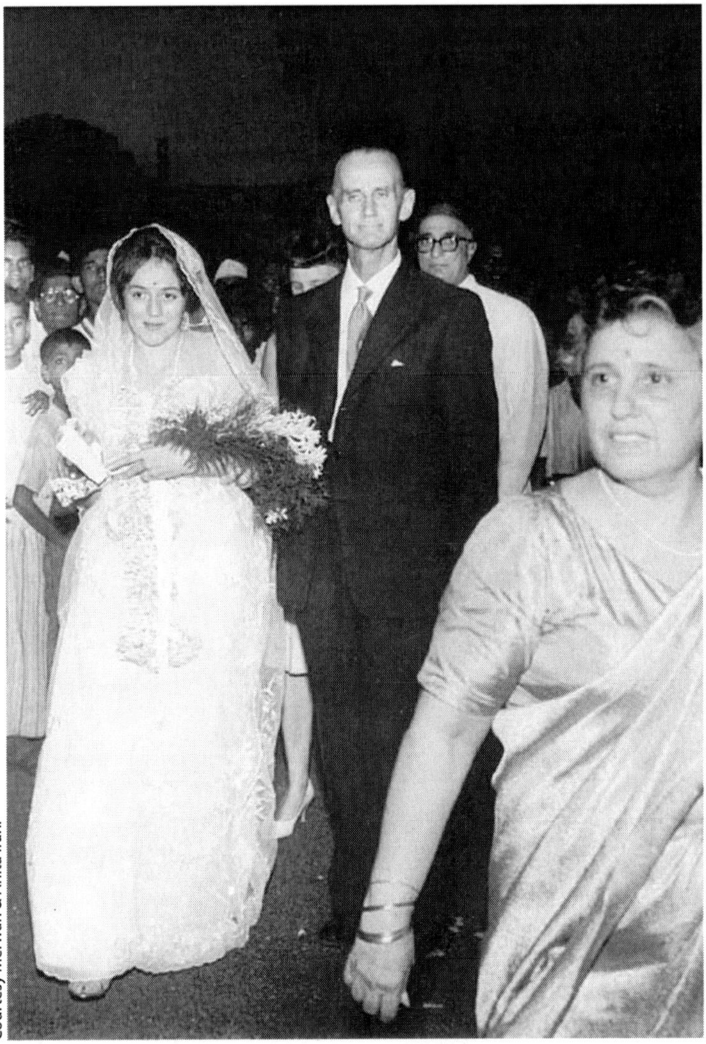

Courtesy Merwan & Anita Irani

William escorts the future Anita Irani down the aisle on the day she married Merwan Irani, son of mandali member Sarosh Irani and his wife Viloo, who is shown in the foreground. Anita had asked that William give the bride away to instill some Western flavour into the June 27, 1963, Indian wedding.

in history an Avatar's birthday was celebrated on the radio in a 10-minute program from the nation's capital.

In Karachi, Pakistan, Baba lovers braved the orthodox Parsi (Zoroastrian) community. Celebrations there included a well-known Baba-lover's lecture tour and the showing of a film on the East-West Gathering on several occasions.

The work to prepare for the World's Fair booth consumed Jane Haynes and others early in 1964. Jane envisioned an array of photographs depicting Baba's work as well as the availability of the Universal Message pamphlets. Some selections for the pamphlet were chosen by those in Myrtle Beach and then sent to India for Baba's approval.

Though the fair opened on April 22, 1964, the pavilion housing the Meher Baba exhibit was not ready for several more weeks. A total of 50 Baba followers volunteered at the booth. Kitty Davy came up from the Meher Center at Myrtle Beach to spend May working at the booth daily from 4 p.m. to 10 p.m.

In her letters, Mani very often skirted the subject of her brother Baba's health or left the topic until after the good news was reported. Baba continued to suffer a great deal from the pain in his hip joint and still depended on a lift-chair.

On the world scene many of his followers were also suffering from various ailments and worry over family matters.

Mani recalled the advice Baba gave to one of his lovers – a police officer – who was facing agonizing family troubles:

"Be courageous. Think more and more of me. I know your love for me and the circumstances you are placed in. Don't wear yourself out with worry."

To another, Baba said, "It is natural at times you feel 100-percent miserable. Be sure that I know everything. When everything goes wrong, the mind becomes helpless and has to rely on the heart.

"These are the moments when you resign to my will and rely solely on my help. When you leave all to Me, I dare not neglect you; and you get relief from your predicaments."[230]

Dr. Goher continued to monitor Baba's health, and she called on William for a consultation, including discussions about Baba's diet.

The year did not pass without another Kalchuri family member getting ill. Bhau caught pleurisy and came under William's care. Because there was no communication between Bhau and his family (Rama, Sheela, and Mehernath) according to Baba's orders, William also served as a messenger by telling Bhau's family that he was being cared for and getting better.

When the family went to Meherazad on a visit, Baba pointedly told them, "If I had written you or you had seen him, what could you have done? Here, I was treating him, so when God is doing everything for him, is there anything more beneficial? I love Bhau a great deal, you know that. Nothing is more important than that. So never worry about him."[231]

Overall, 1964 was another low-key one for Baba. He stipulated there would be no visitors to Meherazad. Exceptions included several East Indian dignitaries as well as a few Westerners – Don Stevens, Stella Kusevich,* and Baba's "sailor boy" Harry Dedolchow. However, most requests were not granted.

Baba responded to a cable sent from Kitty Davy and Elizabeth Patterson seeking permission to visit him in India:

> "Elikit:
> "Your cable made me happy. I am always with you.
> "My love to my Elikitruth.
> "Baba"

The following day Mani sent a more detailed message from Baba:

"I will be in Poona from 1st April to the end of June 1964. For reasons of my own, I will not give darshan to anyone this year. I will be going to Poona for relaxation and want to be left completely undisturbed. Therefore, no one should visit Poona this summer with a view to seeing Me."

Baba seemed to be giving William permission to enjoy some time away from the ashram, for he spent six weeks in Mahabaleshwar during Baba's stay at Guruprasad.

* Stella Kusevich from New York met Baba in 1958. When she unexpectedly arrived at Meherazad in August 1963, she was allowed to see Baba briefly.

In an April 11 letter to his brother and sister-in-law back home, William explains the "holiday":

"Our well at Ahmednagar, ran so ... dry that we decided to empty it and bore down 30 to 40 feet further in hopes of striking water....

"Since it was virtually impossible to restrict the medical work, it was thought best to close down entirely for at least six weeks – till mid-May [or until we get water!]....

"Our water troubles have proven a personal boon to me in the form of a much needed holiday."[233]

William's letter goes on to describe his surroundings at Mahabaleshwar:

"This place is our nearest 'hill-station.' Highest point is 4,710 feet [above sea level] and is 10 minutes' stroll behind the hotel. Plenty of wild beasties such as panther, porcupine, deer, and tiger here and there in remote spots."[234]

Baba publicly acknowledged the death of Jawaharlal Nehru, India's first prime minister, on May 27, 1964. William and Nehru shared the same November 14 birthday. Baba said that Nehru "was matchless as a statesman and that the country has lost its first prime minister who also ranked first in dedicated service to India that he loved so dearly."

On Baba's invitation, William's servant, Motiram, finally got to Guruprasad in the summer of 1964. Baba's question to him showed that the Spiritual Master remained constantly aware of the welfare of his followers.

"He asked me how I was being treated by Dr. Donkin. I told him very well. He told me to stay with Dr. Donkin, which I did. I travelled with him wherever he went," said Motiram.[235]

William's advice and help were still continuously sought on Baba's health issues, and on occasion he would also come to Meherazad to receive Baba's blessing.

Sheela Kalchuri's friendship with William also provided more opportunities for him to see Baba, as the Kalchuri children were favourites with Baba. Sheela recalls one occasion in 1964 when William accompanied them to Meherazad:

"William sometimes drove us; and he too would embrace Baba. William was so tall he would kneel before Baba, kiss both

Baba's cheeks, and then hug him. Sometimes William laid his head on Baba's lap, and Baba would pat his head affectionately."[236]

The spirits of the Westerners were buoyed throughout 1964 with Baba's announcement that there would be another mass darshan for them in 1965. Meanwhile those in the US were still heavily involved in keeping the Baba booth going at the World's Fair in New York. After Mani told her in a letter that "those whose hearts are meant to be touched will be touched," Jane Haynes wrote to Meherazad of the visitors to the booth:

"How can one account for the girls who go by, take the message [printed pamphlet] with a smile, pass on, and in two seconds are back again saying: 'we would like to know more'!

"Or the young man who drives the little Greyhound car that takes people round the Fair, who found himself upstairs standing in Baba's space, asking so many questions....

"Or the man interested in Theosophy who bought a copy of *God Speaks* and left, further along his goal."[237]

Meher Baba's reach was even extending into the presidential White House in 1964. Jane Haynes's son, John, was working in the residence of President Lyndon Johnson. John told the president's daughter Lucy about Baba and gave her some related literature.

In September, William found himself suddenly dispatched to England to deal with a family crisis. His older brother Bryan was dying of cancer and Baba allowed William to go to his brother's bedside to care for him.

While William became a doctor and went off to India to serve his Spiritual Master, his bachelor brother Bryan had followed very much in their father's footsteps. Bryan was a dedicated engineer like his father and many Donkins before him. In his off hours, he was a keen yachtsman and climber, belonging to London's Alpine Club along with William and their other brother John. As the oldest son, Bryan had inherited Winterfold, the family estate in Surrey, after his father's death in 1952.

William's life in India was not a topic of conversation on his occasional visits to his family in England, according to William's twin sister Mary. This posture was probably seeded by the strong disagreement between William and his father over his decision to go to India. In the early years of William's stay in India, his father had persisted in asking him when he was returning to England. William stayed with his sister Mary when not at Winterfold caring for Bryan.

Bryan died in October 1964. On his death his financial wealth and the Winterfold estate were to be divided equally among his surviving siblings – the twins William and Mary and their older brother John. The heirs decided Winterfold should be sold.

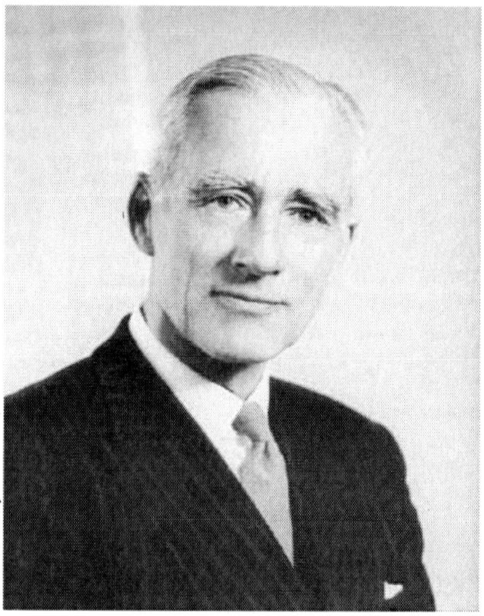
Donkin Family

Bryan Donkin

A friend of Bryan's wrote in the climbing publication *The Alpine Journal* after William's oldest brother's death, "For all his efficiency and social charm, Bryan Donkin did not relax easily in company. But when one had him to oneself in the mountains… he would laugh at nonsense with the rest of us.… I cannot claim that I knew Donkin really well; but then who could? He was really something of an enigma."

That William embodied some of Bryan's traits is shown by an incident during William's visit in England later in the 1960s. His nephew George Mathieson (son of Mary) found William off in another room of the house admiring an antique clock that had come from the Winterfold house. When his sister-in-law Shirley Donkin spotted William and George squirreled off in a corner by themselves during the family party, she commented, "Just like the Donkins – always being anti-social at a social gathering."

The Donkin nature was often fleeting and reclusive. William used the same words many times in the book *The Wayfarers* in describing the God-intoxicated souls he met on the mast tours with Baba.

William's nephew Charles Donkin, a young man at the time, remembers William being involved in the process of getting the Winterfold house ready to sell in the fall of 1964.

"He helped with the packing-up at Winterfold, putting large patches of sticky Elastoplast on antique furniture."

While in England, William also bought a car that he would transport back to India. The car was a Wolseley, maroon in colour.

Nephew George Mathieson recalls his uncle's feelings about the purchase:

"He was very proud of it, polishing it brilliantly. Its colour was officially maroon, but it was certainly a much darker reddish purple, so William called the car, 'the blood clot.'"

George's sister Bridget Barry, the youngest of the children born to William's sister Mary and her husband George Mathieson, remembers William fondly:

"I think it's safe to say that Uncle William was one of the favourite uncles. His general acceptance of us all with our 1960s culture in the UK and later, his loving his fellowman in everyone he met was really quite exceptional."

By December 1964, William was back in India. On December 13 he wrote a letter from Ahmednagar to his older brother John and his wife Shirley, who lived in Birmingham with their three children, giving a brief accounting of some of the items he had removed from Winterfold after Bryan's death. He had taken four of his brother's suits back to India, his father's 8×20 binoculars, and several other things from the workshop and house.

William immediately resumed looking after the medical needs of Baba and his close followers on his return. He was called to examine Baba on December 16. Baba was in pain, and it was thought that perhaps a chip of bone was hurting his hip.

Meanwhile in North America, Elizabeth Patterson and Kitty Davy continued to run Meher Center in Myrtle Beach, while Murshida Ivy Duce oversaw the new Sufism Reoriented organization on the West Coast in California. The women kept in constant touch with Baba in India through personal correspondence from Mani and the quarterly Family Letters, which were distributed to all Baba followers in the nations of the West.

On March 30, Baba and his mandali again travelled from Meherazad to Guruprasad in Poona, following their usual pattern of spending a period of time there each summer because of the cooler climate.

William's servant Motiram recalls that in the summer of 1965, the two of them made another trip to Mahabaleshwar:

"I recall the trip we made. We needed ropes to get down to a special picnic spot at Lingmala Falls. We would go for long walks. William would always carry coffee ... and we always had sandwiches."[238]

The two would stay at a government rest house near Lingmala Falls.

On one occasion, William sent a series of postcards to his family in England offering a birds-eye view of his adventures in Mahabaleshwar. On the back of a postcard showing Lingmala Falls, he drew a sketch of the secret picnic spot he and Motiram discovered behind the 600-foot falls. William wrote on the postcard, "My private and exclusive picnic ledge. It's about 40 feet wide. There's an archway

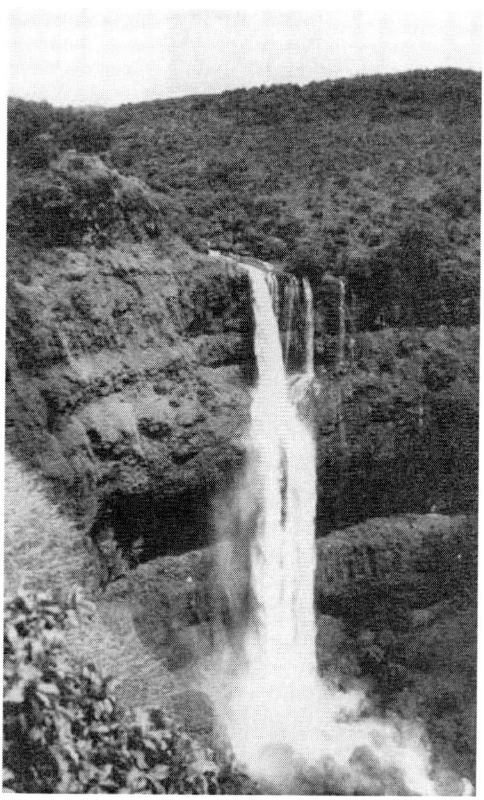

Bif Soper

Lingmala Falls in Mahabaleshwar was a favourite haunt for William Donkin. He even established a secret picnic spot behind the falls that was accessible only by climbing.

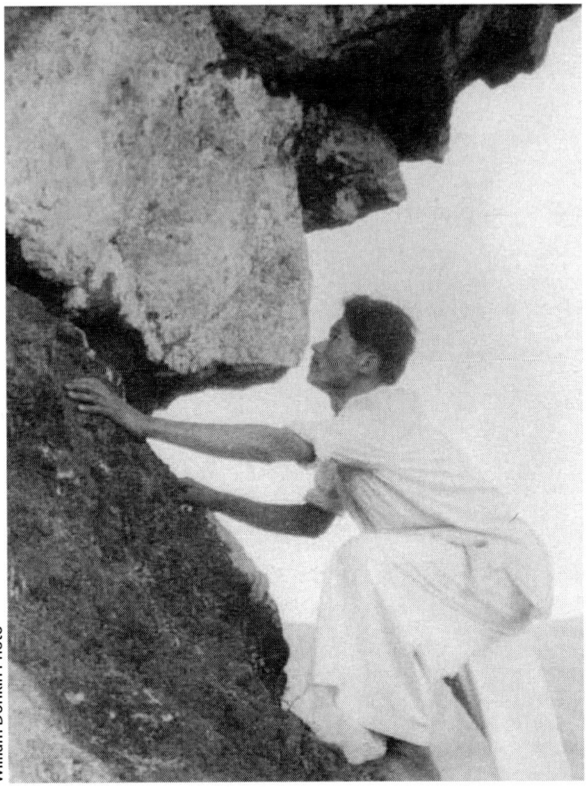

Motiram Kamble scales a cliffside while climbing with William Donkin in Mahabaleshwar in the 1960s. Motiram made a number of trips to Mahabaleshwar with William, where they always went climbing.

and one can sit and have lunch behind the falls in a pleasant, misty spray and very pleasant."

William and Motiram would make another trip to Mahabaleshwar in 1968. William's fondness for the area even prompted Baba to suggest to him that he find some property there, although William never did.

Baba was busy planning yet another darshan for Eastern lovers for Poona, May 1–6, 1965 – six days instead of the original two weeks. Eight people of all ages from Iran also attended this darshan. Two Westerners – Ben Hayman and Harry Kenmore –

were permitted to attend. Other Westerners were assured Baba would hold a darshan for them in December 1965.

Kitty expressed gratitude in a May 16, 1965, letter to Mani after hearing accounts about the Eastern darshan from Kenmore and Hayman when they landed back in the United States.

Baba and the mandali returned to Meherazad from Poona after the darshan and immediately threw themselves into planning the December gathering for the Westerners.

Baba lost a staunch and dedicated British follower in July 1965, when Charles Purdom died in England. Mani wrote at the time, "Dear Charles leaves behind him the finest memorial any man could have in the form of his literary works for Baba, among them *The Perfect Master; God to Man and Man to God*; and *The God-Man*. Charles' passing was a sad loss to all of the Baba family who knew him, and to the English group. "

Baba sent the following message by cable:

"My dear Charles is with me and he is blessed in my eternal Love. My love to Antonia [his wife] and to you all who shared with Charles his service in my cause. Meher Baba."

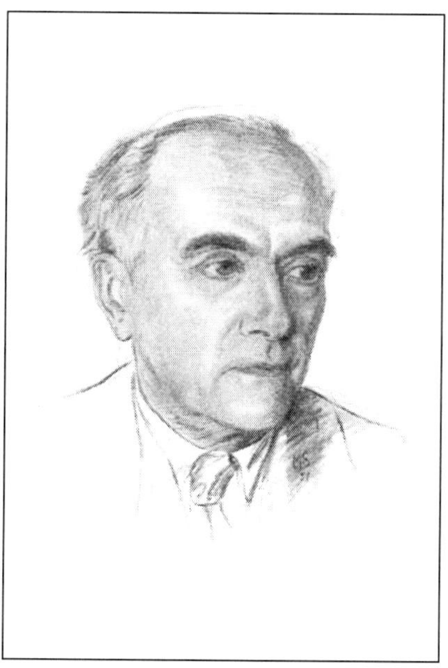

M. Somer Sketch

Charles Purdom wrote the first biography of Meher Baba, which traced the Spiritual Master's life to 1936. He followed this up by writing two other books about Baba – one, a condensed version of the Discourses *in 1955, and the other, an updated biography on Baba published in 1964. A lifelong follower of Baba, Purdom had a full and accomplished career in England as an economist, drama critic, and editor. His youngest son was Hollywood actor Edmund Purdom.*

Delia DeLeon, fellow mandali and friend of Purdom's, wrote from England, "Charles gave of himself unstintingly in his work for Baba; and in spite of ill health these last few years he was determined to get *The God-Man* written – and in doing it, he drew so much closer to Baba and clearer in his understanding. We miss him sorely and are sad for ourselves, but rejoice because he is with Baba."

In the US, the World's Fair booth continued to produce intense activity. Traffic at the booth had resulted in written inquiries asking for Meher Baba book lists, mailings of the Universal Message pamphlet, and a widely circulated photo of Baba holding a lamb.

Kitty, in one of her letters to Mani, mentioned the response to the book *The Prophet*, by Khalil Gibran. The book had soared in popularity since its publication in 1923, when only 1,159 copies sold until the current day when a total of 2,000,000 copies had sold. Kitty pointed out that Norina Matchabelli knew Gibran and that he saw Baba in 1931 – the year he died.

Kitty also reported that 11 guests stayed at the Myrtle Beach Spiritual Center for a week in mid-August. Kitty was also planning a trip to Montreal, with Baba's permission, to stay with her niece, Jenny, and escape the stifling heat that sometimes hits Myrtle Beach in mid-summer.

Those in the West were not prepared for the news that came out of India in September. Baba, without warning, cancelled the anticipated darshan for Westerners that had been planned for December 1965.

In the letter of September 4 to lovers worldwide, Mani wrote of the announcement Baba had made from his armchair in Mandali Hall in Meherazad, "There was a look of infinite fatigue and sorrow in His eyes as he announced this:

"'The world situation is very bad and growing worse daily. The pressure of My universal work is affecting My health tremendously and the pain in my neck is beyond limit. It is the Universal Cross that I bear. I have decided to cancel the Western Sahavas which was to be held in December. I do not in the least like cancelling the sahavas but I have to. I know what I am doing.'"[239]

About 200 to 250 Western lovers had been expected to attend the December sahavas, which would have started on Mehera's birthday. The attendees were to have come from the US, Canada, England, Europe, Australia, Israel, Africa, and a number of other overseas countries. Harry Kenmore had arranged a charter flight from New York to Bombay to carry 132 people, the bulk of the US contingent.

Westerners were to have been put up in hotels in Ahmednagar and to have travelled the nine miles each morning to Meherazad for three hours of darshan from December 23 until 29. Cost of their India stay, including food, 10-day accommodations, and transportation would have been 50 rupees a day or 500 rupees for the 10 days.

Again Baba had stated:

The December Western Sahavas is for Baba-lovers only, and not "meant for the merely interested or curious."

Baba lifted his ban on receiving personal letters after he cancelled the sahavas.

Mani's Family Letter of November 1965 included seven pages of excerpts from Baba-lovers around the world. Many who wrote to him accepted his will, no doubt feeling his pain along with him.

17

Human Frailties and Global Visits

Throughout the 1960s, new Baba centres were opening across India. Because of Baba's precarious health, he usually designated two of the Eastern mandali to attend the official openings.

India's spiritual status was already gaining world attention when the 38th International Eucharistic Council, attended by Pope Paul VI, was held in Bombay on November 28, 1964. At the same time, the Dalai Lama hosted the World Fellowship of Buddhists meeting at Sarnath, near the pilgrim city of Benares in North India.

Despite Baba's strict rules about not allowing visitors, he made an exception when 21-year-old Robert Dreyfuss showed up at the gates of Meherazad to attend the East-West darshan. This American, had hitchhiked from England through 10 countries. He had been on the road for three months and not heard that the darshan planned for December 1965 had been cancelled.

"On both days that he saw Baba, [he] was embraced happily by Him, and received amply of His time and Love," writes Mani in her Family Letter.

Baba instructed Dreyfuss, who had been involved in the drug culture, to return to the US to his family and to the job he had left to come to India. He had looked after violent mental patients in a hospital in Boston. Baba gave Dreyfuss a message and a mission on his departure:

"Go back to the USA, spread my Love among others, particularly among the young and persuade them to desist from taking drugs, for they are harmful – physically, mentally, and spiritually."

Joining Dreyfuss in this work for Baba were Americans Rick Chapman and Allan Cohen. They spread Baba's name and message on drugs across the US, via lectures, interviews, radio shows, college talks, and articles in newspapers and magazines.

William was again allowed to visit his family in England in November 1965 and spent two months there. The trip was a year after his brother Bryan had passed away, and was made in part to deal with the final settlement of the estate. Nephews and nieces had another opportunity to interact with William as shown by their recollections:

"He loved our boyfriends' cars and one year gave us 100 pounds each, I remember it as a large note. I must have been 16 or so," recalls Jane Harding, one of Mary's daughters. "He was glad our boyfriends smoked – and I think relieved to think that we were not as 'strict' about drinking and smoking as our parents were."

John and Shirley Donkin's daughter Jo Storr recalls, "I remember Mum getting very cross with Uncle William for eating too much butter when he was staying with us in Brum [Birmingham].... I also remember him telling me that he had got in a muddle revising for his finals. He had relied on his photographic memory when revising for his anatomy exam – and drew everything onto himself in front of a mirror – it was therefore all back to front. He advised me to take more care with my O Levels."[240]

Life with Baba was again to change for William after he returned from England by ship, landing in India on January 12, 1966. He was called to Meherazad to have a lengthy meeting with Baba on January 20. The gist of the session was William's continued conflict in Meherabad with fellow mandali member Padri. The rift had taken a serious turn, which involved William's friend Sheela Kalchuri. Sheela recalls the incident:

"There was a serious water shortage at Meherabad. Water was their enemy. When I wanted to have a bath there, William suggested that I do so when Padri had his rest," said Sheela. "Unfortunately his servant saw me and told him."

"Padri came and kicked on the door. I was very afraid. Padri went to get a stick and I ran to William and hid there. Padri was shocked to find William watering his garden when he came to find me and told him to stop. He would not. Padri slapped William and William slapped him back."[241]

Sheela said the next day Padri cycled to Meherazad to tell Baba what had happened. Baba called the two men together to sort the conflict out.

Shortly after, it was decided that William should leave Meherabad and take up residence at Khushru Quarters in Ahmednagar. Rooms there had become available.

Sheela says she actually suggested to William the possibility of moving there.

Bhau Kalchuri, in his *Lord Meher* biography series of Meher Baba, gives his opinion of William's situation at the time:

"Although a highly qualified medical doctor, Baba gave Donkin no specific duty, and ... he suffered much frustration, and was often in an irritable mood. It was said that Donkin was never the same after he finished writing *The Wayfarers*."

On occasion, William would throw all of his furniture out of his quarters at Meherabad, sleep on the floor, and then retrieve the pieces and carry them back in the next day. He also sometimes completely dismantled his motorcycle and then put it back together again, which could take up to a month.

Both Baba's sister Mani and Eruch Jessawala's younger brother Meherwan said that in his later years William had become "mast-y" – displaying the qualities of the God-intoxicated souls he had written about in his book.

William's unsettled frame of mind did not make Bhau Kalchuri uneasy, and the two men admired one another. Bhau offered a personal aside about William in a recent interview:

"William went to Baba on my behalf once to tell him I was working too hard and needed rest; that I would collapse if I did not have rest," recalls Bhau. "Baba himself told me that William had intervened and pleaded on my behalf. That was a very caring thing for him to do."

William probably welcomed the move to Ahmednagar. It's certain that Bhau's daughter Sheela was over the moon with happiness that her "best friend" would be living in the same building as her. Sheela explains the process of William's move in her book *Growing Up With God*:

"I liked living in Ahmednagar, but at the same time I missed Meherabad. Most of all I missed my best friend – William Donkin. I was sad not to see William every day, like before. Once William came and said that he too missed me. Judge Khilnani* had been transferred, and he and his family were leaving in a few days, so their rooms would be vacant. I suggested that William move to Khushru Quarters. He asked Baba.

"Adi Sr., too, agreed when William offered to pay rent.

"Padri was happy about it as he had been complaining about William all along.

"Baba later asked me whether I was happy William had moved into the bungalow. I was thrilled. I trusted William implicitly and sought and followed his advice always. I loved William so much, if Baba had told me to stay with him, I would have done so in a heartbeat."

"'You missed him, didn't you?' Baba asked. 'That's why I made him leave Meherabad and stay in Nagar. Because of you.'"

Sheela describes how William, perhaps wanting a touch of the old country, brought rolls of wallpaper from England and tried to paper his new rooms.

"But the paper soon peeled from the uneven surface of the mud walls. He gave up and had them painted."

Sheela would always get a telegram and gift from Baba, who would be in Poona on her May 12 birthday. She remembers sharing the excitement of her birthdays with her friend:

"William would ask me every hour, if any telegram had arrived from Baba. It usually came in the afternoon. A parcel would also arrive ... usually containing a garland that Baba had worn recently. I would hurry to William's room to show him the cable and garland. William would be so happy to see them, repeating over and over how lucky I was. He would close his eyes

---

* Judge Prem Khilnani, his wife Girja, and two sons met Baba in Poona in 1959 and became devoted followers of Meher Baba. They lived for a while in Khushru Quarters in Ahmednagar and later in Bombay. Their son Raj is now a police inspector in Bombay.

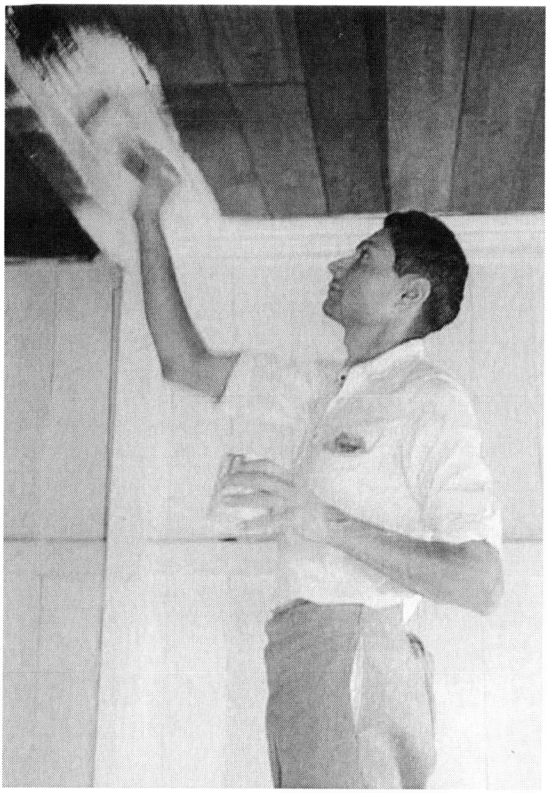

MSI Collection India

Mandali member Padri (Faredoon N. Driver) joined Baba in the 1920s. William and Padri were often at loggerheads over various issues at Meherabad, including the water supply and food quality.

and hold the telegram and garland to his chest so tenderly, since it had come directly from Baba."[242]

There were other incidents that increased the bond between the two. Sheela recalls a family of foxes at Meherabad:

"William studied their habitat. The comings and goings of the mother. William said we can only go and see them at certain times. We fed the young ones milk. When they saw us there they came out of their den."

Sheela saw William as a nature-lover and animal-lover:

"He would even get vaccine for my dog in England. He went to Nagar and learned how to give an IV to a dog from a vet and this helped save my dog."

A serious incident occurred in February 1966 when the dress of Meheru, daughter of Kaikobad, caught on fire while she was cooking. She suffered severe injuries. William treated the wounds, but he could not save her. She died a few days later.

Baba's intuition about the needs of his close followers in both India and beyond was far-reaching and timely.

Kitty Davy, in Myrtle Beach, requested and received directly publications that Baba wrote. The books were placed in Baba's House at Meher Center. Kitty at about this time was suffering from a persistent bronchial sinus condition. Baba, perhaps sensing her distress, dispatched back-to-back telegrams in March:

"March 6, 1966

"Elizabeth:

"I want Kitty to take complete rest. Have all-time nurse for Ruth also extra help for housework. Kitty take long vacation Montreal in May. Keep well and happy. I am with you. My Love to you and Kitty Ruth.

"Meher Baba

"March 7, 1966

"Kitty:

"How are you my dear Kitty. I want you to take good rest and proper treatment. My love to Elizabeth Ruth.

"Meher Baba

Despite Baba's ongoing pain in his hip joint and neck throughout his later lifetime, he could and would reach out to alleviate the sufferings of his lovers in different parts of the world. Even if at times they were suffering in silence.

In a subsequent letter to Mani in Meherazad, Kitty hinted that someone may have "tattled" about her condition to Baba. She pooh-poohed the attention but admitted that a holiday in Montreal might help shake the health problems.

"Baba is right. I need a rest, I think, but not so much because of work as because of some germ I seem to have picked up. Anyway, let's see what the rest will do."[243]

Kitty described the small Baba birthday celebration [attended by 20 people] at Meher Center on February, 25, 1966, as an "intimate, loving occasion."

"Charles [Haynes] read Baba's Prayer beautifully. The film [of Baba] was magnificent, we showed it four times. Then after the film, Frank [Eaton – the Center caretaker] brought out his violin and we sang the four hymns of the booklet *Let Us the People Sing* [by Francis Brabazon]. All enjoyed the singing. We had a lovely birthday cake and lovely ice cream. We ended the film with the Arti [song in praise of Baba]."[244]

On the US West Coast, it was a rough couple of years for Ivy Duce and the Sufis. Like everyone else in the West, Ivy had been looking forward to the Western Darshan and was disappointed by the cancellation. Daughter Charmian was going through a divorce. In late July, Ivy's husband Terry collapsed. He passed away August 15 without ever regaining consciousness. Baba's strong belief in reincarnation may have been tested with Ivy at this time.

"Even when one is aware that a beloved person is about to be ushered by the sentinel of death into another world, one is never actually prepared for the actual event."[245]

Ivy had an opportunity to hint at her close relationship with Baba when a young clergyman came to see her the day before the funeral:

"I immediately reassured him by saying he would not have to hold my hand because I knew perfectly well where my husband was going.... He was intrigued that I might know something of life after death, so I told him that the Church had never been able to answer my questions on this subject and I had gone to India to find out."[246]

While the young clergyman expressed interest in hearing more, saying he would return to visit Ivy after his vacation, it was not to be. On his return he was suddenly married and posted to a church in another part of California.

With the help of her mureeds*, Ivy got moved into a smaller apartment and in 1966 was able to finish a small book, which Baba had approved, titled *What Am I Doing Here?*

The work of Robert Dreyfuss, Rick Chapman, and Allan Cohen was having an impact on the young drug culture. Letters were coming to Meherazad from former drug users:

* "Mureed" is a Sufi term that literally means committed one. A mureed is a person who has committed to a specific Sufi teacher (Murshid).

"Since you sent Bob Dreyfuss to connect us and to stop us from the drug delusion, you have become the most important reality in our lives. Your books fill our shelves, your pictures the walls, and your reality our dreams. We are doing our best to love and understand, believe, and submit.... Obviously it is easier for some than others, and you of course understand this best."[247]

Later in the year Meherazad learned that Baba's reach had even extended to Africa. A Baba-lover in Uganda had celebrated Baba's seventy-second birthday with a gathering at his home with over 400 people, including Africans, Europeans, and Asians of various religions. A sudden downpour of rain accompanied the celebration – always seen as a blessing in Baba's world.

The doors at Meherazad closed tighter again in 1966. In the Family Letter of September, Mani wrote that since mid-August, Baba had put a stop to all visits.

"He makes it emphatically clear that he wants to remain undisturbed until the end of 1967. He tells me to repeat here His oft-repeated wish – that unless Baba on His own sends for someone none should visit him before the end of 1967."

Again, however, an American Baba-lover managed a short visit before the gates to visitors were closed in mid-August 1966.

Rick Chapman, who had led Baba's anti-drug fight in the US, had been successful in being awarded a year's Fulbright Scholarship to teach English in India. While he only spent a few minutes in Baba's company, they were priceless for Chapman:

"Still reeling, I am completely unable to express my happiness at meeting my true Beloved.... Only with Baba's direct support could I walk into and out of the most important event of my life. The secret of it is that there is no sense of walking out of the meeting with Him, but rather He walks with me. How could one bear to meet God, and leave Him?"[248]

Baba's growing popularity in the United States was fuelled by the work of Chapman, Dreyfuss, and Cohen in turning young people away from LSD. Cohen had been closely associated with the psychedelic work of Richard Alpert [later Ram Dass] and Timothy Leary at Harvard University and so had been at the epicentre of the LSD craze of the sixties.

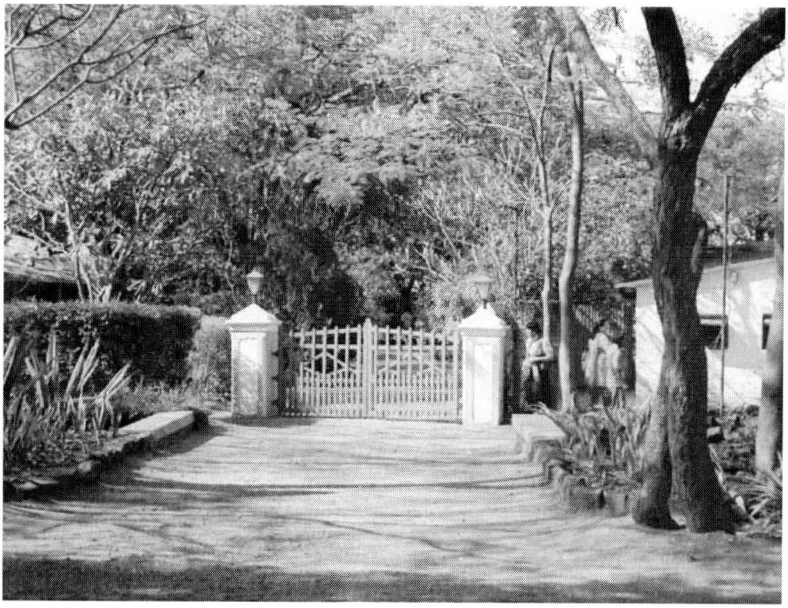
Vishwajeet Parode

These gates provide access to Meher Baba's rural private residence, Meherazad, which was established in 1944. The five-acre residential compound, which today is open to visitors a few times a week, is nine miles north of Ahmednagar.

As the last remaining months of 1966 arrived in Meherazad, the message that Baba wanted to be left alone fell on deaf ears in some cases, with people still showing up at the residential compound gates. In a desperate attempt to stop this, three very visible sign boards in Hindi, Marathi, and English were finally put up. They read, "Avatar Meher Baba has stopped seeing or giving darshan to anyone. By Order"

While William was still called on occasionally for consultations regarding Baba's physical ailments, he was not mentioned as one of the "Baba-lover doctors who are privileged to serve him."

Dr. Ram Ginde, neurosurgeon of Bombay, and Dr. Goher, one of the women mandali and Baba's personal physician, worked together for the most part. Baba's unexplainable neck pain continued to baffle his doctors, as Dr. Ginde explained in a

Family Letters reference, "I got news about Beloved Baba's neck pain from brother Adi, who was with us a day before I left for Delhi; and your letter confirms the same. He also said that you are much worried. I am also in the same predicament. Whatever I know from the knowledge of His cervical condition, I have tried to do in all sincerity. But I must admit, as I have admitted before, my utter failure in regard to relieving Baba's pain."

Baba smiled when he read Dr. Ginde's letter and told Eruch to write Ram and tell him not to be worried and to add, "The root cause of Baba's pain is not physical, but universal, and it will leave Him only in His time."

William certainly had other duties besides occasional consulting on Baba's medical needs. Sheela Kalchuri had seen an ear specialist and William had agreed an ear operation was necessary. Dr. Goher accompanied Sheela to the doctor in Poona, who said she had an infected mastoid [bone] very close to the brain.

There was some fear expressed that Sheela could die even if she had the operation. Baba was involved in the discussions along with Goher and William.

"Baba looked concerned and worried as he examined the x-ray and read Atre's [the doctor's] note. William arrived and conferred with Goher and Baba. It was decided that the operation be done."[249]

Sheela's younger brother Mehernath suffered from acute asthma. William, Padri, and Adi were all involved in treating him, but in the end Baba gave Mehernath a Benadryl (antihistamine) capsule. He instructed Mehernath to continue taking a capsule once a day for three years. At the end of the three years, Mehernath was cured and never had another asthma attack.

Sheela recalls finding herself copying a number of William's habits, including his diligent attitude about cleanliness, which seemed to win her favour with Mehera, Baba's leading woman mandali.

"Because of William's example, I was always washing my hands and cleaning and disinfecting things, which Mehera appreciated."

Sheela's attitude about cleanliness sometimes led to her being teased by other mandali. Once she told the mandali to make sure they dried their hands before coming out of the washroom, fearing that Baba might slip on the dripped water.

"Pendu teased me, saying I was like William.

"'One little thing Baba tells you to do, and you are making such a fuss!' he said.

"I didn't care. I wanted to do it meticulously."

William continued to be involved in Sheela's recovery from surgery, which meant he or Adi Sr. would drive her on the frequent trips to Poona for check-ups.

"When Baba asked William to take me to Poona for my doctor's appointment, the way William replied was as if Baba were doing him a favour by giving him the work.

"'Yes, Baba definitely!' William replied. 'I would love to.'"

"He was beaming, joyous, and proud that Baba was asking him," recalls Sheela. She says William would behave differently with Baba, and that his relationship with Baba was special.

"With me, William was always lively and fun. But in front of Baba, he was quiet, reserved, and polite. He never spoke rudely, argued, or raised his voice with Baba. When called for an embrace, William jumped up and sat on his knees in front of Baba. Baba used to hold William's face between his hands and ask if he would do something for him. William always said yes, and Baba would kiss and embrace him again. At times William would say to Baba, 'I request you to allow me to ...' do some work or pay for something that is needed. He always spoke in that way."[250]

Major celebrations associated with Baba's life were simultaneously celebrated in different parts of the world. India, United States, England, and Australia were the major centres of activities for his followers.

Mirroring Silence Day in India, the activity at Meher Center in South Carolina, on the same day, was at quite a heightened pitch as well. Long-time Baba devotee Wendy Haynes Connor describes the scene at Myrtle Beach on July 10, 1966:

"Many came by bus, car, train, and plane. The Center was all hustle and bustle – the atmosphere was charged with love for the Beloved. Baba's Elizabeth, as always, supervised all the preparations with her usual devotion and care. Kitty and

Jane [Wendy's mother] were seen scurrying here and there and everywhere with suspicious looking bundles in their arms, which of course turned out to be supplies and linens for all the cabins. The telephone was to be heard ringing constantly. Dates were changed, families enlarged and the new arrivals announced every day. Kitty's remarkable vitality was in full force as she juggled room, cabins, and spaces for the visitors. Every nook and corner was used."[251]

Baba would have made use of the enthusiasm which mushroomed on the special days such as his birthday and Silence Day at Baba centres in different parts of the world. Those who fasted and/or remained silent on Silence Day often commented on the heightened energy levels they felt from undertaking silence and fasting.

With the developing ease of world travel, a number of Baba followers in these different countries would from year to year find themselves visiting other continents where Baba followers lived. Even when business prompted these visits, the Baba people often made efforts to seek out the Baba connections, even if it meant only quick visits over a shared cup of tea or coffee.

At the end of 1966, Baba dictated a special message for his lovers, which reads in part,

"Desires and longings are the root cause of all suffering.

"The only Real Desire is to see God, and the only Real Longing is to become one with God....

"To desire the Real Desire and to long for the Real Longing you need My Grace, and you cannot have that until you surrender all other desires and longings to Me...."

Montreal, Canada, was to be the scene of a major world exposition in 1967, and plans were already afoot to create a display on Baba there similar to the one at the New York World's Fair.

Catherine (Cay) Draper, a Baba-lover from Canada, worked closely with Kitty Davy in organizing the booth, and Kitty in turn wrote to Baba's secretary, Adi Sr., about the plan.

Baba gave his approval and blessing to the initiative, which would take Kitty to Montreal on several occasions during the year. Wendy Haynes Connor would accompany her on one trip.

While Baba's seclusion continued and intensified, there were still gaps in the denial of access, perhaps to keep his international following somehow connected and inspired. On February 16, 1967, Bill LePage* came to India from Australia. William, called upon as chauffeur, met Bill on his arrival in Poona and drove him to Meherazad, where he was given a room for 14 days across the hall from fellow Australian and poet Francis Brabazon. Bill recalls his drive to Baba's residence with William:

"I do not remember the journey to Poona [from Bombay], but I do remember lunch with Meherjee and Donkin, and then being driven by Donkin ... a memorable trip, with 'Don' telling me of his meeting with Baba."[252]

Bill met with Baba and the mandali members the next morning.

"It was only after we were all seated that Baba really acknowledged my presence saying, 'Bill seems just like one of the mandali.' That naturally made me happy: I felt comfortable, and, more important, I felt that I was not being intrusive to his comfort.

"I felt no necessity to continually look at Him. I was simply content to be there and do His bidding. I like to think now that a measure of His acceptance of me was that He did not put on any special show for my benefit."

Baba's birthday on February 25, 1967, came and went with fanfare on various levels in different parts of the world.

The scene in Ahmednagar, India – the city that lies between Meherazad (Baba's residential compound) and Meherabad (the tomb and pilgrim centre) reflected Baba's home country's mode of celebration. A letter to Myrtle Beach from Mehera, Baba's chief woman disciple, describes the scene:

"A six-hour procession with 30,000 people, and over 100 gaily decorated bullock carts took place. A full-length, life-size photo of Baba was placed on a jeep, which was decorated to resemble a boat and led the procession. Baba's photo was bedecked

* As a young man, Bill LePage learned of Baba from the Sufis in Australia. He first met Baba in 1954 in India and was ordered by Baba to assist Francis Brabazon in Australia, with duties including building and maintaining Avatar's Abode.

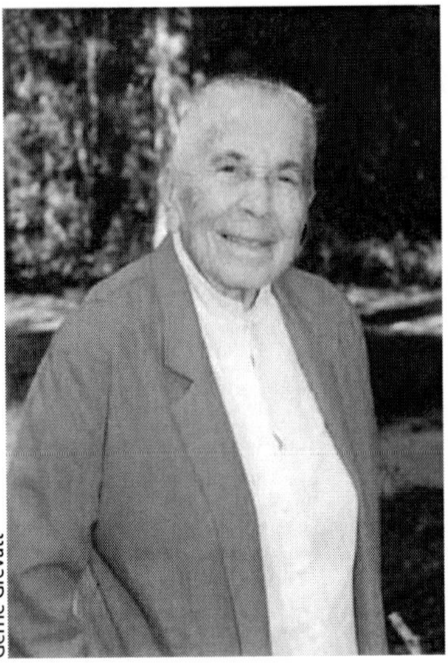
Gerrie Grevatt

British-born Kitty Davy, shown in a photo from the early eighties, continued her mandali work at Meher Spiritual Center in Myrtle Beach, South Carolina, for nearly 40 years. In the early 1960s she expressed worry about the small number of people coming to the Center. This changed dramatically with the rush of the younger generation that was drawn to Meher Baba later in the sixties.

by lights and the various religious symbols were shown. The procession, which went through Nagar's main streets, was accompanied by the chanting of bhajans and prayers sung by the various religious groups, signifying that Baba belongs to all religions, just as all religions belong to Baba."[253]

In March, Baba was consistently experiencing pain in his throat when swallowing. Antibiotics were given, but he did not respond well to them. William was summoned to examine Baba and recommended another treatment.

Kitty was also busy in 1967, planning the design and construction of a new library for Meher Center. The building, made possible through funds from Ruth White, was located on a rise in the Center grounds overlooking the lake and ocean.

Interest in Baba was now growing quickly in the US, which Kitty conveyed in her letters to India. Many newcomers were drawn from university towns and cities in the southern US, including the university towns of Chapel Hill and Durham in North Carolina and Atlanta and other parts of Georgia.

"The search amongst the younger students, men especially, is great and they seem to have so little difficulty accepting Baba – quite a few of the Jewish background amongst them."[254]

While the number of new followers in the USA was more than those in the rest of the Western countries put together, there was new interest in Baba being expressed from European countries such as Germany and Austria.

In India, Baba and the mandali had again adjourned from Meherazad to Poona to take up residence from April through June at the Guruprasad residence, which the Maharani Shantadevi of Baroda provided to him each year.

The luxury Wolseley that William had transported from England for driving Baba was proving popular. The car was used to drive Baba to Poona in April and again for his return trip to Meherazad on July 1. William's fastidious nature in keeping the Wolseley in perfect shape for Baba's journeys was expressed in many other arenas of his life, as Mani recalls:

"Donkin was so particular, so perfect. Once, he was interested in learning about the local birds; he bought books and learned all their names and each one's call. He also knew the names of every hill around Meherazad.

"One day, Baba was joking with the mandali and said something about William, poking fun at him. Francis [Brabazon] joined in, adding something, and everyone laughed. Suddenly Baba said, 'Remember, Francis, [William's] a better man than you any day.'

"Francis nodded, 'I know, Baba.'"[255]

Baba wanted William's book *The Wayfarers* translated into Hindi at this time, and the work began in 1967. Bhau Kalchuri did not have time to start the job while at Meherazad, but he began at once after Baba and the mandali moved to Guruprasad.

Baba instructed Bhau "not to translate William's book literally – as he felt it was too dry [matter-of-fact] an account of the God-intoxicated."[256]

The seesaw of Baba's health continued throughout 1967. The mandali's spirits would be heightened on one occasion to see him actually walking for five minutes. Then a strained back muscle would put him back in a wheelchair. The cervical collar that he had worn at times was almost abandoned during the Poona summer. Baba stated, "Only my lovers' love can help the pain in my neck; it can ease only when my seclusion is undisturbed."

At one point during the year, William's relentless persistence was felt by Eruch Jessawala's family. Driving Sheela Kalchuri to one of her doctor's appointments in Poona, William dropped her off at Eruch's parents' home, known as Bindra House. Before leaving for his hotel, William insisted on seeing where Sheela would be sleeping and asked that another blanket be provided to her because of the cold nights. Gaimai (Eruch's mother) and the others were nervous as William peppered them with questions.

"'Baba told me to take care of Sheela,' he explained. 'So if you cannot look after her properly. I will arrange another room at my hotel.'

"William also asked about the food and returned in the afternoon just to see what had been cooked. 'Is this dish fresh? Or is it left over from yesterday? Sheela's supposed to have eggs.'

"He was back in the evening to check on me, and he telephoned several times to ask whether I was okay.

"Eruch was put off that William had questioned his family's competence, especially Gaimai's. He began remarking that William was cracked; but Baba cut him short, and said that William was obeying him perfectly.

"'This is the way it should be,' Baba stated. 'Don [William] cares about pleasing his Beloved, not about what others will think.'"[257]

Going beyond exquisite maintenance of his automobile, William also installed improvements to the padding and cushions to make sure Baba was comfortable in the car.

One day on a trip to Poona, Adi Sr. noticed William packing six raincoats and six umbrellas. "I get out so many times a day, I need six of each," said William. He would never use the raincoats or umbrellas when they were wet, and would always wipe them off with Dettol to kill the germs in case road water had contaminated them.

Adi Sr. could only shake his head in wonderment at William's precise routines.

Meanwhile, across the world in Myrtle Beach, responsibilities were shifting. The number of visitors at the Meher

Center was increasing and more cabins were added. Kitty's role changed from cabin housekeeping and groundskeeper to that of greeting and helping visitors and guests. She became constantly available to talk about Baba and provide books and information about him. Kitty suggested, and Baba approved, that Jane Haynes take over Kitty's previous duty of showing Baba's House to visitors. Kitty recalled in *Love Alone Prevails* how Baba's message on "Real Work" helped her during this transition:

"It is not a different work to what you have already been doing – it is the same work done in a different way. And that way is the way of effacement, which means the more you work for Me, the less important you feel in yourself. You must always remember that I alone do My work … I allow you to work for Me so that you have the opportunity to use your talent and capacities selflessly and so draw closer to Me."

As 1967 drew to a close, Kitty wrote to Mani, "As I sit on the bed writing, opposite on the wall is a lovely painting of Baba in his well-known pink coat, hand raised in greeting, painted by Lyn Ott.*

"I saw it before his exhibition and snapped it up (agreeing to pay monthly – that little Social Security I have). If Mehera, or any of you ever come this way and like it, then it is for Meherazad; if not it is for the Saroja Reading Room [wing of new Meher Center library]."

The Lyn Ott exhibit, titled "Image of the God-Man – Avatar of the Age," was held in Chapel Hill, North Carolina, from October 28 to November 21, 1967.

Lyn wrote at the time about his location choice for the exhibit, "I feel it appropriate that Chapel Hill should be the place for this exhibition to be shown. Chapel Hill is the place in the West right now where interest and love for Meher Baba has erupted on a momentous scale. In Chapel Hill, love for Baba is literally spilling out on the streets, and I am proud and glad to

---

* Lyn Ott and his wife Phyllis – both painters – were followers of Baba who were allowed to build their home on the grounds of the Meher Center in Myrtle Beach, South Carolina. Lyn continued painting (about 500 paintings), even as he gradually lost his eyesight from the effects of his advancing retinitis pigmentosa.

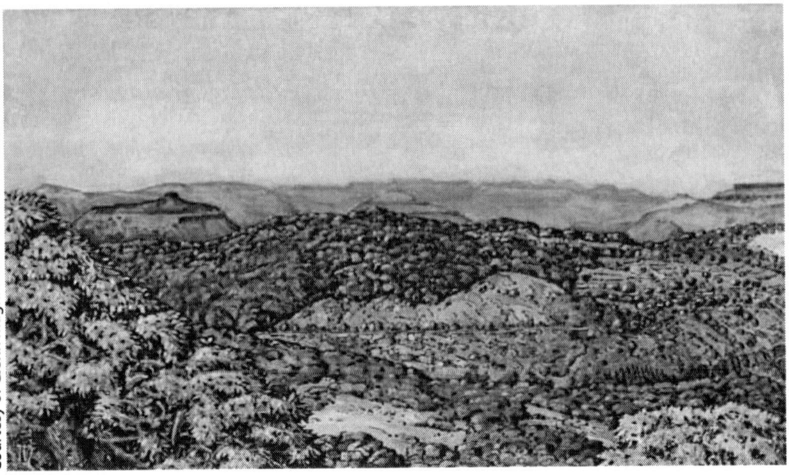

William was an accomplished watercolour artist and made quite a number of scenic paintings while living in India. This painting takes in the mountainous terrain of the Mahabaleshwar/Panchgani area.

be able to lend my work for the advancement of Baba's work in that beautiful and brand-new Baba Center."

In addition to William's other talents, he too was a gifted painter as well as a keen photographer. As a youngster in England, he, his sister, and two brothers had operated their own darkroom at Winterfold, and photography had been a favourite hobby.

When Baba and the mandali went to Poona for the summers, William continued to visit Mahabaleshwar, where he would hike, paint small watercolours, and take photographs. He brought back many photos from these trips and took many candid photos of Baba throughout the years.

As Baba shut the doors further on visiting and promoted independence in his lovers worldwide, he also seemed acutely aware of the pitfalls which might lie before them. Midway through 1968, a stern letter, which Baba's secretary Adi Sr. sent out to only Eastern lovers, was just as meaningful to those in the West. The letter addressed a conflict in one of the Baba enclaves in India.

"Whatever be the cause of the rift, he wants each one to try his best to narrow it down and mend it by forgiving and forgetting one another's trespasses," writes Adi.

The letter went on to point out to followers the importance of holding onto Baba's damaan (hem of garment) very firmly so that it wouldn't slip out of their hands no matter what happened.

Followers were urged not to succumb to lust. Lust, Baba pointed out, is nothing else but the desire for self-happiness, while love is the desire for happiness for others.

Lovers were warned to be wary of persons who claim they are saintly and pious and profess to possess super powers.

Baba was also specific in telling his lovers and workers not to get intimately involved with the family affairs of one another or to get emotionally upset by the personal affairs concerning any of their own families.

The letter closed saying the points raised were "for all his lovers and workers everywhere."

While Baba lovers everywhere were attempting to live up to their Master's expectations, public exposure to Meher Baba was beginning to blossom in unusual and effective ways. In New York State, a quote from Baba's discourse *The New Humanity,* reading "Love is essentially self-communicative," began to appear over windows in buses in more than a dozen of the largest cities.

Mani included this news in her January 25, 1968, Family Letter, citing a letter from Ella Winterfeldt in New York City. "Have just heard from dear Margaret [Craske] that the saying of Baba with his Beloved name is now appearing in all city buses. It is nicely placed above the bus windows, and it is ever, ever so lovely."

Mani reported in the same Family Letter that "England's youth has at last begun to wake up too. The beginning is represented by a heart-warming bunch of artists, musicians, and students who have fallen in love with Baba; who keep bringing their friends, and friends of their friends' friends, to hear of Baba from His old lovers."

Delia DeLeon, from the earliest Baba group in England said, "What a stirring up is taking place! I feel I have plunged into a whirlpool of young people. What is amazing is their natural understanding of Him without wordy explanations, the way they seem to know and accept Him. It is wonderful!"

There were times when Baba appeared to take on the role of referee or school principal in regards to some of the shenanigans going on amongst his mandali. William was often right in the middle of these upheavals.

Sheela Kalchuri Fenster describes one such incident in *Growing Up With God*, involving William's unusual effort at scaring a fellow mandali.

"[William's pranks] provided a rich source of amusing stories to tell Baba. For instance, chipmunks were destroying William's possessions and eating his furniture. One day he killed a chipmunk with a BB gun. He wrote Adi's name on a piece of paper and pinned it to the dead chipmunk, which he hung in front of Adi's office. When Adi discovered it, he started shouting at the top of his voice....William began teasing him.

"Adi threatened, 'Tomorrow I'm going to Meherazad and telling Baba!'

"In Mandali Hall, Baba asked [Sheela] whether there was anything to tell Mehera. I told him what William had done. After lunch, I acted out the scene further between William and Adi. Baba and Mehera laughed a lot!"

Undoubtedly such occasions helped relieve tensions that at times were extreme among Baba's close mandali members.

Along with Mani's Family Letter came news from Baba that he would end his long seclusion on March 25, 1968. But his lovers were reminded that he would still not accept any visitors and they were urged to wait for news from him about another public darshan in the future.

Then, in a typical turnaround, Baba extended his seclusion to end two months later on May 21, 1968.

The usual loosening of seclusion rules, which generally came with Baba and the mandali's move to Guruprasad for April through to June, did not happen in 1968.

Despite his duties, William and Motiram managed to get away again to Mahabaleshwar for a period during the hot summer season.

World events were taking their toll, especially in the United States. "This morning we heard over the radio of the racial violence sweeping across the USA, sparked by the killing of

Dr. Martin Luther King," Mani wrote in an April 6, 1968, letter to Kitty in Myrtle Beach.

Those at Guruprasad essentially experienced a "lock-down" when they arrived at the estate. No one was allowed to leave and no one was allowed to enter. Baba demanded no noise from his mandali while he continued his "universal work."*

Above all, Baba was asking for obedience to his wishes from his lovers:

"Until I announce that I will give my darshan to my lovers, none of you must try to come, none of you must ask to come, none of you must come."

His lovers were also being urged to read the Parvardigar Prayer and Prayer of Repentance daily until July 9, 1968.

One group of Eastern lovers showed up at the gates of Guruprasad "demanding" Baba's darshan. A number of veteran Baba lovers from Poona convinced the group to disperse and leave rather than to defy Baba's wishes.

The Baba bus messages that had become so popular in New York City had also found their way onto the buses in Toronto, Canada, and those of the Indian city of Poona, Meher Baba's birthplace.

Meanwhile Baba's health continued to swing dramatically. One day he would be seen "moving about so swiftly that the mandali have a hard time keeping up with him," and on another day "we see Him weighed down and so infinitely tired, that they move along at a snail's pace to keep in step with him," said Mani in a Family Letter.

William's antics appeared nonstop in the late sixties, according to Sheela Kalchuri:

"Once William scared me. He came to my house wearing a lizard mask with a fake, red tongue attached to it.... William knew I hated lizards, so he hid behind a tree and jumped out when I walked past. I was frightened, but then ... I suggested we use it to scare Adi.

"Early next morning ...I went to Adi's window to tell him I was going to school. Adi was seated next to the window,

* At times Baba would stop and seem far away, rapidly moving his fingers. He said he was doing universal work. What that meant remains a mystery to all.

relaxing and smoking a cigarette.... The next moment William wearing the lizard face popped up from below the window sill. He made a loud hissing noise.... Adi's eyes widened and he choked on his smoke. Then he came outside bellowing curses. He went straight to Meherazad and complained to Baba.

"Next day we were all summoned there. William brought the mask to show Baba, who told him to put it on. Baba laughed and commented, 'Yes, it does look scary. I would be scared too.'

"He told William not to frighten Adi again."[258]

Although it appeared William and Adi Sr. were at loggerheads, Sheela says there was in fact a bond between the two men:

"Adi was one of the few men mandali with a university education like William and they would at times enjoy talking and philosophizing about Baba's discourses. They would even share a drink of whiskey together."[259]

Baba's seclusion did finally end on May 21, 1968, and a little more than two months later Baba declared, "My work is done. It is completed 100 per cent to My satisfaction."

While an opportunity for future darshan was hinted at, Baba said, "Be patient. Wait in My love. Those who wait for Me never wait in vain. You will see Me, but wait till I call. Hold on to My damaan – and wait for My call."

18

Invitation to Darshan, Baba's External Farewell

In a letter to Kitty from Mani on October 12, 1968, the possibility of a darshan in the summer of 1969 was hinted at. William attended a meeting of Baba workers in the same month in Poona. Similar meetings were held by close followers in other parts of India to discuss the possible darshan. Mani also informed Delia DeLeon in England and Ella Winterfeldt in New York of the darshan possibility.

Finally in the Family Letter of November 1, 1968, the long-awaited news came. The darshan for all of his lovers – east and west – would be held in the summer of 1969.

At this point, 100 different books about and by Meher Baba had been published. Baba centres and Baba people all around the world were incorporating "Meher" into centre names, house and cottage names, and names of their children. Businesses as well were popping up with names such as Meher Pharmacy, Meher Tea Shop, Meher Foundry, Meher Market, Meher Café, Meher Academy, and even Meher Poultry Farm.

The dates for the public darshan were set for April 10–June 10, 1969 – a full two months.

Three pages of 26 rules and conditions were circulated around the world. As in the past, Baba expected strict adherence to the 26 stipulations he laid out for the 1969 gathering at Guruprasad in Poona.

Many were familiar, including the stipulation that the darshan was "only for his lovers, old and new, Eastern and Western."

The Westerners would assemble for two hours each morning and the Easterners two hours in the afternoon. Easterners would include those from India, Pakistan, Iran, and Africa. It was expected that 250 people would attend each morning and afternoon session.

The plan was for lovers to rotate through Poona during the two-month period. Westerners were expected to stay only one week and see Baba four times.

He said he would see no one privately nor give private interviews.

Baba wanted all His lovers to return home directly from Poona. If there was any sightseeing to be done, it should occur before they arrived in Poona.

They were told only those who could afford to make the trip without risk to health or livelihood should do so. No one should bring gifts for Him or any of His people.

Group heads oversaw much of the organization of Western and Eastern lovers in co-operation with a few of Baba's key mandali. Indian visitors were divided geographically into 14 different areas of the country and were allowed two to four days of two-hour sessions with Baba. Iranian and African lovers were given two days and all Westerners four days of morning sessions only.

For those who could not attend, Baba said, "Those who want to come and cannot come to Poona ... should not feel upset or disheartened but remain resigned to His Love knowing that 'sometime, somewhere, somehow' His darshan is assured to them also."

His lovers worldwide were in happy shock to receive the darshan news. Ivy Duce describes the response from followers in the United States:

"We of the West immediately began making plans for doing the endless things necessary for a long foreign trip. In order to keep the cost down as much as possible plans were made on each coast to charter planes.... We chartered two planes and went through the most hellish time making all the arrangements, receiving and acknowledging some $200,000 from the charter applicants with the telephones ringing day and night both at the Sufi Center and at my home. I can only hope that in some dim past I have been a travel agent, for I would never willingly go through such an experience again."

Meanwhile in India another event was demanding Baba's presence. On December 23, 1968, Baba's nephew Dara, son of his brother Adi Jr., who was living in London, was to marry Amrit S. Ghildial, daughter of staunch Baba lovers from Dehra Dun, Kumar and Subhadra.

The bride-to-be relates her experience when William and Adi Sr. met her in Bombay to drive her to Ahmednagar:

"They picked me up at the station. I was 18 years old and tired after three days of travelling," says Amrit. "I didn't know these guys. They were speaking in Marathi and Hindi. William spoke to me in my language."

Amrit recalls William's self-effacing humour at the time:

"In introducing himself, he said 'I am William Donkin, but you can call me 'donkey,' – other people do!'"[260]

Amrit drove to the Meher Baba headquarters office in Ahmednagar with the two men and then Adi Sr. drove her on to Meherazad where she stayed.

Baba had arranged the marriage. The ceremony was held in Meherazad. Here Baba took their wedding rings and handed them back to the couple to put on each other's fingers.

"Baba was seated on the veranda of the women mandali's quarters. In the garden facing Him, a colourful tent with rows of chairs accommodated 300 Baba-lovers from Ahmednagar and nearby places, who had been invited for the occasion.

"It was like a small darshan ... Baba looked beautiful in his pink coat, and radiant, but at times there was a great tiredness in his eyes.

Entertainment included a number of favourite gramophone records and Baba's twin nephews singing "There's a Hole in the Bucket," much to Baba's amusement. Women Baba-lovers sang some other songs and Adi Jr. read out a Francis Brabazon poem in honour of Mehera's birthday celebrated on the same day.

"After all had sung the Arti, each guest filed past Baba and bowed before Him – as usual He greeted each with a smile, a caress, a query showing concern over someone's health, a 'don't worry, be happy' message.

"At one time He said to the gathering, 'Look at Me well – when I give My darshan in Poona, you will not be seeing Me as you see Me now.'" The wedding celebration was Meher Baba's last public event.

Late in November, blood and urine samples from Baba had been sent to Ruby Hall Hospital in Poona. The results were not good. Additional samples were sent with William early in December. This time the results were alarming enough that the doctor asked William if the patient was conscious.

William replied that Baba was fully conscious.

Surprisingly, Westerners were still slipping through the cracks and showing up at Meherazad as late as January 1969.

"One of the last visitors to Meherazad while Baba was physically present was an Australian girl named Mary Bennett. She arrived unexpectedly in the afternoon of Sunday, January 5, 1969.

"She was a very simple girl, like a hippie," Mehera recalled. Mary explained that she was hitchhiking in India and had walked barefooted from Ahmednagar to Meherazad.

"Mary had a guitar and Mehera asked her to sing. Since Baba was resting, Mary played softly and sang sweetly. Mehera said Baba would love to hear her also.... "Mary came in and stood a little distance from Baba, who was lying down. He called her near.

"'Go,' said Mehera. 'Baba is calling you.'

"Baba put out his hand to her. She knelt, and Baba patted her on the head and caressed her face. She sang the same song for Baba.

"'Very nice,' Baba said about her song....

"Baba gestured for her to come back in May for the '69 Darshan, but the young woman never returned, and in fact was never heard from again."[261]

Mani's Family Letter of January 26, 1969, quoted an earlier letter she had sent to Fred and Ella Winterfeldt in New York:

"Beloved Baba's health has not been at all good for some time; from the tremendous strain of his seclusion work ... His physical condition is very weak. Goher and the other doctors strongly feel there should be a thorough check-up done. As this is not possible at Meherazad-Ahmednagar, we're trying to persuade Baba to make an early move to have it done in Poona. We are hoping He will agree."

Baba did not agree.

"He refuses moving to Poona before the usual date, which is about the end of March, in time for the darshan beginning April 10."

In the Family Letter, Mani quoted Meher Baba's message which had been issued earlier for his upcoming seventy-fifth birthday on February 25, 1969:

"To love me for what I may give you is not loving Me at all.

"To sacrifice anything in my cause to gain something for yourself is like a blind man sacrificing his eyes for sight.

"I am the Divine Beloved, worthy of being loved because I am Love.

"He who loves me because of this will be blessed with unlimited sight and will see me as I am."

Baba's secretary, Adi, issued a Life Circular at the same time, which stated, "Beloved Avatar Meher Baba wishes all his lovers to know that His three years of intense work has shattered his health. In spite of this He has invited His lovers from all over the world to come to Him for His darshan next summer, for it is time for them to come to Him and receive His Love.

"But with the present condition of His health, how beloved Baba will give His darshan to the thousands who will come, yet remains to be determined; but it will be. He will give His darshan."

Despite assurances, Baba's time on earth in physical human form was running out. There were only days remaining.

An account of Baba's failing health at the beginning of 1969 appears in Naosherwan Anzar's book *The Beloved*:

"In the latter half of January, Baba's health started deteriorating fast. His physical suffering and pain had become more and more evident. On January 30, Baba's body shook with deep spasms. Dr. Keki Byramjee [K.B.] Grant* from Poona and Dr. Ram Ginde from Bombay were called to Meherazad.

Just as Dr. Grant left, Baba told him, "My time has come."

In the early hours of Friday, January 31, 1969, Baba instructed Aloba (one of the mandali) to bring a board at ten in the morning from Mandali Hall to be kept in Baba's room. On the board three couplets of the poet Hafiz were written:

1. Befitting a fortunate slave, carry out every command of the Master, without any question of why and what.
2. About what you hear from the Master, never say it is wrong, because, my dear, the fault lies in your incapacity to understand Him.
3. I am the slave of the Master who has released me from ignorance; whatever my Master does is of the highest benefit to all concerned.

Najoo Savak Kotwal in her book *He Gives the Ocean* recalls sending a letter to her family members covering several days at this time:

"That morning Baba told Dr. Donkin, 'Today is the day of My crucifixion.' You see Beloved Baba was off and on giving hints that he will be no more to the male mandali but not to the ladies because I guess it would involve Mehera."

Again following *The Beloved* book's description:

"[Throughout Friday morning] the spasms continued and his body shook intensely with pain. The allopathic medicines given to him brought no relief. Biochemic pills were given, and when the resident mandali, Dr. Goher, gave him an injection, Baba said, 'Do not forget I am God.'

"At 12:15 p.m. Baba's entire framework shook with severe spasms as he sat on a surgical bed and head raised. His arms flayed and his mouth closed tight. His respiration suddenly stopped. Baba became motionless.

"Eruch Jessawala opened Baba's mouth, put his mouth against it and began breathing into his lungs forcibly. This

* Dr. K.B. Grant founded the Ruby Hall Clinic in Poona in 1959 and brought modern medical care to Poona for decades.

mouth-to-mouth resuscitation was carried on for 30 minutes. Eruch collapsed on the floor out of sheer exhaustion while Dr. Brieseman from Ahmednagar, who had just arrived with Dr. Ginde and Dr. Donkin, gave him (Baba) a cardiac massage.

"Three doctors, Dr. Brieseman, Dr. Donkin, and Dr. Ginde examined Baba's heart. Dr. Ginde checked Baba's eye reflexes. It was pronounced that life was extinct. The Avatar had dropped his body."[262]

Baba-lovers worldwide were not ready for the shocking news. Kitty Davy recalls receiving a call in Myrtle Beach:

"In the early morning hours of January 31, Elizabeth [Patterson] received a telephone call from Fred Winterfeldt in New York with the shocking news that Meher Baba had dropped His physical form. When we were able to get through to Adi Jr., Baba's brother in London, he confirmed the news."

From Adi K. Irani's office in India, a cable was sent out to Baba-lovers all over the world:

> AVATAR MEHER BABA DROPPED HIS PHYSICAL BODY AT TWELVE NOON 31 JANUARY AT MEHERAZAD TO LIVE ETERNALLY IN THE HEARTS OF ALL HIS LOVERS. BELOVED BABA'S BODY WILL BE INTERRED AT MEHERABAD ON 1 FEBRUARY AT 10 A.M. IN THE TOMB HE HAD ORDERED TO BE BUILT LONG AGO

Kitty remembers her feelings:

"I was stunned but I did not experience a loss, I felt strongly that Baba was present where we were. I remembered the words from the Bible that came to remain with me more strongly than ever; words which daily seem a part of my being: 'I live, yet not I, the Christ liveth in me.'

Elizabeth recalled the words that she heard clearly during the night:

"I know that my Redeemer liveth."[263]

Australian Francis Brabazon, who had been living with Baba for 10 years when Baba dropped his body in 1969, later recalled witnessing the departure in a letter to a fellow Baba lover in Australia:

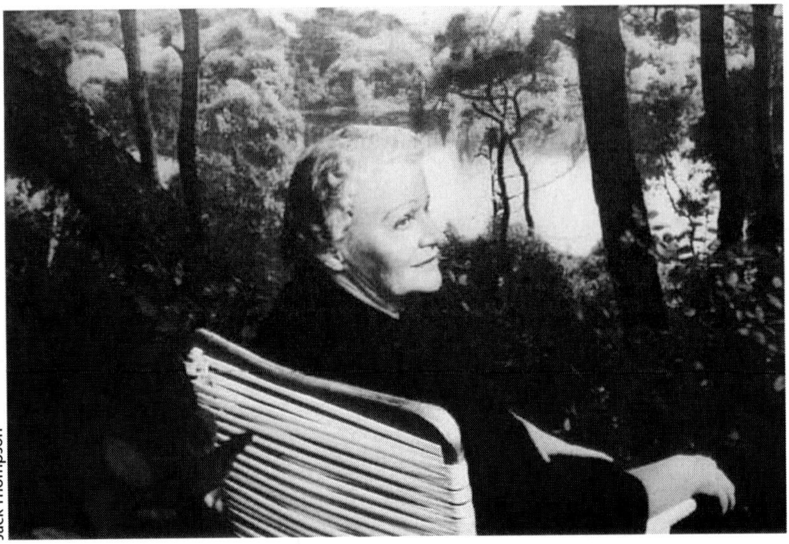

Jack Thompson

Elizabeth Chapin Patterson is shown in a sixties photograph taken at her home – Dilruba – overlooking Long Lake. The house borders Meher Spiritual Center. Meher Baba called the Center his "home in the West" and visited there three times in the 1950s.

"For hours, in relays, we had been pressing His limbs. Suddenly Goher cried, 'No, Baba, no!' And I became aware that our Beloved has stopped breathing.

"Goher recovered sufficiently to prepare and give an injection. Eruch began mouth-to-mouth resuscitation. Mehera came in and collapsed at the head of the bed moaning, 'Baba, Khodai sher [Baba you are God], You can come back if You will.'

"Goher said to me [Francis], 'Why don't you try resuscitation? You know how to do that.'

"I knew nothing would be of any use, yet I kept wondering why the doctors had not come. They would do something; Goher was too distraught to think.

"Then the doctors arrived, and just stood about. I was thinking. Why don't you fellows do something? They gave oxygen and a cardiac injection, apparently in a show of doing something. But the Lord of the universe had finished with His body and did not resume breathing.

"Eruch had collapsed from sheer physical exhaustion, but had soon recovered. He was caressing his Beloved's face and I noticed him lightly pressing His eyelids down; and I wondered why he was doing that; one only did that to someone who had died."[264]

William immediately became part of the decision-making process at Meherazad after Baba dropped the body. He and Eruch agreed that Baba should be interred within 24 hours. Mani arrived shortly after to convey the women's wish that Baba should not be buried for three days. Baba's human form was taken by ambulance to the tomb on Meherabad Hill.

The time before burial was extended when Mehera remembered that Baba had told her that seven days after the end of January He would be well and strong. She now took this to mean that the tomb should be kept open for seven days until February 7 – which would have been His birthday according to the Parsi calendar.

Word of Baba's departure had gotten to Khushru Quarters where Sheela Kalchuri, her mother Rama, and her brother Mehernath were living.

At first the Kalchuris heard a servant crying.

"The servant told us Meher Baba had dropped his body. I didn't believe him," recalls Sheela.

They ran to Adi Sr.'s rooms. They found him seated, holding his head in his hands.

"Rama asked what had happened. Adi did not say a word. He looked up at Rama soulfully, his eyes swollen and red. She repeated what the servant had said. Without answering Adi stood up, put his arms around Rama's neck, laid his head on her shoulders and started bawling loudly.

"Never before had Adi embraced or even touched my mother. He held her and sobbed uncontrollably.

"'What happened Adi? Tell me,' Rama said. 'Why are you crying?'

"Adi couldn't speak. When he calmed down, he said only two words: 'It's true.'

"Then Rama couldn't hold back her own tears. Both began wailing.

"I told them to stop. I still didn't believe it.

"'Take me to Meherazad right now!' I said. 'I'll believe it when I see it for myself.'

"Adi said wistfully, 'No Baby [Sheela], it's true.'

"'I'm going to Meherazad.'"[265]

As when anyone passes away, things began to speed up for some, and come to a complete stop for others.

William suddenly appeared at Khushru Quarters in his Wolseley just as Sheela was boarding a truck for Meherazad. William had already arranged that Baba's body be taken by ambulance to Meherabad Hill.

"Baba is in Meherabad," William told the Kalchuris. He offered to drive Sheela and her family there after he attended to some work. Forever meticulous, William was already organizing a coffin for Baba and wanted to make sure it would be of the highest quality.

After William drove the Kalchuris to Meherabad, he returned to Nagar to fetch blocks of ice to place around Baba's body to slow deterioration. Sheela's family made their way up Meherabad Hill. Baba's body had been temporarily placed in his small cabin. Inside with Him were Mehera, Mani, Goher, and Naja.*

The grief that gripped Mehera was immense. Her tears flowed continuously and she pleaded with Baba to take her with Him. Baba's sister Mani was busy trying to console Mehera. Goher and Naja were standing in the corner weeping. Watching Mehera, Sheela said, "... was the most painful sight I have ever seen in my life.

"The way Mehera was kneeling over Baba's body, sobbing as she kissed his cheek and touched his face – I thought Mehera would not survive. The pain and grief on Mehera's face is something that haunts me to this day."[266]

William and other doctors monitored the condition of the body.

An avalanche of humanity began to make its way to the tomb from across India (and around the world). William would

* Naja, Baba's cousin (sister of Pendu), often cooked for Baba and the women mandali. She, Pendu, and their father Masaji were among Baba's early mandali.

later say to Mani, "Now, Baba is for the world. He is no longer our private Baba. He's for the world now."[267]

The recording of "Begin the Beguine" was played as people filed past Baba's body.

A number of Westerners would come before Baba's body was interred in the tomb. Delia DeLeon, accompanied by Baba's younger brother Adi Jr., came from London. Don Stevens had cabled that he would also come from the United States. On the sixth day, Rick Chapman, Allan Cohen, and Aneece Hassan* arrived from San Francisco.

Late on the night of January 31, Baba's body was moved into the tomb. Cole Porter's song "Begin the Beguine," a favourite of Baba's, was played daily for seven days according to Baba's instructions. On the first day the song was played seven times, first in Baba's bedroom in Meherazad,then at Meherabad in the cabin by the tomb, and later in the tomb.

As the song played, Baba's sister Mani recalled, "It seemed to convey to us His message; that this was not an end but the beginning – the beginning of His completed work bearing fruit."

Blocks of ice were brought daily and placed around Baba's body in the tomb.

Meherwan Jessawala recalls one of the wonderful coincidences that are often experienced by people involved with Meher Baba:

"It was mid-winter. Very hot during the day, but cold at night," said Meherwan. "William went to get ice from Poona. Along the way he came across a big truckload of ice that someone had ordered and then not accepted. William asked if he could buy the entire truckload of ice and he got it."[268]

Mani described the transformation that occurred overnight on January 31, 1969, after Baba's body was placed in the tomb, in a later Family Letter:

"Overnight Meherabad was transformed from an isolated retreat into a crowded pilgrimage ground. It swarmed with people, buses, cycles, taxis, tongas, bullock carts. Padri, who had looked after the place all these years, had a tough job trying to

* Aneece Hassan was with Sufism Reoriented under Ivy Duce and met Baba in 1962 at the East-West Gathering.

accommodate the hourly growing number of lovers. Every foot of indoor and outdoor space was used for their camping in during those days and nights.... A railway track runs between upper and lower Meherabad, and trains obliged by stopping there to disgorge their load of lovers from Bombay and Andhra.... We could hear passing trains give a long whistle as they went by the Hill – the drivers were saluting the Avatar of the Age."[269]

Many followers throughout the world were struggling with whether to go immediately to India. Darwin Shaw, an American disciple living in Schenectady, New York, recalls his own soul-searching at the time:

"Within a couple of days, as I processed what Baba's passing meant in our continuing relationship with him, I began to realize to my amazement that nothing had changed – Baba's presence was the same! My relationship with him had not altered and he was as available as ever. This awareness helped me immensely in my adjustment to the fact that he was no longer physically with us."[270]

William was pouring much of his energy into making sure the coffin for Baba was properly constructed. He and Sheela Kalchuri also shared in the chore of getting new ice blocks for around Baba's body. Sheela recalls in *Growing Up With God* just how meticulous William was in attending to this work:

"William placed the blocks of ice on layers of blankets, so that Baba's body was protected from the melting ice and it wouldn't become muddy under his feet. I raised Baba's feet each day to collect the sawdust* that had been deposited there."

Sheela recalls how William took care even with the ice:

"I was incredulous when William told me that he had paid extra for large blocks of ice to be specially manufactured from boiled water – something unheard of.

"'Why boil the water when the half-melted blocks are being discarded?' I asked.

"William explained that devotees would collect the melting ice and drink it as Prasad. I found this to be true. People

---

* Sawdust sprinkled on ice delays its melting.

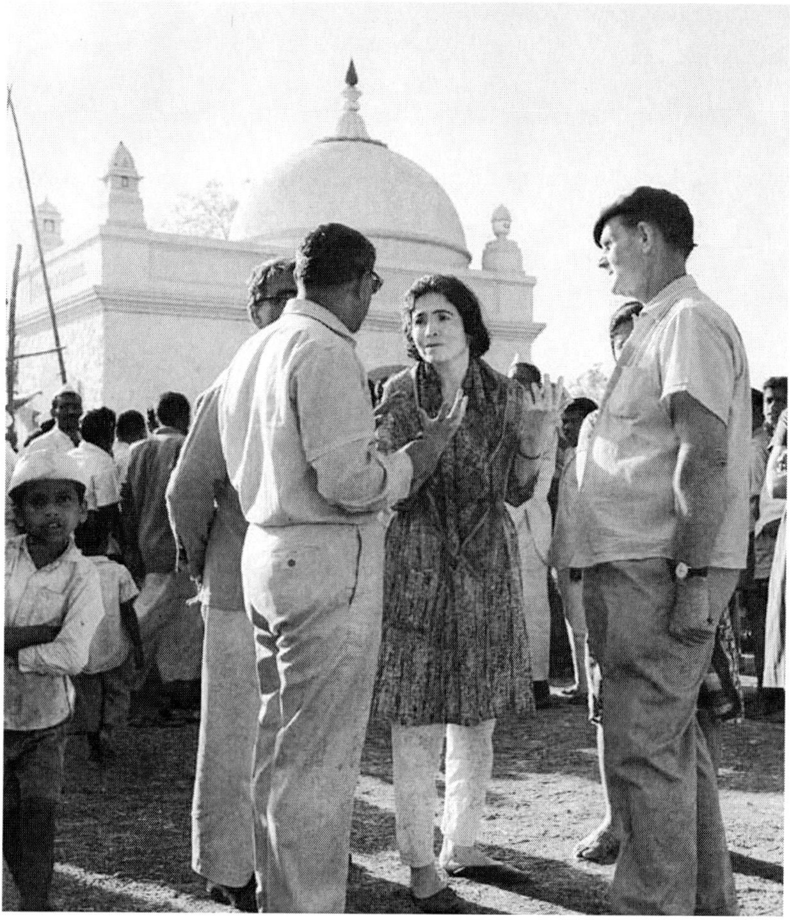

Dr. William Donkin, Meher Baba's sister Mani, Dr. Ram Ginde (back to camera), and Eruch (beside him) talk outside Meher Baba's tomb in Meherabad during the first week of February 1969.

would chip the ice and place the pieces in any container they could find. I was impressed by William's care and forethought."

Meanwhile, the coffin construction was not going as William had hoped. Sheela recalls that William rejected the first coffin saying, "This is not for an ordinary person."

"The next day the carpenter had another sample ready, but it too was rejected. The man said he could rectify the faults

William pointed out, but William insisted he start over, with fresh, seasoned teakwood on all sides.

"A third model was finally approved. The coffin was polished on the outside as well as on the inside according to William's instructions."[271]

William insisted that Sheela be the first one to touch Baba's coffin. Later it was placed on the roof of William's Wolseley, taken to Meherabad. Here William and Sheela carried it to the tin shed.

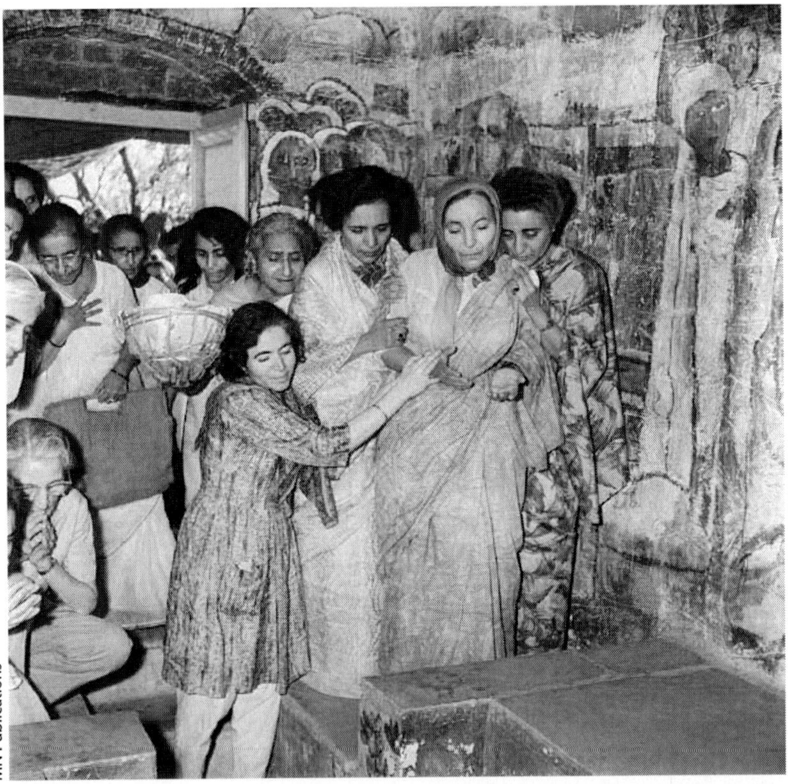

MN Publications

Women mandali members comforting Mehera inside Meher Baba's tomb in February, 1969, include, from left, Mani, Khorshed, Arnavaz, (Mehera), and Katie. Baba's physical form was kept available for seven days, allowing lovers and followers from across India and elsewhere in the world to visit the Samadhi before interment.

At one point Mohammed, the mast who had been a long-time resident of Meherabad came up the hill to the tomb. He was joyful and insisted that Baba was standing right beside everyone, even after he had visited Baba's body in the tomb.

Delia DeLeon had arrived from England and gives her own recollection of what she witnessed:

"I saw Mehera at Meherabad in the morning; all were sitting in the cabin. Mehera was devastated.... Every time we went into the tomb, Mehera sprinkled rose petals on Baba. I remember Mehera saying to most people she greeted, 'Baba is with you.'

"Each time she went into the tomb, however, she broke down.

"'Heart-broken Baba lovers came for this last darshan,' Mehera observed. 'Many with their entire families often arriving at night and not knowing where to go, what to do. The

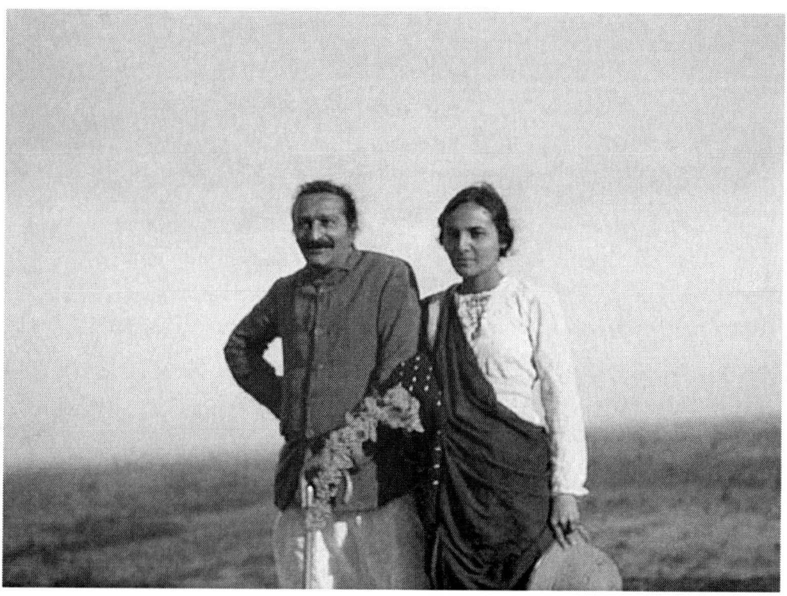

MSI Collection India

Meher Baba and Mehera J. Irani

place was absolutely unprepared to handle this influx, among other inadequacies; there was no electricity, just a few dim kerosene lanterns....'

"'Everyone was in a daze; only knowing that they had to come, they must come. And in the darkest period of our lives, the moon rose shining bright and full for those seven days.'"[272]

Other Westerners arriving from the United States included Rick Chapman, Allan Cohen, and Irwin Luck. Irwin, who had visited India three times in the early sixties, recalls making the sudden decision to go to India:

"'The Western group heads were advising people not to go. Baba treated me like a son coming home when I had visited. I told Fred [Winterfeldt] 'we are family – I am going.'" Irwin was thankful for his determination to get to India; he made it to the tomb on the seventh day, an hour before Baba's body was interred.

William examined Baba every day for those seven days. He would straddle Baba's body and walk forward lifting Baba's arms and legs.

"As William was hovering over Baba's face, he folded his hands to Baba and touched his own eyes in a gesture of reverence. Despite the tragic atmosphere, as William emerged from the Samadhi, he too seemed happy. I had seen that same expression on his face every time he saw Baba at Meherabad and Meherazad. Perhaps he was having some experience of Baba's love and compassion, but I never asked him."[273]

On the final day, February 7, 1969, the ice and sawdust were removed from the Samadhi. Lovers rushed forward to touch the coffin as it was carried from Baba's small cabin.

Mehera descended the steps one final time kissed a large rose and gently tossed it onto Baba's body where it fell perfectly on His heart. Mehera was assured that William had overseen the construction of the coffin so well that it would not break for 100 years and that no earth would ever touch Baba's body.

After Baba dropped the body, William again shifted his primary residence, leaving Khushru Quarters in February to sleep and take his meals at mandali member Sarosh Irani's home, Viloo Villa. There were a main house and three smaller four-room cottages, and William moved into one of the cottages.

In 1969, soon after Baba dropped his body, William moved from Khushru Quarters to Viloo Villa. William Donkin's bungalow at Viloo Villa is pictured today, along with the bedroom he slept in.

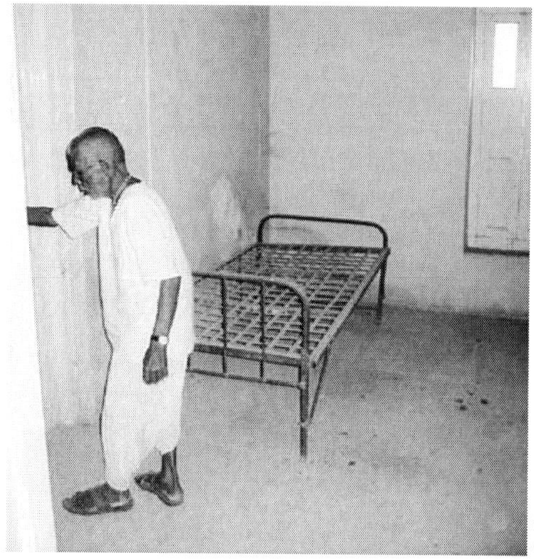

S of L

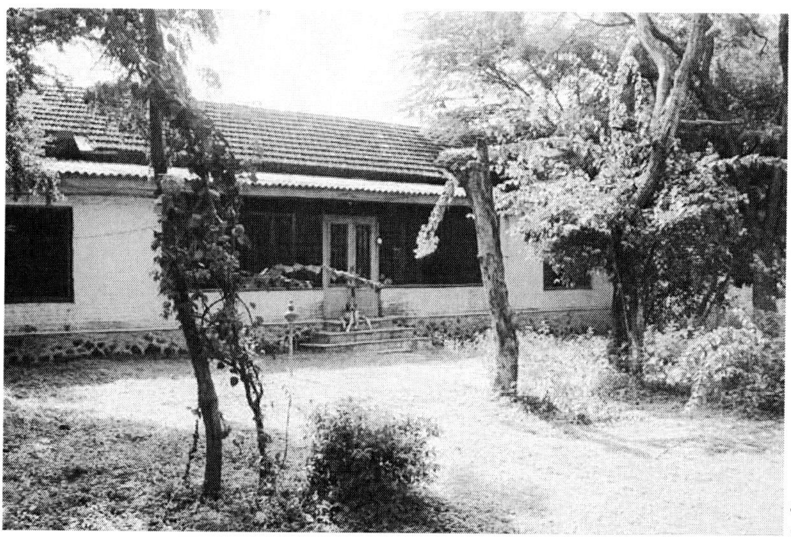

S of L

William's servant Motiram remembers that William had been bothered by the noise from the cinema located next door to Khushru Quarters and saw Viloo Villa as a quieter alternative. Motiram personally "felt lost" without Baba's physical presence. He said the effect on William was perhaps more noticeable:

"William was very disturbed. His fiery temper again was evident."[274]

Baba's nephew, Dara Irani, had spent a part of his early childhood at Viloo Villa before going to England to rejoin his father Adi Jr., who had moved there earlier. He believed William "was at an age where he wanted a little more comfort."

"He would take his meals with Sarosh and Viloo. He would arrive all dressed up for dinner and sit down for a glass of scotch with Sarosh before they ate."

Dara recalls that sometimes after dinner William and Viloo would go next door to a movie at the Military Officers' Club that was part of the Ahmednagar Army Camp complex.

William would still visit Sheela and the other Kalchuri family members each day at his former residence, about a mile and three-quarters away. Sheela recalls one of their conversations, in which William related an experience that influenced his feeling about Baba's physical departure:

"One afternoon when I was with him, we were speaking of Baba and I began crying. William told me not to feel sad, and then he narrated the incident which had taken place a few weeks before Baba dropped his body. Baba was in a critical condition and he told William that he was going to drop his body. William said, 'Baba, I will do my best to treat you and make you well.'

"Baba looked at him pitiably and gestured, 'You have no idea of my suffering.'

"William related, 'When I saw the expression on Baba's face as he said this, tears welled up in my eyes. I saw how much suffering Baba was enduring. That is the reason, when he dropped his body, I didn't cry. Baba is all around us now, ever-present. His physical suffering has ended.'"[275]

19

The Last Darshan, William's Departure

Losing Baba's physical form had hit Sheela's father Bhau very hard. He went into shock immediately. As Baba's long-time night watchman, he continued to carry out his duties even without Baba's physical form to watch over. Sheela travelled almost every day to Meherabad to look after her father.

"I would find Bhau sitting on an iron chair, outside the wooden gate by Baba's cabin, still in shock, totally unresponsive, almost catatonic. It was winter, but Bhau sat outside during the night also, keeping watch. I brought tea and food for him but, again, I had to force-feed him."[276]

Bhau was later diagnosed with typhoid, but he eventually recovered and returned to Meherazad.

The absence of Baba's physical presence caused great heartache among those in his close circle. Mehera cried for days and could hardly be consoled; Eruch, whom Baba had called "his right hand," did not sleep for days; and Bhau was in the coma-like stupor for weeks.

Others were more stoic or had resolved not to break down. Mani, Baba's sister, remained strong, responding to Baba's wish that she should care for and comfort Mehera.

Eruch's younger brother, Meherwan Jessawala, recalls observing William's behaviour after Baba had dropped his body:

"He felt totally lost, and heartbroken."

Despite the pain of the close mandali members, Baba's planned Last Darshan, which he had promised his Eastern and

Western lovers from April through June 1969, was still very much alive. Plans began in earnest for the gathering, and William became one of the key organizers for the event.

The three-month darshan was still to be held at stately Guruprasad. Shortly after Baba's body was interred in the tomb, William went to Poona to make arrangements for those coming from the West.

Baba would have undoubtedly discussed the needs of the Westerners at the April–June 1969 Darshan with William in late 1968. William, always quick to obey, was now anxious to fulfil his Master's wish tenfold – perhaps more so – to honour Baba.

"He went personally to each hotel they would be staying at to ensure it was clean, making the management spray the beds for bedbugs and sterilize the towels, plates, glasses, and utensils."[277]

Meanwhile lovers and followers in the Western world were preparing to go to India, responding to words Baba had issued to his lovers who were concerned about his health before he dropped his body:

"It will be easy for Me to give my lovers My darshan, so you are not to feel concerned about it. I will give darshan reclining and that will be no strain on My body."

Almost 700 men, women, and children representing 16 countries came from the West.

The Myrtle Beach group chose the month of May to attend the darshan in India. One of those attending was 100-year-old Ruth White, whom Baba had called his "soldier."

Australian poet Francis Brabazon, who had lived with Meher Baba in India for the last 10 years, welcomed those attending the darshan.

Lovers from around the world, he said, had come to bow down to Baba in their hearts.

"I have been at mass darshans where tens of thousands came and bowed down to His man-form. But to come thousands of miles to bow down to Him in one's own heart – that is an entirely different order of devotion."[278]

Francis reminded those attending of Baba's compassion and love for them:

"For every step the lover takes to the Beloved, the Beloved takes 10 to the lover. But the lover must continually take that one step. We must practise taking Beloved Baba's darshan, bowing down to Him in our hearts, every day, and then every moment until we have continuous sight of Him."[279]

Wendy Haynes Connor, who had met Meher Baba several times as a child in Myrtle Beach and lives there beside Meher Center today, describes the visit to Baba's Samadhi (tomb) on Meherabad Hill:

"As we walked up Meherabad Hill to sit before the Beloved's resting place, one had the sense that here, more than anywhere, God had suspended time, that there was no beginning, or end, just the eternal now. Each person entered the Tomb to be alone with Beloved Baba and many emerged weeping with the joy of His Love. Suddenly we heard the strains of "Begin the Beguine." A Western Baba-lover, Henry Kashouty, was playing the trombone with all his heart and the notes lingered hauntingly over Meherabad Hill."[280]

Kitty Davy, who was continuing to help Elizabeth Patterson run Meher Center, returned to North America after her trip to India. Only later would she shed tears for Baba:

"After returning from India to the West following the Last Darshan, I had occasion to visit my nieces, Zillah and Jenny in Montreal, and as I sat by the fire one evening, I was able to reflect on Baba's suffering and the culminating events in India of the past year. I recalled His words, 'My suffering is begotten of My compassion and love for mankind.'"

"As I thought of Baba's Love and suffering for all, suddenly tears came – tears that I vowed in India a long time back never to shed except for the beauty of Baba's Love. The moment had come – not in India – not at the Last Darshan – but in the stillness and contemplation of Baba's compassionate Love for all."[281]

William's role in the Last Darshan cannot be underestimated. Not only was he responsible for organizing safe accommodation for the Westerners, but he also suddenly inherited 700 potential patients.

William actually had to provide medical treatment to one of the group members from Myrtle Beach. Brad Gunn, who had a bad case of diarrhoea. He had shifted hotels a couple of times and ended up staying at the Poona Club*, where William was housed, and remembers the experience:

"Physically he was quite a large man, probably six feet tall or more and robust – not huge, but radiating a strong healthy physical appearance. He was wearing a topee, if I remember correctly, along with khaki shorts and a light cotton shirt."

Brad, who had given up drugs after learning about Meher Baba in 1967, continues his description of William:

"He gave the impression of a cross between a retired former professional athlete and a compassionate parish priest. But the most memorable thing about him for me was his vocal delivery. He had a fairly high voice and a posh English accent, but when he was telling a story, as he would approach the punch line, his delivery would become softer and softer until you had to strain to hear what he was saying, and once he delivered the punch line he would laugh and laugh loudly. He gave off a wonderful eccentricity, which I'm sure Baba found to be just delightful. But unfortunately between the accent, his soft delivery, and my feverish condition, I missed most of the punch lines!"

William gave Brad some pills and told him to drink plenty of water. "He said I'd either be dead or better in a day and a half and he was betting on me being better."

"As he had foretold, I was better in a day and a half, though incredibly weak," said Brad. "I had lost 19 pounds since arriving in India, mostly moisture I think, but at least the fever was gone and I no longer had the runs."

"I had missed a couple of days of programs at Guruprasad, though balanced against this was about 20 minutes of Dr. Donkin's caring ministrations. Well worth it in retrospect."[282]

Another Westerner in the Myrtle Beach group, artist David Barison, recalls his first encounter with William:

"I kind of remember this guy at the Poona Club, well-tanned and maybe carrying a tennis racket."

---

* The Poona Club is the oldest and most prestigious club in Poona. It was initiated by royalty and spreads over three premises comprising the Main Club, the Golf Course, and the swimming pool and squash complex.

David says William joined the Western group at their dinner table at the club, and he remembers the moment William sat down next to him:

"He was beside me and suddenly I felt this ray of love coming from him and through me – I actually reeled."

"He said, 'My name is Donkin.'

"And he could tell by the look on my face that I had felt something strong and was actually indicating this.

"'Wow! What was that I felt?' I said to him.

David recalls that William then responded in a proper British accent, "Oh it's not me – it's Baba, you know."

Roy Hayes of Australia also recalls his first encounter with William:

"We were met by Dr. Donkin, one of Baba's mandali, a sweet lovely-mannered man ... he was quite absent minded – there was a good feeling about him."[283]

Another visitor, Leigh Rowan, who arrived in India exhausted, remembers William:

"When we reached the hotel I was taken straight to hospital by Dr. Donkin in his incredible car. The drive there was like a dream. He didn't drive like most people do – he glided. It was like being on a magic carpet. I felt about Donkin that at this time in his life he was almost with Baba. There was a fine veil left that separated him from Baba. He was almost transparent and his eyes were oceans. He was like an elfin lord. He hardly spoke and yet he said everything."[284]

In the midst of darshan activities, William's servant Motiram was married on May 18. The couple visited William in Poona, and William told the hotel management to provide the newlyweds with a meal to celebrate their wedding.

William may not have known it during the April–June darshan sessions, but his own physical life on earth was drawing to a close.

After returning from Poona following the darshan, which included thousands from the East as well as the 700 Westerners, William would have been understandably exhausted.

In early August Harry Kenmore had tea with William and asked him to consider coming to the United States to talk about Baba. William told Harry he would consider it. On August 7 he wrote to Fred and Ella Winterfeldt in Myrtle Beach.

"We are slowly recovering from the shock of January 31st. Physically absent, Baba seems to have made himself available on a greater scale – even to the point of people seeing Him.... Hope you are also travelling on the path of readjustment. I'm sure you are! I suppose soon Baba will compel all of us to go out and tell the world about Him.

"[Signed] ...dear "Donk"

William lived alone in his separate quarters at Viloo Villa in Ahmednagar. His servant Motiram recalls the sequence of events that unfolded on the morning of Saturday, August 9, at William's bungalow at Viloo Villa, "William had asked me to cook for him. He finished his breakfast at 10:30 a.m. I then went to the market to buy food for later in the day."

When Motiram returned, he saw William lying on his bed with a book in his hand. The bedroom door was locked, but Motiram could see inside.

"I thought he was sleeping. I knocked but there was no response."

Concerned, Motiram went to see Adi Sr. to tell him. Adi suspected William was sleeping and told Motiram not to wake him. Later, upon returning to William's bungalow, Motiram became more concerned, and went to see Judge Sanjana, a friend of William's.

"He was Donkin's friend. I told him something had happened. The judge and I came back to Viloo Villa on his motorbike."

Judge Sanjana immediately saw that William was not responding to their calls. He called Adi Sr. immediately and William's bedroom door was finally broken open to get inside.

Sheela Kalchuri Fenster relates the heart-breaking scene that unfolded for her on August 9. They opened the door and saw that William had been reaching for a bottle of heart medication tablets on the table by his bed. No one had known he had a heart condition.

Dr. William Donkin was dead at age 57.

"Since William was a foreigner, a post mortem was mandatory, and his body was taken to the Civil Hospital. Dr. Melvin Brieseman from nearby Booth Hospital knew William well and confirmed that he had heart problems. The official cause of death from the Civil Hospital was given on Sunday, August 10, 1969, as acute cardiac failure (myocardial infarction).

"That evening his body was taken to Meherabad in the back of a soda-bottle delivery rickshaw, without any covering or padding underneath it. We followed in Adi's car," Sheela recalls. "I felt terrible about how William's body was being taken, but no one listened to me."

Sheela cried as William's body was placed in Baba's Interview Cabin at Meherabad.

"But when I went inside the room, I felt as if Baba was standing beside me, I looked around, hoping to catch a glimpse of Baba. The expression on William's face was one of joy. He looked at peace and I felt consoled."

Sheela recalls the last time she saw William alive, the evening before his death:

"William was staying at Viloo Villa. I had an activity after school, so was late, but he waited late for me to come home so he could give me a box of chocolates.

"When he drove away he said 'Good-bye Sheela.'

"I insisted he just say 'Bye Sheela,' like he always did, but he would not and again said 'Good-bye, Sheela.'

"That was the last time I saw him alive."[285]

Sheela and others, including her father Bhau, stayed with William's body the entire night.

"Workers dug the grave [at Meherabad] during the night and William was buried the following [Monday] morning. Eruch, Mani, Adi, Pendu, Aloba, Sarosh, Meherjee, and Meherwan, and a few others attended."

Dr. Harry Kenmore recited Baba's prayers at the graveside service for William. Police held an inquiry a couple of days later and questioned Motiram about details surrounding the day William died.

Mansari Desai*, who looked after Meher Baba's tomb, verified the enchanting details of William's last visit to the Samadhi. She relayed the story in Judith Garbett's book *Lives of Love*:

"It was on 5th August that Dr. Donkin came to Meherabad to visit 'The Boss,' as he always called Baba. After spending time in the Samadhi, he came and talked with me for about two hours on this and that, again went to Baba, and then left. He looked so completely well and healthy that day."

Mansari says that when she went to the tomb the next day, she thought she saw a white sadhra (long muslin garment) pass before the crack in the tomb door before entering. She thought, "Oh, Baba will I find you sitting there, or standing, or what?"

When she went inside, there was no sign of anyone. She noticed that the ground had been disturbed in the place above where Baba's feet would be.

She quickly called Padri, and when they were putting the earth back in place both of them noticed a beautiful fragrance in the air within the tomb. That fragrance persisted over the course of four days and many visitors to the tomb experienced it. On the day William died – Saturday, August 9 – the fragrance suddenly disappeared.

During his 30 years in India, William must have been frustrated on many occasions. From the outset he thought he would be serving Baba as a doctor and would be able to put his six hard years of medical school to work. On at least two occasions others witnessed William's threat to leave Meher Baba's ashram and return to England. But on those occasions, and probably others, Baba quietly "talked" to William, calmed him down, and he stayed.

Even in late 1968, Baba was still telling William he would have important medical work for him to do after his 1969 Darshan duties were complete.

"You will be so busy," Baba told him. "You won't have time to breathe."

---

* Mansari (Mani Desai) met Baba in 1927 after learning of him from her uncle. She became one of the women mandali, but she was ordered by Baba to always stay at Upper Meherabad and was the caretaker of his tomb.

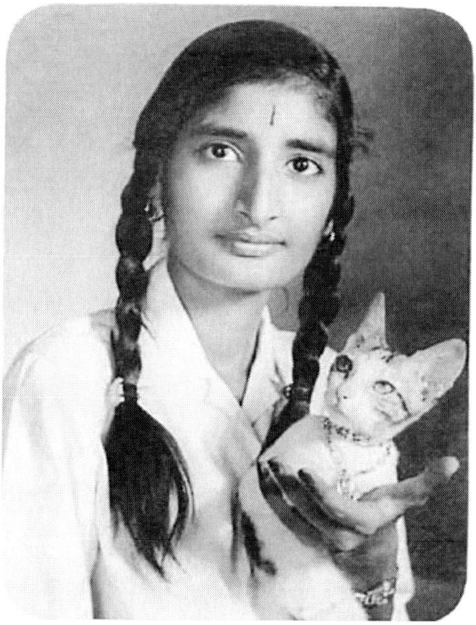

MN Publications

Sheela Kalchuri Fenster considered William Donkin her best friend for over 10 years. Her book, *Growing Up With God,* carries many stories about their special relationship.

Sheela Kalchuri Fenster recalls William's response to Baba at the time:

"William folded his hands to Baba and said, 'I will be very happy to do any work that you give me.'"

William's readiness to do, not necessarily the doctoring associated with his ego, but any work for his Master, would have pleased Baba immensely. At the time Baba called William near him and indicated, "I know how much you love me. Your connection with me is deep. Only I know. Your entire focus is on obeying my orders. Even though you stay in Khushru Quarters, you are pleasing me every moment."[286]

There are those in the Baba community that believe that William Donkin had himself become a mast (God-intoxicated human being) during his life with Baba.

Sheela's father, Bhau Kalchuri, said that William was never the same after writing *The Wayfarers* in the late 1940s, and became like a mast himself in his later life.

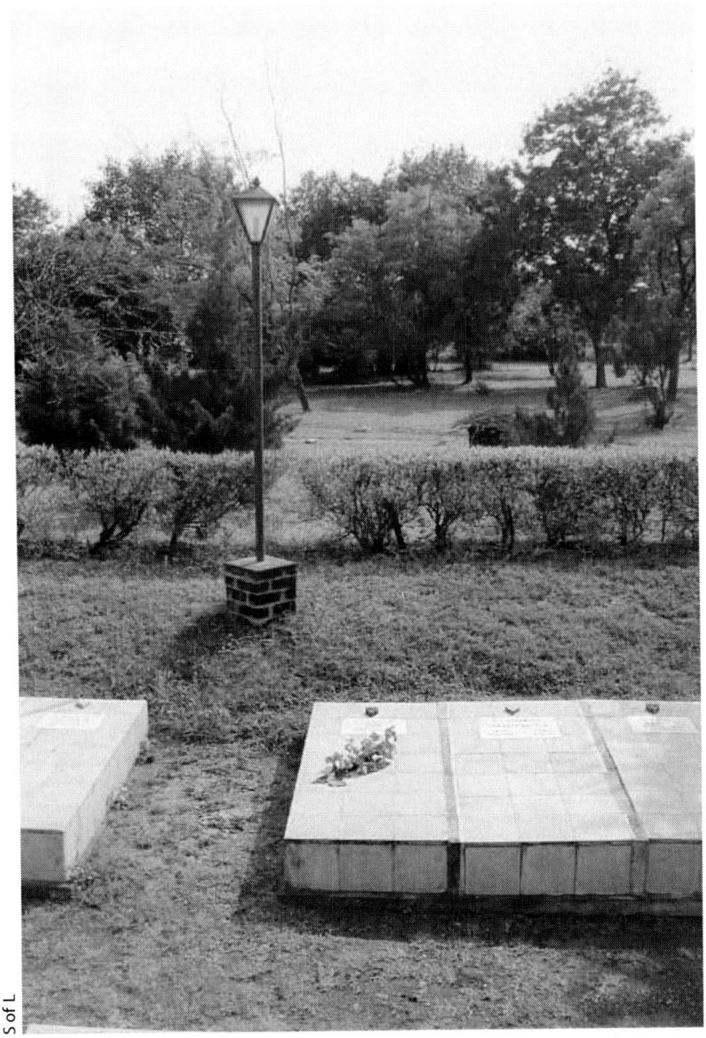

S of L

Dr. William Donkin's gravesite, marked by a sprig of bougainvillea, is located at Lower Meherabad. Other male mandali and two masts are also buried in the cemetery. Female mandali are interred in Upper Meherabad beside Meher Baba's samadhi.

Naosherwan Anzar is author of *The Beloved* (a Meher Baba biography) and founding publisher and editor of *The Glow,* a magazine dedicated to the life of Baba. As a child, Naosherwan knew William in Dehra Dun, where he grew up with his parents who were Baba-lovers.

"He [William] used to take his evening meals with us. I remember him when I was a youngster. He would take walks dressed in his short pants and long socks. He always wore a beret, which I do today...."

Naosherwan witnessed William's erratic behaviour many years later in 1969 after Baba had dropped his body.

"I think he was a mast. We would be having a conversation and right in the middle of it he would throw his head back and begin laughing. He would never finish his sentences."

Ivy Duce, head of Sufism Reoriented, wrote in her book *How a Master Works* that it was "generally conceded among the mandali that Donkin died of a broken heart – his love for Baba was so great."

William did not go softly into the night, however.

Sheela Kalchuri Fenster writes in her book *Growing Up With God* that a mystery still lingers, more than 40 years after his death. According to Sheela, William had completed another book just before Meher Baba dropped his body.

"While he was living at Khushru Quarters, he had finished a manuscript."

According to Sheela, there were many photographs that William had taken of Baba that were pasted down at various places in the handwritten manuscript.

"He told me he was preparing the manuscript for publication in England. The book contained biographical information about William's life, including photos from his childhood of his two brothers and his twin sister Mary, and how he had heard about Meher Baba."

Immediately after William's death, Adi Sr. wrote to William's twin sister Mary and older brother John in England informing them of his death.

Adi Sr.'s letter to the Donkin family reflects his relationship with William:

"Dr. William Donkin, 'Don' as we called him was my brother-disciple to Avatar Meher Baba and lived with me for nearly 24 years.

"I looked after all his interests including his food, stay, and belongings. Being secretary to Avatar Meher Baba, I took all the responsibility of Don's welfare in India for the past three decades.

"Our relationship with each other was like two members of one family by virtue of our common faith and service to Avatar Meher Baba.

"Besides to all Meher Baba followers all over the world, his departure has been a personal loss to me – since he always entrusted to my care everything that belonged to him. During his several trips to England and the USA he made me custodian of all his belongings and left the keys of his house to my care....

"At present, I am in complete custody of all his belongings, which will be disposed of as per the will of the deceased."[287]

William's will soon became a point of contention. Copies of it had been kept at Westminster Bank in England and National and Grindlays Bank in Bombay. In the will, which William had made in 1953, all of his possessions were to be passed on to Meher Baba.

But Meher Baba dropped his body before William did. The will made no stipulations for any other heirs in India, so William's possessions then legally reverted back to his immediate family.

The Westminster Bank, acting as executor of William's estate, asked Adi Sr. to do a thorough search to see if William had possibly made a newer will in the later years. None was located.

Although Adi Sr. insisted that William's intention would surely have been to see his estate channelled into the work of Meher Baba, the Donkin family held firm to the legality that the estate reverted back to them.

At one point Adi Jr. (Meher Baba's younger brother), who was living in England, went to the home of William's twin sister Mary and her husband George Mathieson to plead the case for retaining the proceeds of William's estate in India.

Adi Jr. later wrote to his sister Mani, that while the meeting was cordial, George Mathieson was sticking to the legal interpretation, saying that the family would not relinquish their valid claim on William's estate.

William's estate would have amounted to a sum of money he had inherited from his brother Bryan (less than 100,000 pounds), a number of investment shares which had originated with his family, and his personal property in India including the Wolseley car and a motorcycle. William specifically named all of his nephews and nieces in his will, leaving them each a small amount of money. The rest of his estate was eventually divided equally between his twin sister Mary and brother John.

Although William did not elaborate a great deal on meeting Meher Baba in 1933 at the time, there is a point known which sheds light on the importance of William to Meher Baba.

Artist Phyllis Ott, a long-time lover and devotee of Baba, who lives in a house on Meher Center property in South Carolina, says William was the "only fish caught in the net," in London back in 1933.

What was known as The Circle Editorial Committee, had published a booklet titled *Shri Meher Baba, The Perfect Master, Questions and Answers* in 1933 and made it available to anyone who visited the committee's office at 50 Charing Cross Road, London, SW1. The booklet was a very detailed document with tough spiritual questions and answers. While William may not have been the only person to see the booklet, he certainly was the one whose life was changed the most after seeing it.

"Dr. Donkin picked up the booklet and eventually ended up at Kitty Davy's parents' house to meet Baba," says Phyllis. "He really was the only fish they caught from publishing that booklet."

Sheela Fenster had questioned William about the details of his first 1933 meeting with Baba at the time she viewed his mysterious manuscript, but William said he had included this in his new book, which she could later read.

Sheela referred specifically to photo albums William had:

"One of William's hobbies was photography. He spent hours carefully cataloguing his collection of photos and placing them in albums.

"'No one has these photos of Baba,' William remarked to me once, as he had the photos printed in Poona and did not make copies. He had a box camera and others with interchangeable lenses. He liked to take candid shots of Baba, the mandali, and darshan programs."

According to Sheela, William also travelled around India retracing Baba's historic footsteps and taking photos of bungalows and rest houses where Baba and the mandali had stayed. He told Sheela, "It's important to keep a record for posterity."

"William maintained files full of correspondence between himself and Baba, neatly kept in chronological order. After Baba dropped his body, William would take out his files and read through them, and perhaps some of these were to be included in the new manuscript."

In showing the manuscript to Sheela, William would make sure they both wore rubber gloves so the pages would not be stained.

"We would look through his collection of photographs, deciding where to insert them. William had drawn the title of the book and his own name in calligraphy on the front page (I don't recall the title). There was even a page of the manuscript in Baba's own handwriting.

"'This page Baba himself wrote,' William told me.'"[288]

Just as Meher Baba wrote a mystery book in 1925 that had disappeared, William's second book has not surfaced in the more than 40 years since his passing.

Was it perhaps discarded by a servant who cleaned out William's room after his death? Perhaps someone who knew William took it. William might have hidden it away for safekeeping or shipped it off to a British publisher before he died.

"The book was to be a surprise to everyone. He hadn't told the others he was writing it. I asked if he had told Baba, and he said he had. I had suggested he ask Baba to dictate an introduction, and William said he planned to. But Baba had become ill by then, and William never got the chance."[289]

Baba's sister Mani reflected on the death of William and what it meant to the fellow mandali members in her August 26, 1969, Family Letter to the West:

"On the 9th of this month, Don [William] passed away of a heart attack. It was as sudden as it was unexpected. On Wednesday he had tea with Dr. Harry Kenmore, one of Baba's intimate mandali, who has come to stay for a month at Meherazad....

"Among our many dear remembrances of Don, dearest is his unwavering fidelity to His Master whom he served 'to the end,' sticking by Baba through the roughest years of our life with Baba, Don was the only Western disciple chosen to accompany Baba in the New Life as one of His 'Companions.' And now Don has started out on his true New Life. To the Mandali it means the loss of a very 'dear brother.'"

Woman mandali Meheru Irani recalled that "Baba thought very highly of him."

Eruch Jessawala, Baba's "right hand," who had interpreted Baba's gestures for so many years, also remembered William's sense of duty and service:

"You may not have heard how in '69 Donkin saw to it that the Westerners who came for the big darshan in Poona should stay healthy.

"On his own, he would inspect the kitchens or the hotels where the Westerners would be staying to make sure that proper sanitary procedures were followed. Don took this duty so seriously that he cleaned the latrines of the hotels himself to make sure they were done properly.

"That was Don's nature. People would come here and think Don was a servant, never realizing that he was one of Baba's close ones and a British gentleman – an orthopaedic surgeon.

"This was his way. He would never push himself forward, he would always be in the background seeing to everything himself. What a gem he was. It is too bad you didn't get to meet him. Then you would know what real service is like."

As stated many pages ago, William may well still be a mystery to many.

The words the 25-year-old medical student wrote from London to Meher Baba on September 6, 1937, may provide a clue to his beautiful, steadfast, inspiring dedication:

"Dearest Baba:

"Please may I love you a thousand times more than I do now? I feel as cold and empty at times and if only I could be on fire loving you then perhaps I could forget my petty self a bit.

"I am so looking forward to coming back to you dearest. I am so looking forward to coming back to you....

"You are so pure, and so lovely.... Life back here seems so pointless....

"I do long to come back to you....

"Yours always,

"Will Donkin"

Dr. William Donkin – a Divine gem indeed.

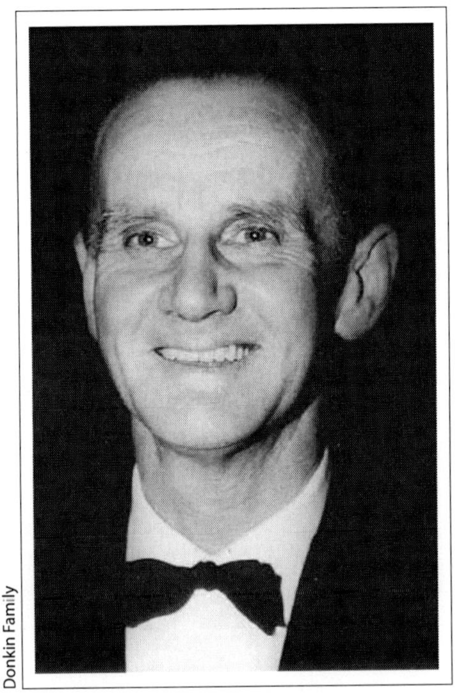

Donkin Family

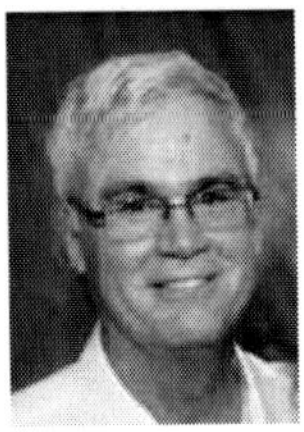

Bob Mossman is a retired Canadian journalist. He has been a follower of Meher Baba since 1967 and lives by the ocean, dividing his time between Nova Scotia and South Carolina.

Works Cited

Books

Anzar, Naosherwan. The Beloved: The Life and Work of Meher Baba. North Myrtle Beach, SC: Sheriar Press Inc., 1974.

Baba, Meher. Discourses. Edited by Ivy Duce and Don Stevens. 3 vols. San Francisco CA: Sufism Reoriented, 1967.

Davy, Kitty. Love Alone Prevails, A story of life with Meher Baba. North Myrtle Beach, SC: Sheriar Press Inc., 1981.

DeLeon, Delia. The Ocean of Love: My life with Meher Baba. North Myrtle Beach, SC: Sheriar Press, Inc., 1991.

Donkin, William. The Wayfarers: Meher Baba with the God-Intoxicated. San Francisco, CA: Sufism Reoriented, 1948.

Duce, Ivy. How A Master Works. Walnut Creek. CA: Sufism Reoriented, Inc., 1975.

Fenster, David. Mehera-Meher: A Divine Romance. 3 vols. Ahmednagar, Ms. India: Meher Nazar Publications, 2003.

Fenster, Sheela Kalchuri. Growing Up With God. Ahmednagar, Ms. India: Meher Nazar Publications, 2009.

Garbett, Judith. Lives of Love. The Women Mandali of Avatar Meher Baba. Woombye, Queensland AU: Woombye Word Design, 1998

Grant, John. Practical Spirituality with Meher Baba. Sydney, AU: Merwan Publications, 1987.

Irani, Mani S. 82 Family Letters, To the Western Family of Lovers and Followers of Meher Baba (1956–1969). North Myrtle Beach, SC: Sheriar Press, 1976.

Irani, Mehera J. Baba Loved Us Too, Stories of Meher Baba and His Pets. North Myrtle Beach, SC: Sheriar Press, 1989.

Jessawala, Eruch. The Ancient One. Edited by Naosherwan Anzar. Englishtown, NJ: Beloved Books, 1985.

Kalchuri, Bhau. Lord Meher. Myrtle Beach, SC, USA: Manifestation Inc., 1986–1997.

Kalchuri, Bhau. Meher Baba's New Life. Pune, India: Ed Flanagan, Walter & Kim Witowski, Daniel Ladinsky, Barry & Katherine Beckett, Ava Craig, John & Anita Dennison; 2008.

Knowles, Charmian. Spread My Love. Walnut Creek, CA: Sufism Reoriented, 2004.

Kotwal, Najoo Savak. He Gives the Ocean, Stories of the Savak Kotwal's Family Life with Meher Baba. Myrtle Beach, SC: Sheriar Foundation, 2006.

LePage, Bill. The Turning of the Key: Meher Baba in Australia. Myrtle Beach, SC, USA: Sheriar Press, 1993.

LePage, Bill (Compilation and Editing). The Narrow Lane. Bombay, India: Meher House Publications / Meher Baba Foundation, Australia, 1979.

Natu, Bal. Glimpses of the Godman. 5 Vols. Walnut Creek, CA: Sufism reoriented; Meher House Publications, Bombay, India; Sheriar Press and Sheriar Foundation, Myrtle Beach, SC: 1977–1994.

Purdom, Charles. The God-Man, The Life, Journeys and Work of Meher Baba with an Interpretation of his Silence and Spiritual Teaching. Crescent Beach, SC: Sheriar Press, 1979.

Purdom, Charles / Schloss, Malcolm (Compiled). Three Incredible Weeks with Meher Baba. North Myrtle Beach, SC: Sheriar Press, 1979.

Shaw, Darwin. As Only God Can Love. North Myrtle Beach, SC: Sheriar Foundation, 2003.

Other Sources

Donkin, William – Personal Diaries, India, 1939–1945.

[The diaries have recently been published in book form as Donkin's Diaries, Travels in India with Meher Baba, 1939-1945; editor, Sarah McNeill; North Myrtle Beach, SC: Sheriar Foundation, 2011.]

Meher Baba Journal (Magazine). Meher Editorial Committee, Ahmednagar, India, 1938–1942.

The Awakener Magazine, A Journal Devoted to Meher Baba. Editor, Filis Frederick, Seattle WA: Warren C. Healy Press, 1953–1986.

The Life Circulars of Avatar Meher Baba. Editor, Adi K. Irani, Meher Vihar Trust, Hyderabad, India:,1968.

Glow International, A Journal Devoted to Meher Baba. Editor Naosherwan Anzar, Beloved Archives Inc., New Jersey, USA: current quarterly magazine founded in 1966.

Notes

Chapter 1

1 The Wayfarers: pg 6

2 Ibid

3 "A Camel Journey from Tugurt to Kana": by Norman Pearn and William Donkin, The Geographical Journal, Vol 83, No 5 (May, 1934), pg 399–409

4 Ibid

5 Ibid

6 The Awakener. Vol 20, No 2. A journal devoted to Meher Baba published from 1953 to 1986

7 Avatar Meher Baba Trust Archives

Chapter 2

8 Avatar Meher Baba Trust Archives

9 Ibid

10 Avatar Meher Baba Trust Archives

11 Ibid

12 Mehera-Meher, A Divine Romance: by David Fenster, pg 393

13 William Donkin Diary: Aug 4, 1939

14 Love Alone Prevails: by Kitty Davy

15 William Donkin Diary: Aug 2, 1939

16 Ibid

17 Mehera-Meher: Vol II, pg 20

Chapter 3

18 Lord Meher: Vol 7, pg 2517

19 William Donkin Diary: Nov 14, 1939

20 William Donkin Diary: Oct 11, 1939

21 William Donkin Diary: Dec 4, 1939

22 Ibid: Dec 18, 1939

23 Mehera-Meher: Vol II, pg 42

24 The Wayfarers: pg 103

25 Ibid

26 The Wayfarers: pg 65

Chapter 4

27 Mehera-Meher: Vol II, pg 43

28 Gift of God, pg 57

29 William Donkin Diary: June 3, 1940

Chapter 5

30 The Wayfarers: pg 73

31 Ibid: pg 75

32 Ibid: pg 76

33 William Donkin Diary: Dec 12, 1940
34 Ibid: Dec 31, 1940
35 Ibid: Dec 31, 1940
36 The Wayfarers: pg 105

Chapter 6

37 William Donkin Diary: May 19, 1941
38 Ibid: July 7, 1941
39 Ibid: Nov 18, 1941
40 Avatar Meher Baba Trust Archives
41 William Donkin Diary: Aug 5, 1942
42 Ibid: Oct 22, 1942
43 Avatar Meher Baba Trust Archives
44 William Donkin Diary: April 30, 1943
45 Lord Meher: Vol 8, pg 2868
46 William Donkin Diary: May 23, 1943
47 The Beloved: by Naosherwan Anzar
48 William Donkin Diary: April 4. 1944
49 Ibid: Oct. 10, 1944
50 William Donkin Diary: Feb 12, 1945
51 Glimpses of the Godman: Vol 8
52 Glimpses, Vol 1, pg 91–92
53 William Donkin Diary: May 1, 1945
54 Ibid: May 14, 1945
55 Ibid: June 4, 1945
56 Lord Meher: Vol 8, pg 3050
57 William Donkin Diary: July 14, 1945
58 Lord Meher: Vol 8, pg 3053
59 William Donkin Diary: Oct 8, 1945

Chapter 7

60 Messages
61 Mehera-Meher: Vol 11, pg 304
62 Ibid
63 Ibid: pg 305
64 Glimpses: Vol 1, pg 142
65 Ibid
66 "Awakening to God," The Glow Magazine, Aug 1998
67 Mehera-Meher: Vol 11, pg 308
68 Ibid
69 Ibid pg 309–10
70 Ibid
71 Lord Meher: Vol 9, pg 3142
72 The Wayfarers: pg 10–11
73 Mehera-Meher, Vol 11, pg 320
74 Ibid
75 Avatar Meher Baba Trust Archives

76 How a Master Works: by Ivy Duce
77 Ibid: pg 43
78 Ibid: pg 28
79 Ibid: pg 42
80 Ibid: pg 43

Chapter 8
81 Ibid: pg 279
82 Glimpses; Vol I, pg 279
83 The Wayfarers: pg 32
84 The Wayfarers: pg 1, Extra Supplement
85 Ibid: pg 2
86 The Wayfarers: Pamphlet 1, pg 14
87 Ibid
88 The Wayfarers: Pamphlet 2, pg 8
89 Ibid: pg 10
90 The Wayfarers: Pamphlet 2, pg 14
91 Mehera-Meher: Vol II, pg. 357
92 The Wayfarers: Pamphlet 2, pg 16
93 Author interview 2010
94 The Wayfarers: Pamphlet 2, pg 22
95 Ibid
96 The Wayfarers: Pamphlet 2, pg 23–24
97 Mehera-Meher: Vol II, pg 374
98 Author interview 2010
99 The Wayfarers: Pamphlet 2, pg 26–27

Chapter 9
100 The Ancient One: Eruch Jessawala
101 Ibid: pg 40
102 Love Alone Prevails: Kitty Davy, pg 334
103 Ibid: pg 335
104 Meher Baba's New Life: Bhau Kalchuri
105 Ibid
106 Ibid
107 Meher Baba's New Life
108 Ibid
109 Ibid
110 How a Master Works: pg 66
111 New Life Circular, No 5, March 10, 1950; also New Life Circular, No 17, Sept 11, 1950
112 Lord Meher: Volume 10, pg 3454
113 The Awakener: Volume III, No 1, (1960), pg 20
114 Meher Baba's New Life
115 Ibid
116 Glimpses: Vol II, 5, pg 171
117 Lord Meher: Vol 10, pg 3511

118 Ibid: pg 3524
119 Ibid
120 Glimpses: Vol II, pg 195
121 Meher Baba's New Life
122 Lord Meher: Vol 10, pg 3548
123 Meher Baba's New Life
124 He Gives the Ocean
125 New Life Circular: No 4, pg 44
126 New Life Circular: No 7, pg 90
127 How A Master Works: pg 70
128 The Awakener: Vol 2, No 1, pg 19
129 New Life Circular: No 7, pg 102–3
130 Lord Meher: Volume 10, pg 3592
131 New Life Circular: No 8, pg 184–5

Chapter 10
132 The New Phase of Baba's Life: Appendices I–XXVIII
133 Love Alone Prevails: pg 346
134 Love Alone Prevails: pg 349
135 Baba's New Life
136 Glimpses: Volume II, pg 321
137 New Life Circular: No 25
138 Love Alone Prevails: pg 356–7
139 Glimpses: Volume II, pg 343
140 Glimpses: Volume II, pg 365
141 "Baba's Orders" by Dr. William Donkin, Meher Baba Journal, Dec 1941
142 Love Alone Prevails: pg 357
143 Meher Baba's New Life
144 Glimpses: Volume II, pg 398

Chapter 11
145 "Recollections," The Awakener, Volume 6, pg 25 (1960)
146 Love Alone Prevails: pg 385
147 How a Master Works: pg 84
148 Mehera-Meher: Vol III, pg 29
149 Ibid
150 Glimpses: Vol III, pg 30
151 Ibid: pg 31
152 Love Alone Prevails: pg 392
153 Ibid: pg 393
154 Glimpses: Vol III, pg 55
155 Ocean of Love: by Delia DeLeon
156 Mehera-Meher: Vol III, pg 50
157 Mehera-Meher: Vol III, pg 51
158 Ibid: pg 65
159 How a Master Works: pg 104

160 Ibid: pg 105
161 Love Alone Prevails: pg 402
162 How a Master Works: pg 138
163 Spread My Love: by Charmian Duce Knowles
164 How a Master Works: pg 145
165 Mehera-Meher: Vol III, pg 92
166 Glimpses: Vol II, pg 94
167 Spread My Love
168 How a Master Works: pg 15
169 Love Alone Prevails: pg 414–15

Chapter 12

170 Glimpses: Vol III, pg 107
171 The Beloved: by Naosherwan Anzar
172 Glimpses: Vol III, pg 134
173 Glimpses: Vol III, pg 221
174 Lord Meher: Vol 9–10, pg 4043
175 Glimpses: Vol III, pg 272
176 Glimpses: Vol IV, pg 11
177 Glimpses: Vol IV, pg 40
178 The God Man: by Charles Purdom, pg 212–13
179 Ibid: pg 215

Chapter 13

180 Author interview: October 2010
181 The God-Man: pg 235
182 How a Master Works: pg 188–89
183 As Only God Can Love: by Darwin Shaw, pg 193
184 He Gives The Ocean: by Savak Kotwal

Chapter 14

185 How a Master Works: pg 203
186 Ibid: pg 213
187 Lord Meher: Vol 13, pg 4750
188 Love Alone Prevails: pg 449
189 Mehera-Meher: Vol III, pg 168–69
190 Lord Meher: Vol 15, pg 5145
191 Author Interview, 2010
192 Love Alone Prevails: Page 486
193 He Gives the Ocean
194 Lord Meher: Volume 15, pg 5213
195 Ibid: Volume 15, pg 5241
196 82 Family Letters: pg 29
197 Lord Meher: Vol 15, pg 5358
198 Growing Up With God: by Sheela Kalchuri Fenster, pg 59–60
199 Ibid: pg 69
200 As Only God Can Love: by Darwin Shaw, pg 438

201 Love Alone Prevails: pg 527
202 Ibid: pg 532
203 Practical Spirituality with Meher Baba: by John Grant
204 Ibid
205 Ibid
206 Ibid

Chapter 15

207 82 Family Letters: pg 54
208 Love Alone Prevails: pg 550
209 Ibid
210 82 Family Letters: pg 63–64
211 Growing Up With God: pg 143
212 Ibid: pg 144
213 Ibid: pg 146
214 Author interview: October 2010
215 82 Family Letters: pg 178
216 Author Interview, Oct 2010
217 How A Master Works: pg 343
218 Lord Meher: Volume 17, pg 5885
219 82 Family Letters: pg 127
220 How a Master Works: pg 346
221 Ibid: pg 347
222 82 Family Letters: pg 145
223 How a Master Works: pg 362
224 Love Alone Prevails: pg 593-96

Chapter 16

225 82 Family Letters: pg 151
226 82 Family Letters: June 12, 1963
227 82 Family Letters: Aug 9, 1963
228 Love Alone Prevails: pg 607
229 82 Family Letters: Oct 3, 1963
230 82 Family Letters: Sept 26–Oct 3, 1963
231 Growing Up With God: pg 282
232 82 Family Letters: Dec 10, 1963
233 Donkin Family Papers
234 Ibid
235 Author interview: October 2010
236 Growing Up With God: pg 312-13
237 82 Family Letters: Aug 20, 1964
238 Author interview: October 2010
239 82 Family Letters: Sept 8, 1964

Chapter 17

240 Donkin Family Remembrances, 2009
241 Author Interview, Oct 2010

242 Growing Up With God: pg 365
243 Love Alone Prevails: pg 637
244 Ibid
245 Ibid
246 Ibid: pg 409
247 82 Family Letters: pg 251, Feb 16, 1966
248 Ibid: pg 260
249 Growing Up With God: pg 372
250 Ibid: pg 531
251 Love Alone Prevails: pg 641
252 The Turning of the Key: by Bill LePage, pg 185
253 Ibid
254 Love Alone Prevails: pg 652
255 Mehera-Meher: Vol III, pg 39
256 Lord Meher: Vol 20, pg 6589
257 Growing Up With God: pg 532
258 Growing Up With God: pg 637–38
259 Author Interview

Chapter 18

260 Author Interview
261 Mehera-Meher: Vol III, pg 468–69
262 The Beloved: pg 103
263 Love Alone Prevails: pg 673–74
264 The Turning of the Key: by Bill LePage, pg 230–31
265 Growing Up With God: pg 721-22.
266 Ibid: pg 723 and 725
267 Mehera-Meher: Vol III, pg 489
268 Author interview, October 2010
269 Family Letters: pg 344
270 As Only God Can Love: by Darwin Shaw
271 Growing Up With God: pg 734
272 Ibid: pg 736
273 Mehera-Meher: Vol III, pg 500
274 Author interview, October 2010

Chapter 19

275 Growing Up With God: pg 742
276 Ibid
277 Ibid: pg 743
278 Love Alone Prevails: pg 676
279 Ibid: pg 677
280 Ibid: pg 678
281 Ibid: pg 679
282 Remembrance courtesy of Brad Gunn
283 The Empty Chair: Meher Baba's 1969 Darshan: by Barbara Bamberger Scott

284 Ibid
285 Author Interview
286 Growing Up With God: pg 746
287 Avatar Meher Baba Trust Archives
288 Growing Up With God: pg 744
289 Ibid

Index